Updates in Hypertension and Cardiovascular Protection

Series editors
Giuseppe Mancia
Milano, Italy

Enrico Agabiti Rosei
Brescia, Italy

The aim of this series is to provide informative updates on both the knowledge and the clinical management of a disease that, if uncontrolled, can very seriously damage the human body and is still among the leading causes of death worldwide. Although hypertension is associated mainly with cardiovascular, endocrine, and renal disorders, it is highly relevant to a wide range of medical specialties and fields – from family medicine to physiology, genetics, and pharmacology. The topics addressed by volumes in the series Updates in Hypertension and Cardiovascular Protection have been selected for their broad significance and will be of interest to all who are involved with this disease, whether residents, fellows, practitioners, or researchers.

More information about this series at http://www.springer.com/series/15049

Costas Tsioufis • Roland E. Schmieder
Giuseppe Mancia
Editors

Interventional Therapies for Secondary and Essential Hypertension

European Society of Hypertension

Springer

Editors
Costas Tsioufis
First Cardiology Clinic
National and Kapodistrian
University of Athens
Athens
Greece

Giuseppe Mancia
IRCCS Istituto Auxologico Italiano
University Milano-Bicocca
Milano
Monza
Italy

Roland E. Schmieder
Department of Nephrology and
Hypertension, University Hospital
Friedrich-Alexander University
Erlangen-Nürnberg
Erlangen
Germany

ISSN 2366-4606 ISSN 2366-4614 (electronic)
Updates in Hypertension and Cardiovascular Protection
ISBN 978-3-319-34140-8 ISBN 978-3-319-34141-5 (eBook)
DOI 10.1007/978-3-319-34141-5

Library of Congress Control Number: 2016947840

Printed on acid-free paper

This Springer imprint is published by Springer Nature
The registered company is Springer International Publishing AG Switzerland

Foreword

This book *Interventional Therapies for Essential and Secondary Hypertension*, co-edited by Costas Tsioufis from the University of Athens, Rolland Schmieder from the University of Erlangen, and Giuseppe Mancia from the University of Milan, is part of the series on Hypertension and related sequelae published by Springer with the official endorsement and collaboration of the European Society of Hypertension.

The identification of secondary forms of hypertension in everyday clinical practice is essential but troublesome; thus, a significant portion of such patients remains undiagnosed. Furthermore, therapies that are successfully targeted towards these secondary forms can improve, apart from blood pressure control, cardiovascular and renal outcomes. During the last years, interventions for essential hypertension have been introduced and evolved, and currently the status regarding their safety and efficacy draws research and clinical interest.

In this publication, a significant effort was made to integrate all available information for the pathophysiology, diagnosis, and treatment for secondary hypertension. This is not an easy task due to the wealth of data in this setting rendering expert analysis and critical approach for delivering best care to these patients. Regarding the other important pillar of this book, the innovative therapeutic modalities of neurohumoral modulation, they are presented in a comprehensive and up-to-date manner disseminating current evidence and providing in-depth approach to this lively area of research and clinical management of essential hypertension.

On behalf of the European Society of Hypertension, we would like to thank Springer for this important effort to improve information and education on hypertension. Also, our special thanks go to Professors Costas Tsioufis, Rolland Schmieder, and Giuseppe Mancia who have provided us this excellent work on the major topic of interventional therapies for essential and secondary hypertension. We hope that the readers will find this European Society of Hypertension/Springer scientific cooperation rewarding and useful in clinical practice.

Brescia, Italy — Enrico Agabiti Rosei

Preface

Blood pressure lowering is the main and most important mechanism of cardiovascular protection in hypertension. For more than half a century, antihypertensive drugs of different classes demonstrated their safety and efficacy to achieve blood pressure control in numerous randomized clinical trials. However, in the usual clinical practice, blood pressure control by applying the traditional antihypertensive treatment added on top of lifestyle changes resulted quite poor, and only 35 % of hypertensive patients remain within the target. Also, among patients with uncontrolled hypertension, secondary forms of the disease are increasingly being diagnosed because of both more accurate clinical approach being pursued and more refined diagnostic procedures being applied.

In this book *Interventional Therapies for Essential and Secondary Hypertension*, as editors, we sought to integrate evidence and critically review treatment modalities in such a diverse spectrum of disease entities. In the first four chapters of this publication, the reader can find answers to "when and how" best therapies in secondary forms of hypertension can be provided by experts in the field.

In the latter years, novel interventional techniques have been introduced either to reduce the burden of uncontrolled essential hypertension despite optimal ongoing pharmacological treatment (e.g., renal sympathetic denervation, carotid baroreceptor stimulation, etc.) or to reduce the additional cardiovascular risk of conditions strongly associated with essential hypertension (e.g., continuous positive airway pressure in sleep apnea).

Given the scientific debate on the effectiveness of interventional approaches to uncontrolled hypertension in the relevant 18 chapters of this book, the available data are presented with veracity and clarity in order to form the modern concept for these promising therapies.

Our primary goal was to provide the updated clinical context of interventional therapies for secondary and essential hypertension hoping that the readership can grasp and place in perspective their potential applications. Each chapter was written by experts in hypertension, and a clinical orientation to tackle the stated problems was largely aimed. All aspects are addressed in a comprehensive and practical manner trying to answer current questions of treating physicians. We would like to thank all contributors of this book for their intellectual work inspired by their high-level professional skills. However, we believe that the success of each book, as always happens, is based on the judgment of the readers.

Athens, Greece — Costas Tsioufis
Erlangen, Germany — Roland E. Schmieder
Milano, Italy — Giuseppe Mancia

Contents

Part I

Interventions for Secondary Hypertension

Interventions for Renovascular Hypertension

1

Thomas Zeller, Ulrich Beschorner, and Elias Noory

Abbreviations

BP	Blood pressure
DUS	Duplex ultrasound
e-GFR	Estimated glomerular filtration rate
FMD	Fibromuscular dysplasia
PTRA	Percutaneous transluminal renal angioplasty
RAS	Renal artery stenosis
RI	Resistive index

1.1 Introduction

The term renal artery stenosis (RAS) summarizes different causes of vascular lesions resulting in impaired blood flow to the kidney. Accounting for approximately 90% of RAS atherosclerosis is the most common etiology and is most often caused by plaque progression from the aortic wall into the renal artery origin resulting in the typical appearance of the ostial atherosclerotic RAS with additional diffuse atheroma of the abdominal aortic wall (Figs. 1.1 and 1.3). The prevalence of atherosclerotic RAS increases with age, risk factors, and concomitant diseases like

The authors do not have any conflict of interest with the content of this manuscript.

T. Zeller, MD (✉) • U. Beschorner, MD • E. Noory, MD
Abteilung Kardiologie und Angiologie II,
Universitäts-Herzzentrum Freiburg – Bad Krozingen,
Suedring 15, Bad Krozingen 79189, Germany
e-mail: thomas.zeller@universitaets-herzzentrum.de

C. Tsioufis et al. (eds.), *Interventional Therapies for Secondary and Essential Hypertension*, Updates in Hypertension and Cardiovascular Protection,
DOI 10.1007/978-3-319-34141-5_1

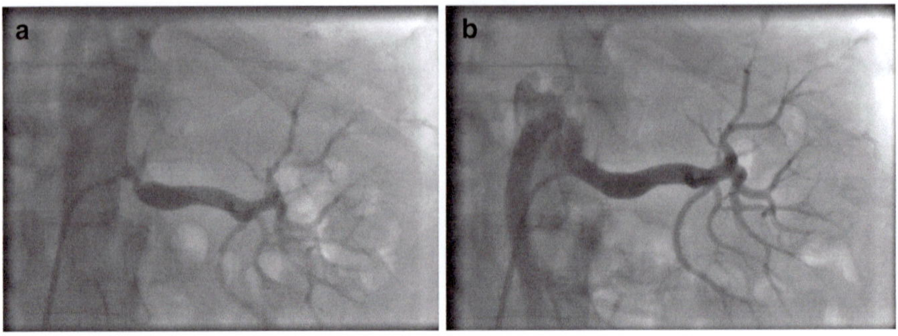

Fig. 1.1 Tight ostial stenosis of the left renal artery prior (**a**) and after 7-mm stent placement (**b**). Note: poststenotic enlarged vessel diameter, stent diameter matches to the diameter of the distal renal artery segment

diabetes mellitus, hyperlipidemia, hypertension, and aorto-iliac type of peripheral occlusive disease, and coronary artery disease [1, 2]. Atherosclerotic RAS is a progressive disease; even if more current literature suggests lower rates due to a more widespread use of statins progression, total occlusion was reported in the DRASTIC trial in 18 % within 1 year [3–6]. There is a close association between severity of RAS and kidney atrophy that may lead to ischemic nephropathy [7, 8]. The exact etiology of ischemic nephropathy is still unknown, the loss of kidney filtration capacity in RAS is not only due to hypoperfusion, but also because of recurrent micro-embolism and other not yet completely understood mechanisms [9, 10].

Fibromuscular dysplasia (FMD), as the second frequent etiology of RAS, is a collection of vascular diseases that affects all the three layers of the arterial vessel wall and is of unknown etiology. FMD accounts for less than 10 % of cases of RAS and rarely leads to vessel occlusion or ischemic nephropathy [11–13]. FMD tends to affect mainly younger women, is most commonly located at the distal half of the renal artery trunk or the side branches, and is characterized by a beaded, aneurysm-like appearance on angiography (medial dysplastic type, Figs. 1.2a and 1.9c, d). Less frequently seen are ostial locations, angiographically hard to distinguish from atherosclerotic disease. Intravascular ultrasound shows a marked reduction of overall vessel diameter, the affected vessel segment is shrunken, and the lesion is of fibrotic nature (intimal fibroplasia, Fig. 1.2b). Other potential causes of RAS are, in particular in Asia, vascular inflammatory disease, e.g., Takayasu's arteritis [12] and RAS following implantation of an abdominal endoprosthesis for the treatment of abdominal aortic aneurysm.

1.2 Indications for Intervention

Patient's individual characteristics, such as life expectancy, comorbidities, quality of blood pressure (BP) control, and renal function are key aspects for indicating a revascularization procedure. However, evidence supporting benefit

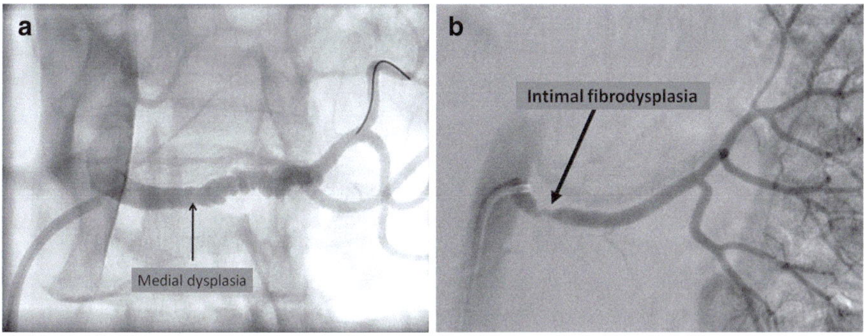

Fig. 1.2 (**a**) Left renal artery with characteristic angiographic "string of beads" appearance representing the most common type of fibromuscular dysplasia, the medial type; (**b**) left caudal renal artery angiogram showing the more rare type of intimal fibrodysplasia located close to the renal artery origin

of aggressive diagnosis and timing of renal revascularization still remains sparse. Among patients receiving medical therapy alone, there is the risk for deterioration of kidney function with worsening morbidity and mortality in particular in bilateral severe RAS. Under dedicated conditions, renal artery revascularization can provide immediate improvement in kidney function and BP; however, as with all invasive interventions, renal artery revascularization may result in mortality or substantial morbidity in a small percentage of patients [14, 15]. Due to outcome of the latest randomized controlled trials [14–16], general consensus exists that renal revascularization should be reserved for patients with anatomically significant RAS who present with particular clinical scenarios such as recent onset of hypertension or "flash" pulmonary edema or congestive heart failure with preserved left ventricular function or acute oligo-anuric renal failure with global kidney ischemia [17]. However, no consensus exists about the definition anatomically significant RAS. None of the randomized controlled trials including ASTRAL and CORAL did include diagnostic methods for evaluation of the significance of RAS before randomization [14–16]. Verification of significance of RAS should be performed either by duplex ultrasound and/or by invasive pressure gradient measurement even if this diagnostic step is not reimbursed in all health-care systems.

Potential benefits of RAS renal revascularization Reperfusion of the ischemic kidney results in a reduction of renin secretion, which decreases angiotensin and aldosterone production, thereby decreasing peripheral arterial vasoconstriction and promoting hypervolemia. Improvement in renal perfusion enhances glomerular filtration and therefore promotes natriuresis. Moreover, reduction of humoral activation might result in reduction of left ventricular mass and improvement of diastolic dysfunction [18, 19]. Lastly, BP control should become improved.

1.3 How Do the Study Results Look Like?

1.3.1 Impact of Revascularization on BP Control

Until 2007, 21 uncontrolled cohort studies of stenting/angioplasty were published in a total of 3,368 patients. Cure, improvement, or worsening of arterial hypertension was documented to range from 4 to 18 %, 35 to 79 %, and 0 to 13 %, respectively [5, 6]. Two studies reported a statistically significant reduction in the New York Heart Association Functional Class of congestive heart failure after stent placement in patients with global kidney ischemia – either bilateral disease or stenosis to a solitary functioning kidney. These patients with congestive heart failure not associated to coronary artery disease and repeated admissions for pulmonary edema had improved volume management, restored sensitivity to diuretics, and lowered rehospitalization rates, suggesting that some individualized patient categories benefit substantially from renal revascularization [17, 18, 20–22].

Three randomized controlled trials compared plain balloon percutaneous transluminal renal angioplasty (PTRA) to medical treatment with ≥6 months of follow-up. Notably, these trials were small and had no adequate power for clinical outcomes. All three studies concluded that PTRA in unilateral atherosclerotic RAS has some drug-sparing potential [4, 23, 24], but previous uncontrolled studies overestimated the potential for lowering BP. However, significantly improved diastolic and systolic BP in the angioplasty cohort was the result of a meta-analysis of those three trials [25].

The three recent randomized trials comparing stent angioplasty combined with medical therapy compared to medical therapy alone ("The angioplasty and stenting for renal artery lesions trial" (ASTRAL [15]), the "Stent placement in patients with atherosclerotic renal artery stenosis and impaired renal function trial" (STAR [14]), and the "Cardiovascular Outcomes in Renal Atherosclerotic Lesions" (CORAL [16])) did not result in significant differences in BP outcomes, whereas the daily drug dose was reduced in the ASTRAL trial.

1.3.2 Impact of Revascularization on Renal Function

In the ASTRAL trial, 806 of initially planned 1000 patients with atherosclerotic RAS, in whom the need for revascularization was uncertain, were enrolled. Fifty-nine percent of patients were reported by the investigators to have RAS > 70%, and 60 % had a serum creatinine of ≥150 μmol/L. At a mean follow-up of 34 months, differences in renal function, kidney, and cardiovascular events were insignificant including all subgroups such as patients with global ischemia or impaired or rapidly decreasing kidney function. The primary study endpoint, the decline in renal function over time (mean slope of the reciprocal of the serum creatinine level over time), was significantly slower in the revascularization group (-0.07×10^{-3} vs. -0.13×10^{-3} L/μmol/year, P=0.06 [15]).

The STAR multicenter trial enrolled 140 patients to detect a 20 % or greater decrease in creatinine clearance [14]. At 2 years, the primary endpoint was reached in 16 % of patients in the stented group and 22 % of patients in the medical treatment group without statistical significant. Noteworthy, more than 50 % of the patients randomized to stenting had a less than 70 % diameter stenosis and 28 % of patients did not receive a stent mainly because of the false diagnosis of RAS by MRA. This largely underpowered trial showed that deterioration of renal function may progress despite successful revascularization, underscoring the complex cause of ischemic nephropathy with an important parenchymal component affected by risk factors for atherosclerosis. It also showed that if technical skills are insufficient, a considerable number of stent-related complications including two procedure-related deaths can occur.

The CORAL trial included 947 patients with an angiographic >60 % RAS taking at least 2 antihypertensive drugs. There was similar decrease in estimated glomerular filtration rate (eGFR) over time [16]. Over a median follow-up period of 43 months, the rate of the primary composite endpoint (death from cardiovascular or renal causes, myocardial infarction, stroke, hospitalization for congestive heart failure, progressive renal insufficiency, or the need for renal-replacement therapy) did not differ significantly between stented patients and those who received medical therapy alone (35.1 % and 35.8 %, respectively; hazard ratio with stenting, 0.94; P = 0.58). During follow-up, there was a consistent modest difference in systolic BP favoring the stent group (−2.3 mmHg; 95 % CI, −4.4 to −0.2; P = 0.03) despite an increase in the mean number of antihypertensive drugs from 2.1 to 3.5 in the control cohort. The study was flawed by including a high percentage of patients who have been enrolled with moderate degree of RAS only; the corelab adjudicated mean percentage diameter stenosis was 67 % only.

1.3.3 Impact of Revascularization on Survival

In the ASTRAL, STAR, and CORAL trials no difference was seen in the secondary endpoints cardiovascular and renal morbidity and death [14–16]. A recent comparison of two consecutive registries comparing conservative treatment with revascularization resulted in a 45 % reduction of mortality for the revascularization cohort [21]. To date, no major differences in survival are evident between patients undergoing either surgical or endovascular procedures, although only a few studies addressed this issue directly.

Predictors of Clinical Success of Endovascular Revascularization

- Global renal ischemia defined as significant bilateral RAS or RAS of a solitary kidney was identified in several studies as an independent predictor for improved BP control [20, 26–28].
- Elevated pulse pressure has been shown to be predictive of outcome regarding stabilization of renal function and improved BP control following renal stent placement [29]. It seems as if a wide pulse pressure reflects a more advanced

Table 1.1a Impact of pulse pressure and BP response following renal stenting [29]

	BP improved	BP unchanged	BP worsened	P value
Mean pulse pressure	47 ± 15 mmHg	82 ± 10 mmHg	111 ± 14 mmHg	<0.05

Table 1.1b Correlation between pulse pressure and renal function response following renal stenting [29]

	Renal function stable/improved	Renal function worsened	P value
Mean pulse pressure	53 ± 20 mmHg	107 ± 18 mmHg	<0.05

stage of vascular stiffness and renal disease identifying patients less likely to respond to renal revascularization (Tables 1.1a and 1.1b).

- Irreversible microvascular kidney disease secondary to longstanding (uncontrolled) hypertension results in glomerulosclerosis and nephrosclerosis increasing the flow resistance in the affected and unaffected kidneys. An increased intrarenal resistance serves as a marker of structural alterations of the renal microvasculature. This increased vascular resistance can be determined by color duplex ultrasound [30–33]. An increased resistance index exceeding 0.8 was predictive for a treatment failure [34], whereas another study still resulted in a treatment benefit regarding BP reduction and stabilization of renal function; however, this effect was less pronounced with a resistance index >0.8 as compared to below 0.8 [35].
- Preinterventional pressure gradient measurement: This procedure is recommended in particular in uncertain cases and not as routine procedure because a reliable determination of the gradient requires a dedicated pressure-wire, which is expensive and extends procedure time and potential complications. While the measurement of a resting pressure gradient was not predictive for the BP response, Leesar et al. have found the best correlation with BP response after successful revascularization with baseline hyperemic translesional pressure gradient [36]. Hypertension improvement at 1 year occurred in 84 % of those with hyperemic translesional pressure gradient ≥21 mmHg compared to 36 % with hyperemic translesional pressure gradient <21 mmHg ($P < 0.01$). These results need to be confirmed in a larger series of patients including clinical endpoints. De Bryune et al. found an increase in ipsilateral renal vein renin release starting with a distal lesion to aortic systolic pressure ratio of 0.9 and below [37].
- Mahmud et al. reported a decreased renal perfusion as measured by renal frame counts and renal blush grade [38]. Renal frame count is increased in significant RAS. Clinical responders tended to have higher baseline renal frame counts as compared to nonresponders and had significantly greater improvement in their renal frame count values following stenting. Three quarters of the BP responders had a baseline renal frame count ≥25, and of those patients with an increase in renal frame count >4, 79 % were responders to revascularization. Renal frame count adds a functional assessment to the morphologic assessment of RAS. The application of renal blush grade as an indicator of microvascular flow might be helpful for evaluating the efficacy of embolic protection devices.

Several factors may argue against renal revascularization or predict poorer outcomes, including the presence of proteinuria >1 g/24 h, renal atrophy, severe renal parenchymal disease, and severe diffuse intrarenal arteriolar disease. Moreover, adverse consequences of renal atheroembolization at the time of surgical revascularization have been documented [33, 39]. Similarly, atheroembolization may be provoked by percutaneous revascularization [14, 40].

In summary, based on clinical experience despite the lack of positive randomized controlled trials, indications and contraindications for renal revascularization are the following:

1.3.4 Indications for PTRA

Hemodynamically relevant (≥70 %) unilateral and bilateral RAS with arterial hypertension and normal or impaired renal function, with a life expectancy of at least 2 years after the intervention

Hemodynamically relevant unilateral and bilateral RAS or renal artery occlusions in acute or subacute terminal renal insufficiency

1.3.5 Contraindications Against PTRA

Hemodynamically not relevant RAS <70 % (duplex: no side difference in resistive index (RI), no increase in acceleration time; angiography: ratio of invasively measured pressure distal to stenosis; aortic pressure >0.9)

Life expectancy markedly reduced due to concomitant diseases

Chronic dialysis

"Hostile aorta" (relative contraindication, Fig. 1.3)

1.4 How to Diagnose a Hemodynamically Significant RAS

Prior to renal artery revascularization, a proper patient examination is mandatory including a complete cardiovascular status, the exploration of potential life expectancy limiting concomitant diseases, a 24-h BP monitoring, a renal duplex scan, and blood and urine chemistry [5]. Key noninvasive diagnostic tool for determination of the hemodynamic relevance of a RAS is duplex ultrasound.

Color-coded duplex ultrasound (DUS) DUS is a noninvasive frequently repeatable bed-side examination and is currently the only noninvasive diagnostic method to reliably determine the significance of a RAS using the side-to-side difference of the intrarenal resistance index. There is a highly specific correlation between a side difference of the RI of >0.05 and an at least 70 % angiographic diameter stenosis [30, 31, 41]. The same holds true for an extended acceleration time of more than 70 ms. All other duplex parameters like a peak systolic flow

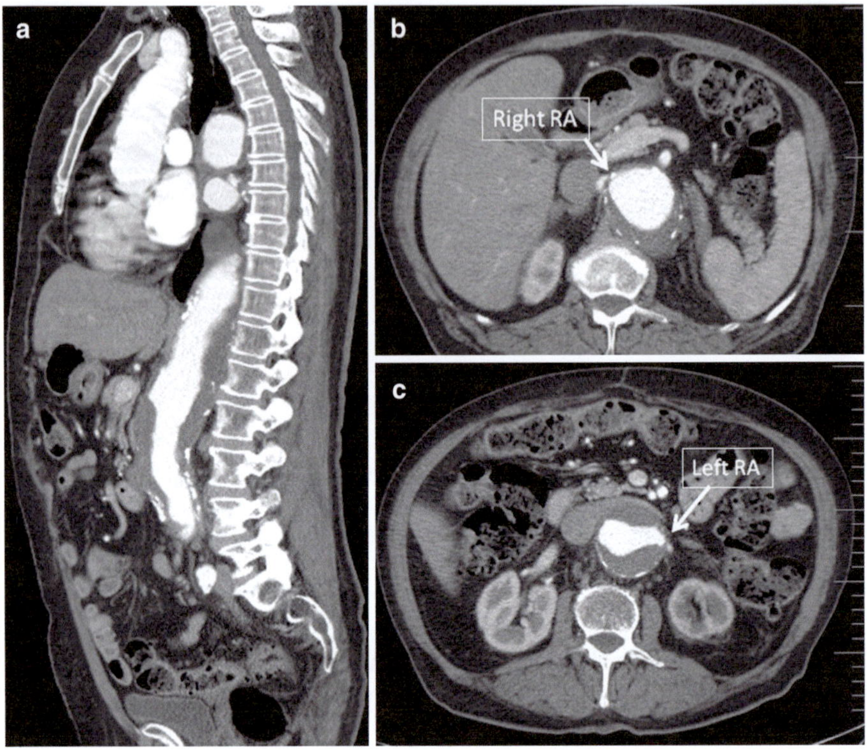

Fig. 1.3 (**a**–**m**) Abdominal and left iliac artery aneurysm with diffuse thrombus and atheroma ("hostile aorta", **a**–**f**); subtotal ostial occlusions of both renal arteries (**b**, **c**, **g**, **i**); double wire technique ("no touch", **f**); predilatation (3 mm) left renal artery (rigid lesion, balloon waist, **j**); 6/10-mm stent placement left renal artery (**k**); final result after bilateral 6-mm stent placement (**h**, **l**, **m**). Note: A 45-cm long sheath is used together with a 6 F renal double curve guiding catheter due to the tortuous access arteries

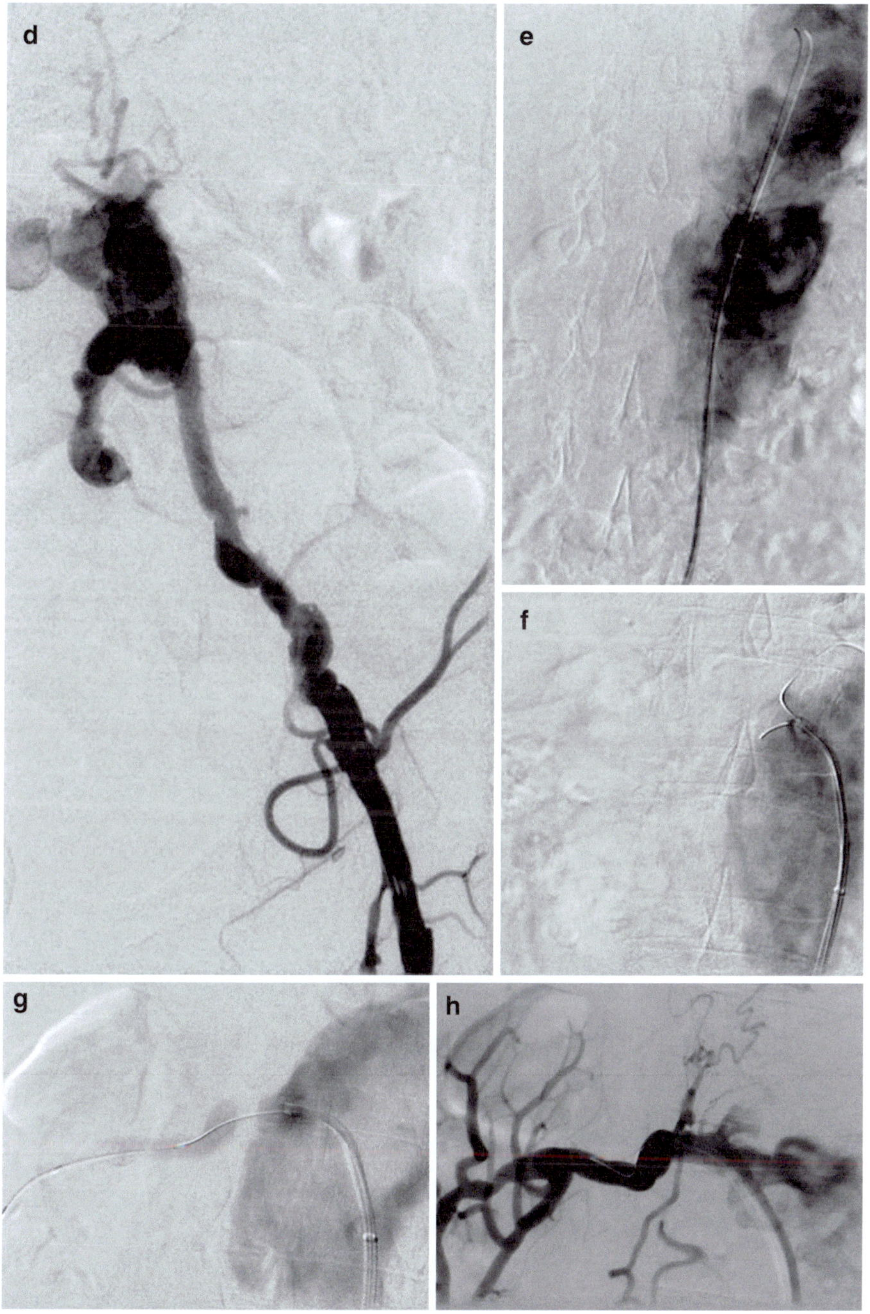

Fig. 1.3 (continued)

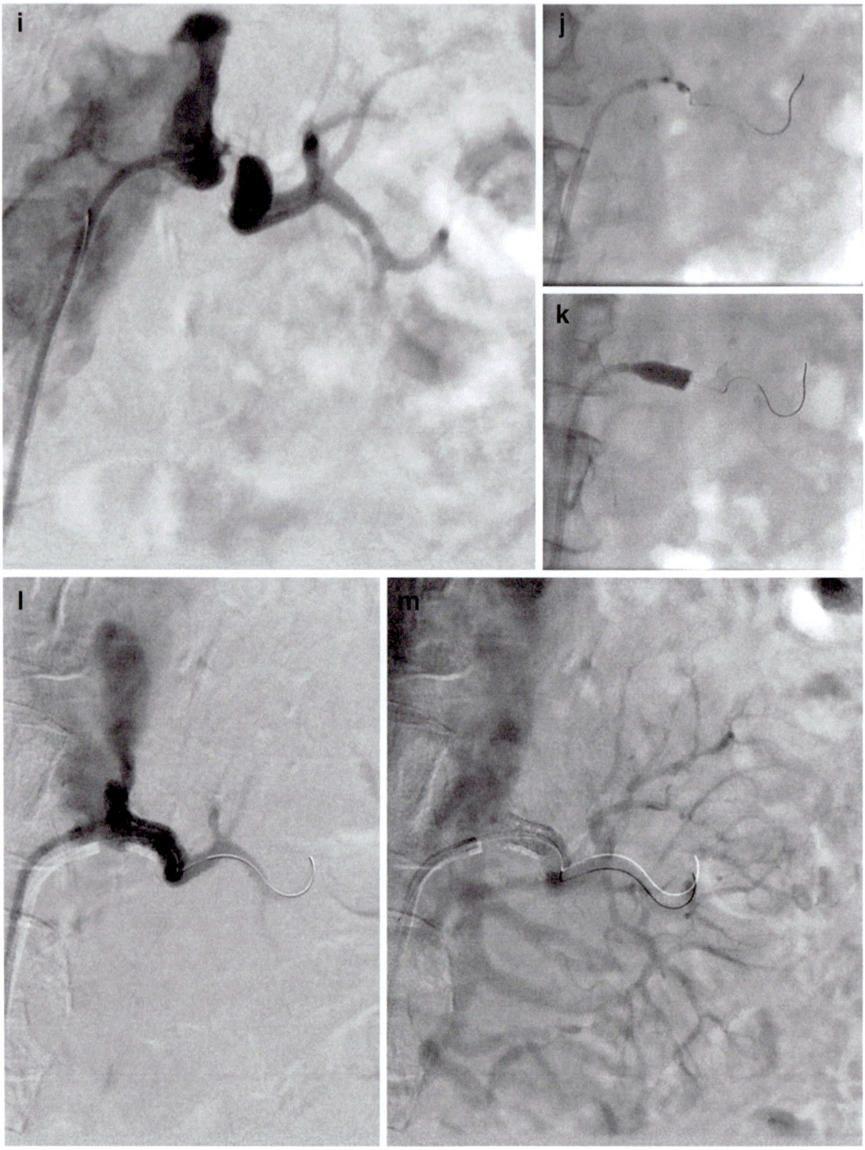

Fig. 1.3 (continued)

velocity >200 cm/s or a renal aortic flow velocity ratio >3.5 are correlated to a 50 or 60 % angiographic diameter stenosis and offer therefore indeed a high sensitivity in terms of detecting a RAS [30, 42]; however, the specificity detecting a hemodynamically relevant RAS is low. Provided that DUS is performed by an experienced physician with an adequate ultrasound machine, it should be the preferred imaging method.

1.5 Procedural Aspects

The first renal artery angioplasties were performed by the pioneers Felix Mahler in Berne and Andreas Grüntzig in Zurich in 1977 [43, 44]. Plain balloon PTRA was the only method of percutaneous treatment for RAS with satisfying acute and long-term results for angioplasty FMD and atherosclerotic RAS of the renal artery trunk until the 1990s [45, 46]. However, acute and chronic outcomes of PTRA of ostial atherosclerotic RAS were limited due to dissections, elastic recoil, and rigidity of the lesion [45, 47]. Since stenting became established, percutaneous renal revascularization is considered first-line therapy for the treatment of atherosclerotic RAS [20, 35, 45, 47–51]. In the era of low-profile premounted renal stent systems, atherosclerotic RAS can be treated successfully in almost all cases with restenosis rates ranging from 0 to 23 % depending on the renal artery diameter [20, 35, 47–50, 52–54].

1.5.1 Techniques and Devices for Endovascular Treatment of RAS

Patient preparation Part of preprocedure, predischarge, and follow-up visits should be:

Renal functional parameters (serum creatinine concentration, serum urea, at least an eGFR, or preferably creatinine clearance measured using 24-h urine; the role of cystatin C is uncertain).

Ambulatory 24-h BP monitoring.

DUS of the renal arteries with measurement of renal–aortic flow velocity ratios, intrarenal RI, and kidney size.

Analysis and documentation of antihypertensive medication.

The patient should provide informed consent at least 1 day before the procedure.

Fasting 6 h before the procedure.

Prehydration with intravenous iso-osmotic saline or orally (mineral water, tea) in patients with advanced renal insufficiency (eGFR <60 mL/min).

Preprocedure computed tomography or magnetic resonance tomography angiography might be helpful for interventional access route considerations.

1.5.2 Pre- und Postprocedure Medication

Dual antiplatelet therapy: In case of chronic pretreatment with aspirin, the prescription should be continued 100 mg/day for life and oral bolus of 500 mg aspirin should be given before the procedure; clopidogrel 600 mg given as a loading dose on the day of the procedure or the day before followed by 75 mg/day for 4 weeks.

After placement of the sheath, administration of a heparin bolus of 5000 IU.

There is controversy regarding the administration of acetylcysteine to capture free radicals, at a dosage of 2×600 mg (1200 mg) on the day before the procedure and on the day of the procedure.

Statins might reduce kidney fibrosis in chronic hypertensive individuals [55] and should be prescribed as part of the general secondary preventive medical treatment of atherosclerotic RAS.

In a small randomized trial, nebivolol given prior to the intervention has shown improved renal function outcomes as compared standard drug regimen [56].

1.5.3 Access Route

1.5.3.1 Femoral Access

The femoral access is the standard access route provided patent aorto-iliac access arteries and the absence of marked tortuosity of the pelvic arteries or an acute caudal angled course of the renal artery. The guiding catheter technique has replaced the original guidewire technique, as it is easier and safer to use.

The interventional sequence is as follows:

Following local anesthesia, a 6- or 7-F sheath (11 cm long) with a hemostatic valve is placed in the common femoral artery. If there is tortuosity in the access arteries (Fig. 1.3g), a 23-cm or even 45-cm long sheath may be helpful.

Introduction of a 0.035″ or 0.038″ standard J guidewire into the thoracic aorta.

The nonselective diagnostic angiogram can be either performed via a 6-F pigtail diagnostic catheter or the guiding catheter. Using a diagnostic catheter, the catheter is advanced to the level of the 12th thoracic vertebral body with a C-arm position at 20° left anterior oblique projection. Using a guiding catheter for diagnostic angiography, the guidewire is advanced up to the descending aorta and the guiding catheter (55 cm in length) is positioned at the level of the L1/L2 interlumbar space and, with the wire in place keeping the tip of the guiding catheter away from the aortic wall, the nonselective angiography of the renal arteries is performed by injecting 10 cc of contrast agent in DSA technique.

Following identification of the origin of the affected renal artery, the guiding catheter tip is positioned slightly above the renal artery ostium. The guidewire should still be exposed to the aorta in order to avoid aortic wall contact of the guiding catheter tip during manipulation. Thereafter the guidewire is removed. The guiding catheter tip usually "falls" into the ostium of the renal artery needing only mild corrections without significant risk of plaque embolization. Prior to the first selective dye injection, the guiding catheter should be cleared of any plaque and thrombus material that may have been collected in its tip during the probing process. This can be achieved either by aspiration via the Tuohy-Borst valve, or by simple back bleeding through the open valve (Fig. 1.4; [41]). Depending on the anatomical conditions, a guiding catheter with an internal mammary artery (approximately 90 %), renal double curve, hockey stick, or Judkins right configuration is used.

Alternatively, a Vista BriteTip IG™ "guide sheath" (Cordis – Cardinal Health, Fremont, CA, USA) is available, combining a 55-cm long guide catheter with a hemostatic valve. This saves 1 F in the outer sheath size.

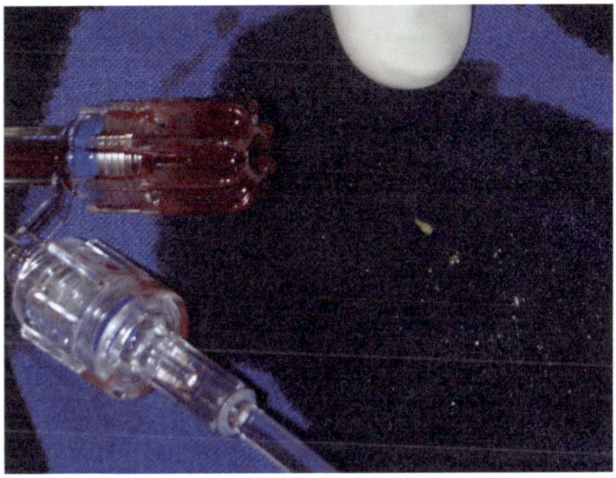

Fig. 1.4 Atheroma originating from the aortic wall collected after retrograde bleeding through the guiding catheter with opened hemostatic valve

1.5.3.2 Brachial or Radial Access

Bilateral brachial or radial access routes are feasible, but the left side is preferable in order to avoid passage across the cerebral arteries. Moreover, the distance to the renal arteries is shorter from the left arm. In most cases, a 6-F sheath or alternatively a 7-F guide sheath is placed in the brachial (radial) artery in a retrograde fashion. After placement of a 0.035″ guidewire with hydrophilic coating at the level of L1, nonselective imaging of the origins of the renal arteries is carried out, followed by placement of the guiding catheter as described above for the femoral access [41].

Materials required for the brachial access are a 7-F guide sheath, 90 cm long, with a multipurpose configuration; guiding catheter: 6 F, 100 cm long, with a multipurpose or right Amplatz configuration; and a Terumo 0.035″ stiff J wire. For a radial access, dedicated 120-cm long guiding catheters are mandatory.

1.5.4 Preprocedural Angiography

Before starting the intervention, the RAS has to be nonselectively and selectively imaged using angiography. With normal aortic anatomy, the renal artery origins are best assessed using a 20° left anterior oblique projection. In approximately 15 % of the normal population, the kidneys have multiple arteries, and the accessory arteries sometimes have atypically positioned origins (e.g., the distal infrarenal abdominal aorta, proximal common iliac artery). Attention should therefore be given to ensure that the renal artery does supply the entire renal contour; otherwise, accessory arteries should be sought.

1.5.5 Procedure

1.5.5.1 Atherosclerotic RAS

After selective exploration of the renal artery, a 0.014″ extra support guidewire with a nonhydrophilic coated tip is introduced across the RAS as far as the segmental arteries (*caution:* the parenchyma should not be damaged).

Markedly calcified RAS and stenoses ≥90% require predilatation with a coronary balloon catheter at least 3 mm in diameter (Fig. 1.5). Otherwise, the premounted stent systems can also be used for direct stenting.

If there is an ostial stenosis (defined within 10 mm distal from the origin), the stent should completely cover the renal artery ostium and extend 1–2 mm into the aortic lumen (Figs. 1.1a and 1.5a).

The ratio of the stent to the diameter of the renal artery should be 1:1–1.0:1.2. *Caution:* oversizing can lead to aortic wall rupture or aortic dissection in particular in eccentrically calcified lesions.

There is controversy regarding the use of distal protection systems, and in the authors' view, distal protection should not be done routinely until manufacturers are able to supply dedicated systems for renal application.

A technique to avoid renal embolism is the "no-touch" technique which is illustrated in Fig. 1.6a–d [57]. Basically, a 1 F larger guiding catheter has to be used (7 F) for exposing a second 0.014″ guidewire to the suprarenal aortic wall in order to keep the tip of the guiding catheter away from the renal artery origin.

The use of covered stents (e.g., Advanta V12, Atrium Medical, Hudson, NH, USA) and drug-eluting stents is usually limited to the treatment of in-stent restenosis or small arteries with a diameter ≤4 mm and still investigational.

"Hostile aorta" The term "hostile aorta" describes a rare condition of a diffuse soft atheroma in the aortic wall in particular around the renal artery origins which can be present in normal aortic diameters but preferably in ecstatic or aneurysmatic abdominal aortas (Fig. 1.3). This high soft plaque burden dramatically increases the peri-interventional embolic risk. Proper planning of the interventional strategy is mandatory including a preinterventional computed tomography – or magnetic resonance angiography (Fig. 1.3a–c, [58]) is mandatory in order to limit guiding catheter manipulations to a minimum. A "no-touch" technique is highly recommended and such procedures should be performed only by experienced operators and in desperate clinical conditions.

1.5.5.2 Dedicated Interventional Tools

"Non-flip-tip" technology In bended arteries, dedicated renal stent devices with a long so-called anti-flip tip of the stent carrying balloon catheter facilitates the introduction of the stent into the lesion even without predilation. The Hippocampus™ 0.014 Balloon Expanding Rapid Exchange Renal Stent System (Medtronic Corp., Concesio Brescia, Italy [59]) device consists of a long "non-flip-tip" with minimal entry profile. Since the system shows a progressive flexibility, the guidewire will not be straightened and possibly flipped out of the origin. As soon as the balloon segment with the crimped stent is advanced through the curve of the guiding catheter or introducer sheath, the long balloon catheter tip is already inserted in the renal artery trunk reducing the risk of flipping the guidewire back into the aorta.

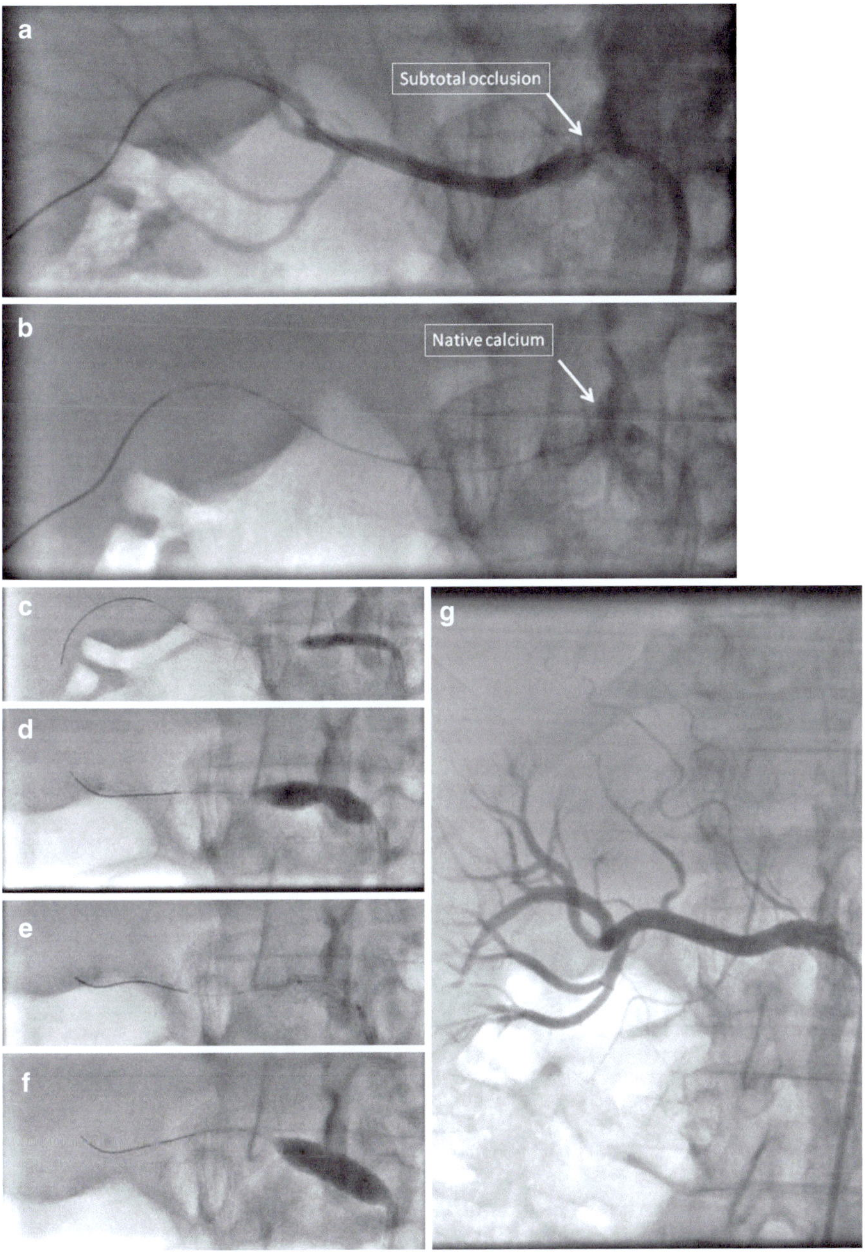

Fig. 1.5 Subtotal calcified ostial right renal artery stenosis (**a**); native calcium (aortic wall calcium) at the renal artery origin (**b**); step-wise predilatation with 2.5 mm (**c**) and 4-mm coronary low profile balloons; placement of a 6/12-mm stent, low pressure with remaining waist (**d**, **e**) in order to avoid renal artery rupture or dissection at the stent edge due to stent oversizing; full stent expansion with slightly removed balloon catheter (**f**); final result, stent reaching into the aortic lumen (**g**)

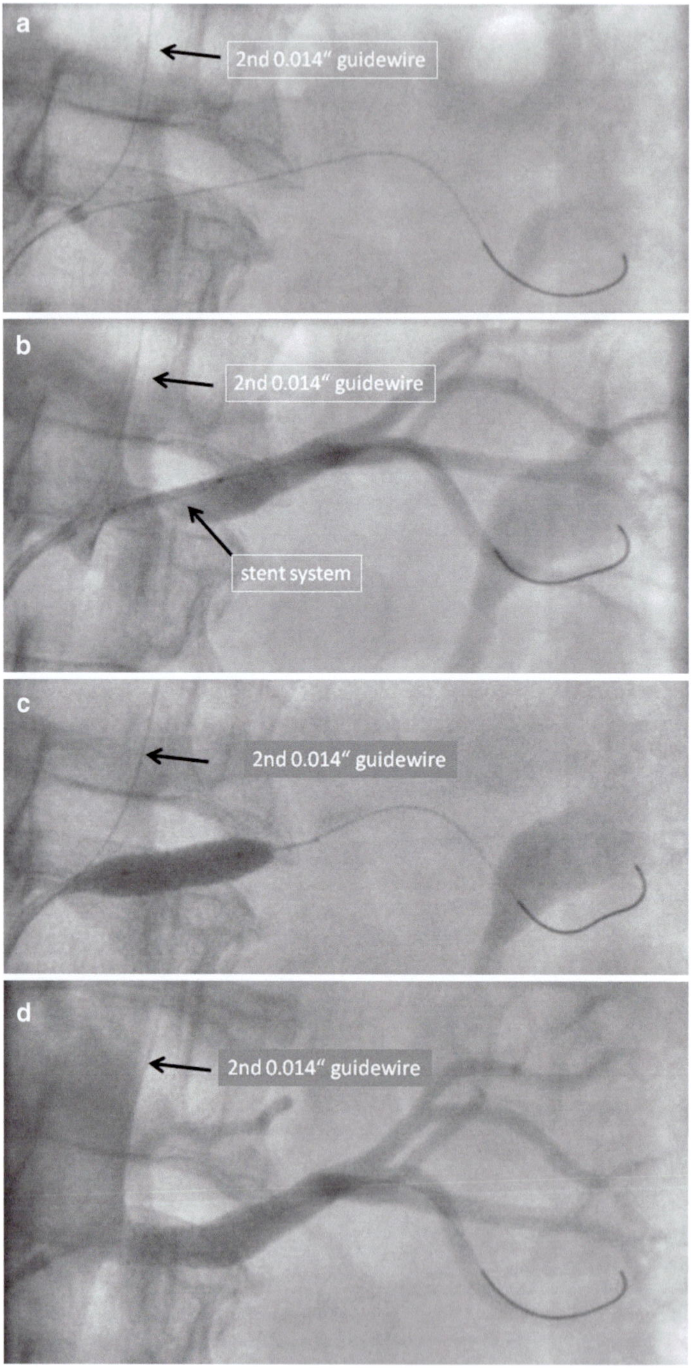

Fig. 1.6 (**a**–**d**) "No-touch technique": stenting of left renal artery using a modified "no-touch" technique. (**a**) One 0.014″ guidewire each in the renal artery and the suprarenal aorta. (**b**) Placement of the stent, aortic guidewire still in place. (**c**) Release of the stent, aortic wire still in place. (**d**) Final result [41, 57]

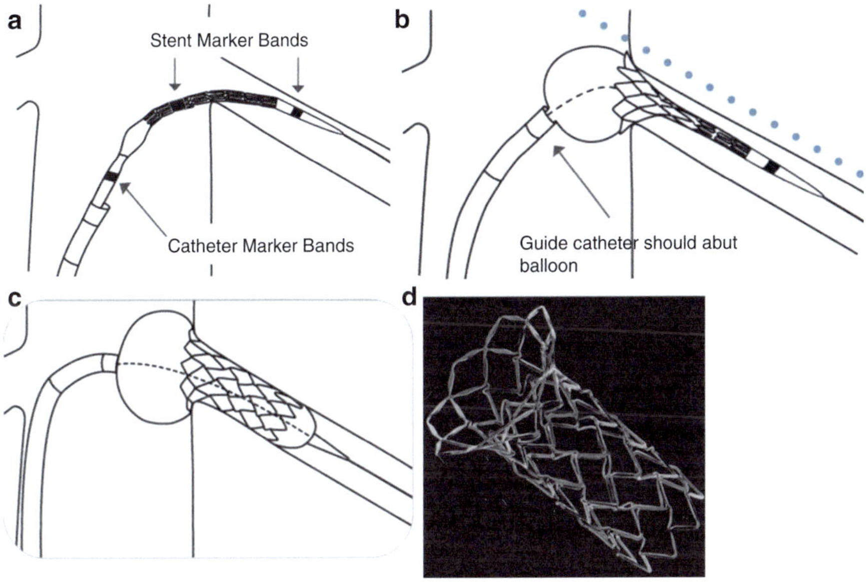

Fig. 1.7 (**a–d**) The dual-balloon delivery system (**a**) enables rapid, precise placement of the stent with the initially inflated locator balloon, which physically stops at the ostium and visually confirms the right position (**b**). Inflating the second balloon results in stent placement and further increasing the pressure in the locator balloon results in a flaring of the proximal stent end (**c**). The flared stent conforms anatomically to the aorto-ostial junction resulting in increased proximal scaffolding and ostial coverage (**d**)

In ostial atherosclerotic RAS, balloon-expandable stents are mandatory to resist the acute vessel recoil at the origin. Several stents like the Hippocampus™ show a progressive radial strength towards the proximal end which covers the renal artery origin.

Ostial flared stent technology: A stent device dedicated to ostial stenting represents the ArchStent® (Eucatech, Rheinfelden, Germany/Ostial Corporation, Mountain View, CA, USA; Fig. 1.7a–d). The dual-balloon delivery system enables rapid, precise placement of the stent with the initially inflated locator balloon, which physically stops at the ostium and visually confirms the right stent position. Inflating the second balloon results in stent placement and further increasing the pressure in the locator balloon results in a flaring of the proximal stent end. The flared stent conforms anatomically to the aorto-ostial junction resulting in increased proximal scaffolding and ostial coverage. Thus the aortorenal plaque is completely attached to the vessel wall and recrossing the stent in case of restenosis can easily be performed. A pilot study (BOSS-I) showed a 100 % acute technical success rate.

Self-expanding stents: In distally located lesions, low-profile self-expanding stents fitting through a 6-F guiding catheter (e.g., Xpert™, Abbott Vascular, Diegem, Belgium or Maris deep™, Medtronic, Fig. 1.8) should be used because of the high mechanical forces exposed to the renal artery trunk during respiration resulting in significant vessel kinking imposing the risk of stent fracture with consecutive abrupt vessel occlusion resulting in functional kidney loss.

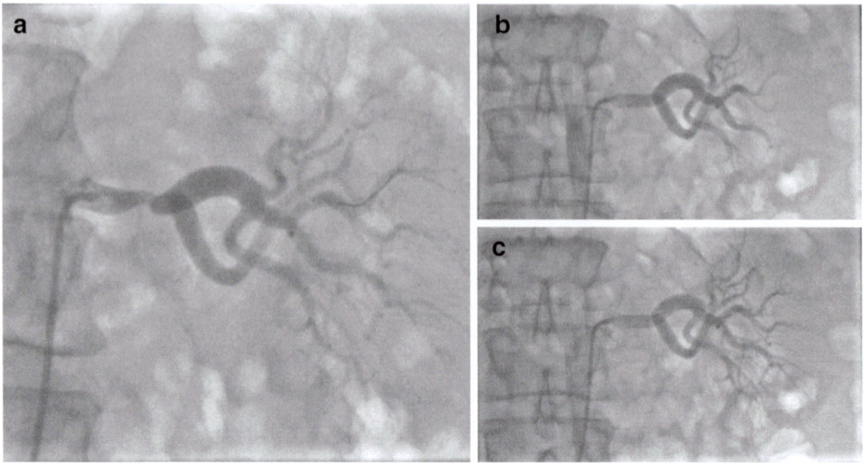

Fig. 1.8 High-grade stenosis of the distal left renal artery trunk (**a**); result after placement of a 6/20-mm 4-F sheath (6-F guiding catheter) compatible nitinol stent (**b**, **c**)

1.5.5.3 Nonatherosclerotic RAS

- Stenting is usually only indicated in ostial atherosclerotic RAS. In all other locations and etiologies, balloon angioplasty with provisional stent placement is still regarded as standard of care [11–13, 60] using a balloon diameter with a 1: 1 to 1: 1.2 ratio compared to the reference vessel diameter for the treatment of trunk and branch artery lesions. For verifying the appropriate balloon size, the artery dimension can either be measured using onsite programs or using a background image ("overlay function", Fig. 1.9c, d).
- In FMD, stenoses usually result from membranes (Figs. 1.2a and 1.9a, b) or – if located at the renal artery origin – of a shrunken dysplastic vessel wall with high rigidity (Fig. 1.2b). In both anatomical conditions, Cutting Balloon (Boston Scientific, Galway, Ireland) or scoring balloon angioplasty (Spectranetics, Colorado Springs, CO, USA) with a balloon diameter about 0.5–1.0 mm smaller than the reference vessel diameter either effectively disrupts the membrane or increases vessel compliance in ostial lesions. Following Cutting Balloon angioplasty, a properly sized regular balloon can be used for further optimization of the acute angioplasty result (Fig. 1.9d).
- Direct stenting of FMD ostial RAS should be avoided because of the risk for incomplete stent expansion due to the limited vessel wall compliance.

1.5.6 Postprocedural Follow-Up

Monitoring of cardiovascular parameters for 12 h is recommended, as excessive drops in BP may occur in individual cases, particularly in younger patients (<50 years of age). Particularly in patients with preprocedural renal insufficiency, function parameters must be repetitively checked, at least until 48 h after dye exposure.

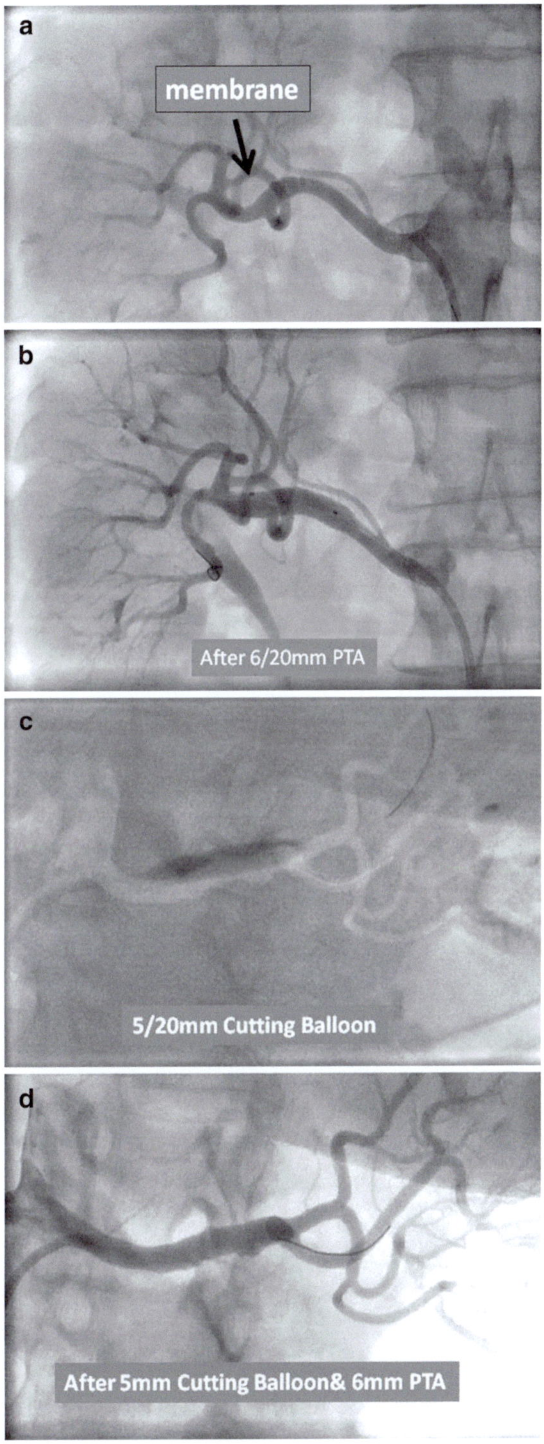

Fig. 1.9 Right renal artery with distal high-grade renal artery stenosis caused by a membrane (*arrow*, (**a**)), result after 6/20-mm balloon angioplasty, balloon shoulders visible like a foot print (**b**). Figure 1.8 shows the same lesion as Fig. 1.2a, 5/20-mm Cutting Balloon angioplasty using a background image for orientation ("overlay") (**c**) followed by a 6/20-mm regular balloon angioplasty with the final result (**d**)

1.5.7 Potential Risks of the Procedure

General potential interventional risks are:

Renal (cholesterol) embolization with subsequent deterioration in renal function, potentially progressing to terminal renal insufficiency ("hostile aorta").

Contrast-induced nephropathy: the risk increases along with the initial degree of renal dysfunction.

Renal artery and aortic dissection or rupture.

Incorrect stent placement.

Local vascular complications at the puncture site, such as false aneurysm, arteriovenous fistula, hematoma requiring transfusion, etc.

1.5.8 Recommended Equipment Checklist

Table 1.2 summarizes access and lesion-specific tools that should be available on stock for renal interventions.

1.6 Patient Follow-Up

After discharge, we recommend outpatient clinic follow-up examinations at 6 and 12 months post procedure and annually thereafter. Follow-up examinations should include – besides a physical examination – analysis of the antihypertensive and secondary preventive medication, ambulatory 24-h BP measurement, office-based BP measurement, and blood chemistry including serum creatinine, urea, and potassium. DUS has been shown to be a reliable screening method for detection of renal artery restenosis in particular following stent placement [31, 64–66]. In general, significant restenosis following renal artery stenting is a rare event ranging from 0 to 23 % depending on the renal artery diameter with highest restenosis rates in small diameters of 4–5 mm [20, 35, 47–50, 52–54]. Restenosis following balloon angioplasty is usually treated with stent placement; for the treatment of in-stent restenosis, a variety of treatment options are recommended including the placement of either a covered stent or a drug-eluting stent or in recent times using drug-eluting balloons ([61, 62, 64], Table 1.2). Plain balloon angioplasty or even cutting balloon angioplasty is associated with high recurrence rates of in-stent restenosis [61, 62].

Table 1.2 Summary of recommended devices

Special situation	Tool	Device example(s)
Brachial access	Diagnostic (4/5 F) or guiding catheter (6 F)	Multipurpose, Amplatz right, Judkins right
Femoral access	Diagnostic catheter (4/5 F)	SIM 1 or SOS Omni (diagnostic catheter)
	Guiding catheter (6/7 F)	IMA, Judkins right, hockey stick, RDC
Standard lesion	Guidewire	0.014″ extra support nonhydrophilic guidewire (e.g., Galeo ES™, Biotronik; BMW™, Abbott Vascular)
Subtotal occlusion/irregular lesion	Guidewire	0.014″ extra support hydrophilic coated (e.g., Pilot™ 150, Abbott Vascular)
"Undilatable" lesion	Plaque modulation device	AngioSculpt (AngioScore/Spectranetics)
FMD		Cutting Balloon (Boston Scientific)
Ostial lesion	Balloon-expandable stent	For example, Hippocampus™ stent (Medtronic) Dynamic renal™ (Biotronik) Herculink Elite™ (Abbott Vascular) Express™ SD (Boston Scientific) ArchStent™ (Ostial Solutions)
Acute angle of the renal artery origin	"Anti-flip-tip" balloon/stent device	Hippocampus™ stent (Medtronic)
In-stent restenosis [61, 62]	Drug-eluting stent	Promus™ (Boston Scientific)/Xience™ (Abbott Vascular), etc.
	Covered stent	Be Graft (Bentley-Innomed GmbH) Advanta V12/ICAST (Atrium)
	Drug-eluting balloon	Falcon® (Medtronic) Sequent Please® (B. Braun) In. Pact Pacific® (Medtronic)
Chronic total occlusion	Guidewire	For example, Asahi™ series (Asahi Intecc/Abbott Vascular) or Victory™ (Boston Scientific)
	Crossing device	Excimer laser (Spectranetics)
Thrombus-containing lesion	Distal protection devices	Filters (e.g., Emboshield pro™, Abbott Vascular, Fibernet™, Lumen Biomedical, Plymouth, USA) Distal occlusion balloon (Percusurge™, Medtronic [63])
Renal artery perforation	Main artery	Covered stent (Be Graft™)
	Segmental artery	Microcoils (e.g., Trufill, Cordis – Cardinal Health)

References

1. Harding MB, Smith LR, Himmelstein SI, Harrison K, Phillips HR, Schwab SJ, Hermiller JB, Davidson CJ, Bashore TM (1992) Prevalence and associated risk factors in patients undergoing routine cardiac catheterization. J Am Soc Nephrol 2:1608
2. Missouris CG, Buckenham T, Cappuccio FP, MacGregor GA (1994) Renal artery stenosis: a common and important problem in patients with peripheral vascular disease. Am J Med 96:10–14
3. Zierler RE, Bergelin RO, Davidson RC, Cantwell-Gab K, Polissar NL, Strandness DE Jr (1996) A prospective study of disease progression in patients with atherosclerotic renal artery stenosis. Am J Hypertens 9:1055–1061
4. van Jaarsveld BC, Krijnen P, Pieterman H, Derkx FH, Deinum J, Postma CT, Dees A, Woittiez AJ, Bartelink AK, Man in 't Veld AJ, Schalekamp MA, for the Dutch Renal Artery Stenosis Intervention Cooperative Study Group (2000) The effect of balloon angioplasty on hypertension in atherosclerotic renal-artery stenosis. N Engl J Med 342:1007–1014
5. Baumgartner I, Lerman LO (2011) Renovascular hypertension: screening and modern management. Eur Heart J 32(13):1590–1598
6. Tendera M, Aboyans V, Bartelink ML, Baumgartner I, Clement D, Collet JF, Cremonesi A, De Carlo M, Erbel R, Fowkes FGR, Heras M, Kownator S, Minar E, Ostergren J, Poldermans D, Riambau V, Roffi M, Röther J, Sievert H, van Sambeek M, Zeller T (2011) ESC guidelines on the diagnosis and treatment of peripheral artery diseases: document covering atherosclerotic disease of extracranial carotid and vertebral, mesenteric, renal, upper and lower extremity arteries. Eur Heart J 32:2851–2906
7. Rimmer JM, Gennari FJ (1993) Atherosclerotic renovascular disease and progressive renal failure. Ann Intern Med 118:712–719
8. Caps MT, Zierler RE, Polissar NL, Bergelin RO, Beach KW, Cantwell-Gab K, Casadei A, Davidson RC, Strandness DE Jr (1998) Risk of atrophy in kidneys with atherosclerotic renal artery stenosis. Kidney Int 53:735–742
9. Shanly PF (1996) The pathology of chronic renal ischemia. Semin Nephrol 16:21–32
10. Border WA, Noble NA (1998) Interactions of transforming growth factor-beta and angiotensin II in renal fibrosis. Hypertension 31:161–188
11. Persu A, Touze E, Mousseaux E, Barral X, Joffre F, Plouin PF (2011) Diagnosis and management of fibromuscular dysplasia: an expert consensus. Eur J Clin Invest 42:338–347
12. Gottsäter A, Lindblad B (2014) Optimal management of renal artery fibromuscular dysplasia. Ther Clin Risk Man 10:583–595
13. Trinquart L, Mounier-Vehier C, Sapoval M, Gagnon N, Plouin PF (2010) Efficacy of revascularization for renal artery stenosis caused by fibromuscular dysplasia: a systematic review and meta-analysis. Hypertension 56(3):525–532
14. Bax L, Woittiez AJ, Kouwenberg HJ, Mali WP, Buskens E, Beek FJ, Braam B, Huysmans FT, Schultze Kool LJ, Rutten MJ, Doorenbos CJ, Aarts JC, Rabelink TJ, Plouin PF, Raynaud A, van Montfrans GA, Reekers JA, van den Meiracker AH, Pattynama PM, van de Ven PJ, Vroegindeweij D, Kroon AA, de Haan MW, Postma CT, Beutler JJ (2009) Stent placement in patients with atherosclerotic renal artery stenosis and impaired renal function. Ann Intern Med 150:840–848
15. ASTRAL Investigators, Wheatley K, Ives N, Gray R, Kalra PA, Moss JG, Baigent C, Carr S, Chalmers N, Eadington D, Hamilton G, Lipkin G, Nicholson A, Scoble J (2009) Revascularization versus medical therapy for renal-artery stenosis. N Engl J Med 361:1953–1962
16. Cooper CJ, Murphy TP, Cutlip DE, Jamerson K, Henrich W, Reid DM, Cohen DJ, Matsumoto AH, Steffes M, Jaff MR, Prince MR, Lewis EF, Tuttle KR, Shapiro JI, Rundback JH, Massaro JM, D'Agostino RB, Dworkin LD, for the CORAL Investigators (2014) Stenting and medical therapy for atherosclerotic renal-artery stenosis. N Engl J Med 370:13–22
17. Messerli FH, Bangalore S, Makani H, Rimoldi SF, Allemann Y, White CJ, Textor S, Sleight P (2011) Flash pulmonary oedema and bilateral renal artery stenosis: the Pickering Syndrome. Eur Heart J 32:2231–2237

18. Kane GC, Xu N, Mistrik E, Roubicek T, Stanson AW, Garovic VD (2010) Renal artery revascularization improves heart failure control in patients with atherosclerotic renal artery stenosis. Nephrol Dial Transplant 25(3):813–820
19. Zeller T, Rastan A, Schwarzwälder U, Müller C, Frank U, Bürgelin U, Sixt S, Schwarz S, Noory E, Neumann FJ (2007) Regression of left ventricular hypertrophy following stenting of renal artery stenosis. J Endovasc Ther 14:189–197
20. Zeller T, Frank U, Müller C, Bürgelin K, Bestehorn HP, Cook-Bruns N, Schwarzwälder U, Neumann FJ (2003) Predictors of improved renal function after primary stenting of severe atherosclerotic ostial renal artery stenosis. Circulation 108:2244–2249
21. Kalra PA, Chrysochou C, Green D, Cheung CM, Khavandi K, Sixt S, Rastan A, Zeller T (2010) The benefit of renal artery stenting in patients with atheromatous renovascular disease and advanced chronic kidney disease. Catheter Cardiovasc Interv 75:1–10
22. Gray BH, Olin JW, Childs MB, Sullivan TM, Bacharach JM (2002) Clinical benefit of renal artery angioplasty with stenting for the control of recurrent and refractory congestive heart failure. Vasc Med 7(4):275–279
23. Plouin PF, Chatellier G, Darne B, Raynaud A (1998) Blood Pressure outcome of angioplasty in atherosclerotic renal artery stenosis: a randomized trial. The EMMA-study group. Hypertension 31:823–829
24. Webster J, Marshall F, Abdalla M, Dominiczak A, Edwards R, Isles CG, Loose H, Main J, Padfield P, Russel IT, Walker B, Watson M, Wilkinson R (1998) Randomised comparison of percutaneous angioplasty vs continued medical therapy for hypertensive patients with atheromatous renal artery stenosis. Scottish and Newcastle Renal Artery Stenosis Collaborative Group. J Hum Hypertens 12:329–335
25. Nordmann AJ, Woo K, Parkes R, Logan AG (2003) Balloon angioplasty or medical therapy for hypertensive patients with atherosclerotic renal artery stenosis? A meta-analysis of randomized controlled trials. Am J Med 114:44–50
26. Rocha-Singh KJ, Mishkel GJ, Katholi RE et al (1999) Clinical predictors of improved long-term blood pressure control after successful stenting of hypertensive patients with obstructive renal artery atherosclerosis. Catheter Cardiovasc Interv 47:167–172
27. Watson PS, Hadjipetrou P, Cox SV, Piemonte TC, Eisenhauer AC (2000) Effect of renal artery stenting on renal function and size in patients with atherosclerotic renovascular disease. Circulation 102:1671–1677
28. Kawarada O, Yokoi Y, Morioka N, Shiotani S, Higashimori A (2010) Cardiac benefits of renal artery stenting. EuroIntervention 6(4):485–491
29. Dieter RS Darki A, Nanjundappa A, Chhokar VS, Khadim G, Morshedi-Meibodi A, Freihage JH, Steen L, Lewis B, Leya F (2009) Usefulness of wide pulse pressure as a predictor of poor outcome after renal artery angioplasty and stenting. Am J Cardiol 104(5):732–734
30. Radermacher J, Chavan A, Schäffer J, Stoess B, Vitzthum A, Kliem V, Bleck J, Gebel MJ, Galanski M, Brunkhorst R (2000) Detection of significant renal artery stenosis with color Doppler sonography: combining extrarenal and intrarenal approaches to minimize technical failure. Clin Nephrol 53(5):333–343
31. Zeller T, Bonvini RF, Rastan A, Sixt S (2008) Colour-coded duplex ultrasound for diagnosis of renal artery stenosis and as follow-up examination after revascularization. Catheter Cardiovasc Interv 71:995–999
32. Krumme B, Blum U, Schwertfeger E, Flügel P, Höllstin F, Schollmeyer P, Rump L (1996) Diagnosis of renovascular disease by intrarenal and extrarenal Doppler scanning. Kidney Int 50:1288–1292
33. Radermacher J, Weinkove R, Haller H (2001) Techniques for predicting a favourable response to renal angioplasty in patients with renovascular disease. Curr Opin Nephrol Hypertens 10(6):799–805
34. Radermacher J, Chavan A, Bleck J, Vitzthum A, Stoess B, Gebel M et al (2001) Use of Doppler ultrasonography to predict the outcome of therapy for renal-artery stenosis. N Engl J Med 344:410–417

35. Zeller T, Müller C, Frank U, Bürgelin K, Horn B, Cook-Bruns N, Schwarzwälder U, Neumann FJ (2003) Stent-angioplasty of severe atherosclerotic ostial renal artery stenosis in patients with diabetes mellitus and nephrosclerosis. Catheter Cardiovasc Interv 58:510–515
36. Leesar MA, Varma J, Shapira A, Fahsah I, Raza ST, Elghoul Z, Leonard AC, Meganathan K, Ikram S (2009) Prediction of hypertension improvement after stenting of renal artery stenosis: comparative accuracy of translesional pressure gradients, intravascular ultrasound, and angiography. J Am Coll Cardiol 53:2363–2371
37. De Bryune B, Manoharan G, Pijls NHJ, Verhamme K, Madaric J, Bartunek J et al (2006) Assessment of renal artery stenosis severity by pressure gradient measurements. J Am Coll Cardiol 48:1851–1855
38. Mahmud E, Smith TW, Palakodeti V, Zaidi O, Ang L, Mitchell CR, Zafar N, Bromberg-Marin G, Keramati S, Tsimikas S (2008) Renal frame count and renal blush grade: quantitative measures that predict the success of renal stenting in hypertensive patients with renal artery stenosis. JACC Cardiovasc Interv 1:286–292
39. Krishnamurthi V, Novick AC, Myles JL (1999) Atheroembolic renal disease: effect on morbidity and survival after revascularization for atherosclerotic renal artery stenosis. J Urol 161(4):1093–1096
40. Cooper C, Haller S, Colyer W, Steffes M, Burket MW, Thomas WJ, Safian R, Reddy BK, Brewster PS, Ankenbrandt M, Virmani R, Dippel EJ, Rocha-Singh K, Murphy TP, Kennedy DJ, Shapiro JI, D'Agostino R, Pencina MJ, Khuder SA (2008) Embolic protection and platelet inhibition during renal artery stenting. Circulation 117:2752–2760
41. Zeller T (2014) Renal artery stenosis. In: Zeller T, Cissarek T, Gray WA, Kröger K. Vascular medicine – therapy and practice, 2nd ed. Thieme. Stuttgart, New York, Delhi, Rio ISBN: 313176841X
42. Staub D, Zeller T, Trenk D, Maushart C, Uthoff H, Breidthardt T, Klima T, Aschwanden M, Socrates T, Arenja N, Twerenbold R, Rastan A, Sixt S, Jacob AL, Jaeger KA, Mueller C (2010) Use of B-type natriuretic peptide to predict blood pressure improvement after percutaneous revascularisation for renal artery stenosis. Eur J Vasc Endovasc Surg 40:599–607
43. Grüntzig A, Vetter W, Meier B, Kuhlmann U, Lütolf U, Siegenthaler W (1978) Treatment of renovascular hypertension with percutaneous transluminal dilatation of a renal artery stenosis. Lancet 1:801–802
44. Mahler F, Krneta A, Haertel M (1979) Treatment of renovascular hypertension by transluminal renal artery dilatation. Ann Intern Med 90:56–57
45. Baert AL, Wilms G, Amery A, Vermylen J, Suy R (1990) Percutaneous transluminal renal angioplasty: initial results and long-term follow-up in 202 patients. Cardiovasc Interv Radiol 13:22–28
46. Bonelli FS, McKusick A, Textor SC, Kos PB, Stanson AW, Johnson CM, Sheedy PF 2nd, Welch TJ, Schirger A (1995) Renal artery angioplasty: technical results and clinical outcome in 320 patients. Mayo Clin Proc 70:1041–1052
47. Dorros G, Prince C, Mathiak L (1993) Stenting of renal artery stenosis achieves better relief of the obstructive lesion than balloon angioplasty. Catheter Cardiovasc Diagn 29:191–198
48. Blum U, Krumme B, Flügel P, Gabelmann A, Lehnert T, Buitrago-Tellez C, Schollmeyer P, Langer M (1997) Treatment of ostial renal-artery stenoses with vascular endoprotheses after unsuccessful balloon angioplasty. N Engl J Med 336:459–465
49. Dorros G, Jaff M, Mathiak L, Dorros II, Lowe A, Murphy K, He T (1998) 4-year follow-up of Palmaz-Schatz stent revascularisation as treatment for atherosclerotic renal artery stenosis. Circulation 98:642–647
50. White CJ, Ramee SR, Collins TJ, Jenkins JS (1999) Renal artery stent placement: utility in lesions difficult to treat with balloon angioplasty. J Am Coll Cardiol 30:1445–1450
51. van de Ven PJ, Kaatee R, Beutler JJ, Beek FJ, Woittiez AJ, Buskens E, Koomans HA, Mali WP (1999) Arterial stenting and balloon angioplasty in ostial atherosclerotic renovascular disease: a randomised trial. Lancet 353:282–286
52. Zeller T, Rastan A, Kliem M, Schwarzwälder U, Frank U, Bürgelin K, Schwarz T, Amantea P, Müller C, Neumann FJ (2005) Impact of carbon coating on restenosis rate after stenting of atherosclerotic renal artery stenosis. J Endovasc Ther 12:605–611

53. Sapoval M, Zähringer M, Pattynama P, Rabbia C, Vignali C, Maleux G, Boyer L, Szczerbo-Trojanowska M, Jaschke W, Hafsahl G, Downes M, Beregi JP, Veeger N, Talen A (2005) Low-profile stent system for treatment of atherosclerotic renal artery stenosis: The GREAT Trial. J Vasc Interv Radiol 16:1195–1202
54. Lederman RJ, Mendelsohn FO, Santos R, Phillips HR, Stack RS, Crowley JJ (2001) Primary renal artery stenting: characteristics and outcomes after 363 procedures. Am Heart J 142: 314–323
55. Keddis MT, Garovic VD, Bailey KR, Wood CM, Raissian Y, Grande JP (2010) Ischaemic nephropathy secondary to atherosclerotic renal artery stenosis: clinical and histopathological correlates. Nephrol Dial Transplant 25:3615–3622
56. Duranay M, Kanbay M, Akay H, Unverdi S, Sürer H, Altay M, Kırbaş I, Covic A, Zoccali C (2009) Nebivolol improves renal function in patients who underwent angioplasty due to renal artery stenosis: a pilot study. Nephron Clin Pract 114(3):c213–c217
57. Feldman RL, Wargovich TJ, Bittl JA (1999) No-touch technique for reducing aortic wall trauma during renal artery stenting. Catheter Cardiovasc Interv 46:245–248
58. Lin J, Li D, Yan F (2009) High-resolution 3D contrast-enhanced MRA with parallel imaging techniques before endovascular interventional treatment of arterial stenosis. Vasc Med 14(4):305–311
59. Rastan A, Krankenberg H, Müller-Hülsbeck S, Sixt S, Tübler T, Müller C, Schwarzwälder U, Frank U, Schwarz T, Leppaenen O, Neumann FJ, Zeller T (2008) Improved renal function and blood pressure control following renal artery angioplasty: the renal artery angioplasty in patients with renal insufficiency and hypertension using a dedicated renal stent device study (PRECISION). EuroIntervention 4(2):208–213, Erratum in: EuroIntervention. 2008 Nov; 4(3): table of contents
60. Cluzel P, Raynaud A, Beyssen B, Pagny JY, Gaux JC (1994) Stenoses of renal branch arteries in fibromuscular dysplasia: results of percutaneous transluminal angioplasty. Radiology 193:227–232
61. Zeller T, Rastan A, Schwarzwälder U, Müller C, Schwarz T, Frank U, Bürgelin K, Sixt S, Noory E, Beschorner U, Hauswald K, Branzan D, Neumann FJ (2007) Treatment of instent restenosis following stent-supported renal artery angioplasty. Catheter Cardiovasc Interv 70:454–459
62. Zeller T, Sixt S, Rastan A, Schwarzwälder U, Müller C, Noory E, Bürgelin K, Schwarz T, Hauswald K, Brantner R, Neumann FJ (2007) Treatment of reoccurring instent restenosis following reintervention after stent-supported renal artery angioplasty. Catheter Cardiovasc Interv 70:296–300
63. Henry M, Klonaris C, Henry I, Tzetanov K, Le Borgne E, Foliguet B, Hugel M (2001) Protected renal stenting with the PercuSurge GuardWire device: a pilot study. J Endovasc Ther 8:227–237
64. Del Conde I, Galin ID, Trost B, Kang J, Lookstein R, Woodward M, Gustavson S, Cambria RP, Jaff MR, Olin JW (2014) Renal artery duplex ultrasound criteria for the detection of significant in-stent restenosis. Catheter Cardiovasc Interv 83:612–618
65. Chi YW, White CJ, Thornton S, Milani RV (2009) Ultrasound velocity criteria for renal in-stent restenosis. J Vasc Surg 50(1):119–123
66. Fleming SH, Davis RP, Craven TE, Deonanan JK, Godshall CJ, Hansen KJ (2010) Accuracy of duplex sonography scans after renal artery stenting. J Vasc Surg 52(4):953–957; discussion 958

Primary Aldosteronism: A Field on the Move

2

Michael Doumas and Stella Douma

Abbreviations

ARR	Aldosterone-renin ratio
CT	Computed tomography
dRHTN	Drug-resistant hypertension
HTN	Hypertension
MRI	Magnetic resonance imaging

2.1 Introduction

Arterial hypertension (HTN) is a multifactorial disease, and its etiology remains unknown in the majority of patients, the so-called "essential hypertension" population [1]. Primary aldosteronism is the most common form of secondary HTN; however, its exact prevalence remains unknown [2]. It has to be acknowledged however that higher prevalence rates (up to 30% of hypertensive patients) are subject to referral bias and probably overestimate the true prevalence of primary aldosteronism.

Accumulating evidence indicates that primary aldosteronism is highly prevalent in patients with drug-resistant hypertension (dRHTN). Small clinical studies reported

M. Doumas (✉)
2nd Propedeutic Department of Internal Medicine, Aristotle University of Thessaloniki, Thessaloniki 54124, Greece

Hippokration General Hospital, 49, Konstantinoupoleos Street, Thessaloniki 54643, Greece
e-mail: michalisdoumas@yahoo.co.uk

S. Douma
3rd Department of Internal Medicine, Aristotle University of Thessaloniki, Thessaloniki 54124, Greece

C. Tsioufis et al. (eds.), *Interventional Therapies for Secondary and Essential Hypertension*, Updates in Hypertension and Cardiovascular Protection,
DOI 10.1007/978-3-319-34141-5_2

prevalence rates of up to 25 % [3–6], while more recent studies point toward lower prevalence rates of 11–15 % [7, 8]. The accurate and prompt detection of primary aldosteronism in patients with dRHTN has recently gained wide scientific interest, due to the introduction of interventional methods for the management of dRHTN: renal sympathetic denervation and carotid baroreceptor stimulation [9–13]. Patients with primary aldosteronism are not likely to respond to such interventional therapy, and is thus of utmost importance to exclude such patients in clinical studies evaluating the effects of interventional therapy.

The diagnosis of primary aldosteronism in real life is time consuming and might be tricky [14]. Clinical judgment based on appropriate training and long-term experience is required to evaluate controversial test results, overcome the uncertainty, and appropriately manage "gray-zone" patients: to offer surgical cure when indicated and avoid unnecessary and inappropriate operation when it is not indicated [2, 15].

The aim of this chapter is to provide the basis for detecting primary aldosteronism in dRHTN in the interventional era; to summarize the magnitude of the problem; to critically discuss available tests for the screening, confirmation, and lateralization of primary aldosteronism; to present the therapeutic options; and to propose a simple algorithm for the diagnosis and management of primary aldosteronism.

2.2 Importance of Detecting Primary Aldosteronism in the Interventional Era

Resistant or difficult to control hypertension is partially attributed to undiagnosed cases of secondary HTN [16, 17]. Primary aldosteronism is without doubt the most common form of secondary HTN in this patient population, accounting for up to 25 % in patients with dRHTN [3–6]. We have recently reported a much lower prevalence of primary aldosteronism (11 %) in a large sample of more than 2000 patients with dRHTN [7]. In the RESIST-POL study, primary aldosteronism was detected in 15.7 % of patients with dRHTN [8], confirming that although the prevalence of primary aldosteronism in resistant hypertension is lower than traditionally believed, primary aldosteronism affects a considerable portion of such patients. This portion of patients is of paramount clinical importance in the era of interventional management, mainly for two reasons: (a) because HTN can be effectively cured in patients with primary aldosteronism, either with adrenalectomy in unilateral adenomas or medical therapy in bilateral hyperplasia, avoiding the detrimental cardiovascular sequelae of primary aldosteronism, and (b) because patients with primary aldosteronism are unlikely to respond to interventional management of dRHTN through either renal sympathetic denervation or carotid baroreceptor stimulation.

Up to now, secondary dRHTN was an exclusion criterion in all studies evaluating the effects of renal denervation and baroreceptor stimulation [18–21]. This, along with the conduction of these studies in highly specialized centers provided the impression that appropriate exclusion of primary aldosteronism has been performed before intervention. However, no study has reported either the diagnostic algorithm (screening and confirmation) used for primary aldosteronism or the percentage of patients diagnosed and subsequently excluded from the study, raising doubts about the appropriate exclusion of patients with primary aldosteronism in conducted studies. The potential inappropriate inclusion of patients with primary aldosteronism in previous studies would have blurred the findings of the studies, due to the anticipated inefficacy of interventional techniques to lower blood pressure in these patients.

Future studies should incorporate a simple diagnostic work-up, specifically for the exclusion of primary aldosteronism. Such a diagnostic algorithm could include the conduction of aldosterone-renin ratio (ARR) in all patients deemed potentially eligible for the study, and a confirmatory test (intravenous saline load or captopril) for the accurate diagnosis of primary aldosteronism. The appropriate exclusion of primary aldosteronism, a condition found in 10–25 % of patients with dRHTN, is expected to uncover the true effect of interventional therapies.

Another issue that needs to be highlighted is the effect of mineralocorticoid receptor antagonists in patients with dRHTN and primary aldosteronism. Based on studies reporting a similar efficacy of spironolactone in patients with dRHTN both with and without primary aldosteronism [22], many primary care physicians are confused, and therefore screening for primary aldosteronism is of minimal clinical value. The truth however is different. Spironolactone is effective in dRHTN when added on top of a multidrug regime, including renin-angiotensin system blockers, calcium antagonists, and diuretics. In contrast, spironolactone is highly effective in primary aldosteronism as monotherapy in most cases or combined with a second drug in the minority of the cases [7]. It is not uncommon for patients with uncontrolled HTN using 5–7 antihypertensive drugs, to withdraw all prior medication and have their blood pressure controlled with small doses of spironolactone alone. Moreover, the identification of aldosterone-producing adenomas can be followed by adrenalectomy, and subsequent surgical cure, avoiding excessive target organ damage and cardiovascular morbidity and mortality associated with primary aldosteronism.

2.3 The Magnitude and the Consequences of the Problem

Primary aldosteronism is the most common form of secondary hypertension; however, the exact prevalence rates of this condition remain controversial. Whatever the prevalence, there is no doubt that primary aldosteronism is associated with increased cardiovascular morbidity and mortality, partly due to the effects of elevated aldosterone levels on the human vasculature.

2.3.1 Prevalence

Jerome Conn described primary aldosteronism in 1955 and speculated that this clinical entity might account for as much as 20 % of hypertensive patients [23]. However, several observational studies dampened the initial enthusiasm pointing toward a much lower prevalence of less than 1 % [24–27], establishing a general belief that prevailed for almost four decades [28]. A second epidemic of primary aldosteronism was initiated by the Brisbane group, which reported a prevalence of 8.5 % in a sample of almost 200 hypertensive patients [29], and leaded to prevalence rates of up to 39 % [30]. A recent survey of 18 studies revealed a wide variation in prevalence rates, ranging from 1.4 to 32 %, for a median of 8.8 % of studied hypertensive patients [31]. The US guidelines for primary aldosteronism estimate the overall prevalence of primary aldosteronism at 6.1 % in the general hypertensive population, acknowledging that the prevalence is higher than 10 % in specialty settings [32].

Up to now, the largest study specifically aimed to evaluate the prevalence of primary aldosteronism in the general hypertensive population comes from Italy. The Primary Aldosteronism Prevalence in Hypertensives (PAPY) study included 1125 hypertensive patients and reported a prevalence of 11.2 % [33]. However, study participants were referred to specialized centers by general practitioners, raising the possibility of selection bias. Indeed, a marked heterogeneity in prevalence rates across participating centers was observed, and exclusion of two centers with the highest prevalence rates resulted in a significant drop of prevalence from 11.2 to 7.4 %. Two other studies claiming unselected population reported a prevalence rate of 3.8 % for primary aldosteronism and 1.5 % for aldosterone-producing adenomas, respectively [34, 35].

The wide variation in the prevalence of primary aldosteronism between different studies is probably ought to differences in patient selection, employed diagnostic methodology (the tools used to screen and confirm the diagnosis), and the severity of HTN in study participants. Indeed, the prevalence of primary aldosteronism depends strongly on the latter parameter. Primary aldosteronism was found in 2 % of patients with Stage I hypertension, while the corresponding rates in Stage II and Stage III hypertension were 8.5 and 13.5 %, respectively [36]. The PAPY study confirmed these findings, reporting a prevalence of 7.2 % in patients with Stage I HTN and 19.5 % in patients with Stage III HTN [33].

2.3.2 Cardiovascular Consequences

Accumulating evidence strongly indicates that primary aldosteronism is associated with greater target organ damage and increased rates of cardiovascular morbidity and mortality compared to patients with essential HTN and similar blood pressure levels [37, 38], suggesting an additive effect of aldosterone excess on tissue damage, independent of and beyond blood pressure elevation per se. Indeed, primary aldosteronism is associated with a twofold increase of left ventricular hypertrophy [39], increased arterial stiffness [40], higher carotid intima-media thickness [41], microalbuminuria [42], endothelial dysfunction [43], myocardial fibrosis and stiffening [44], prolonged QT interval [45], arrhythmias [46], atrial fibrillation [39], coronary artery disease and nonfatal myocardial infarction [39], cerebrovascular disease [46], heart failure [39], metabolic syndrome [47], and altered glucose homeostasis [46, 48]. It therefore seems of utmost importance to recognize primary aldosteronism promptly, before the development of target organ damage and the cardiovascular sequelae.

Cardiovascular complications seem to be dependent on serum potassium levels. In the German Conn's registry, the largest available registry for primary aldosteronism, it was found that patients with hypokalemia had significantly higher cardiovascular morbidity and mortality than patients with normokalemia [38]. Although most studies report higher mortality rates in patients with primary aldosteronism compared to patients with essential HTN, a recent report from the same registry revealed that all-cause mortality was not significantly different between patients with primary aldosteronism and patients with essential HTN, when adjustments for confounding factors were made [49].

2.4 Diagnosis

The diagnostic work-up for primary aldosteronism follows the typical diagnostic flow-chart of an endocrine disorder: screening, confirmation, and localization. What is specific for primary aldosteronism is that the localization is very important due to the different management of disease subtypes (bilateral hyperplasia, and adenoma).

2.5 Screening

Arterial HTN is found in one fourth to one third of the adult population, currently affects more than one billion individuals worldwide, and is expected to affect about 1.5 billion people at the end of next decade [50]. Given the enormous number of affected individuals, the most important question from the clinical point of view is who to screen for primary aldosteronism without performing unnecessary and costly tests in every hypertensive patient (Table 2.1). The obvious question that comes next is how to screen selected individuals, in order to detect primary aldosteronism without missing diseased patients [14].

2.5.1 Who to Screen

The Japanese guidelines [51] recommend screening for all patients with arterial HTN, while the US guidelines [32] recommend screening in selected group of patients: patients with dRHTN, patients with severe and moderate HTN, patients with hypokalemia (spontaneous or diuretic-induced), and patients with adrenal incidentaloma. Patients with a family history of primary aldosteronism or onset of HTN

Table 2.1 Who to screen for primary aldosteronism

Resistant hypertension
Moderate and severe hypertension
Hypokalemia (spontaneous or drug induced)
Adrenal incidentaloma
Family history of primary aldosteronism

before the age of 40 years have also been proposed as candidates for screening, and this recommendation seems rational. Further patient populations proposed for screening include patients with metabolic syndrome, diabetes mellitus, and obstructive sleep apnea [52]. However, this proposal increases exponentially the number of patients to be screened, and seems to reach Japanese guidelines that recommend screening for all hypertensive patients.

Several factors limit the implementation of these recommendations in everyday clinical practice, including the cost, the manpower, and the hospital amenities [14]. The cost of measuring plasma renin activity and plasma aldosterone is very high in the US ($420); although the cost is lower in Europe, it still remains considerably high if ARR is going to be performed in all hypertensive patients.

2.5.2 Aldosterone to Renin Ratio (ARR)

The ratio of plasma aldosterone to plasma renin activity (ARR) was introduced 35 years ago as a screening test for primary aldosteronism [53]. The subsequent wide application of this screening test led to an almost tenfold increase of disease detection [54]. This test unveils the autonomous production of aldosterone, independent from the renin-angiotensin system, which characterizes primary aldosteronism. A ratio of more than 30 (when plasma aldosterone is expressed in ng/dl and plasma renin activity is expressed in ng/ml/h) is suggestive but not diagnostic of primary aldosteronism. Some centers use either lower (20) or higher (40–50) ARR cutoff values, in the effort to minimize either missing cases of primary aldosteronism or false-positive results, respectively.

The use of ARR as a screening test has offered a "great forward thrust" in the primary aldosteronism field and acted as the driving force for uncovering the magnitude of the problem. However, ARR is not devoid of significant limitations, and several factors need to be taken into account when performing and evaluating ARR as a screening test for the diagnosis of the disease.

First, the ARR is a ratio, and its value greatly depends on the denominator, the plasma renin activity values. Therefore, the ARR might be high (>30) in patients with low renin hypertension, a condition that accounts for up to 30 % of hypertensive patients, and is much more common in older subjects [55] and patients with dRHTN [7]. It therefore seems wise to use an elevated serum aldosterone value (>15 ng/dl in most centers, >12 ng/dl in some centers) as an additional criterion to high ARR, in order to consider this test indicative of primary aldosteronism [7].

Second, the accuracy of renin determination decreases with decreasing values, and the measurement of renin becomes less accurate in low and especially in very low renin levels. Such levels are observed in patients with primary aldosteronism and low-renin essential hypertension. In order to avoid ARR overestimation in such cases, one can use the arbitrary value of at least 0.2 ng/ml/h for plasma renin activity to be used for ARR determination in very low renin levels.

The most common and important parameter affecting ARR determination regards antihypertensive therapy. Apart from alpha-blockers and non-dihydropyridine calcium antagonists, all other antihypertensive drugs exert a major effect on ARR determination. Beta-blockers and centrally acting agents increase significantly the ARR by suppressing renin levels and result in false-positive findings. In contrast, diuretics, ACE inhibitors, and angiotensin receptor blockers decrease the ARR by increasing renin levels and result in false-negative findings.

Therefore, antihypertensive therapy needs to be – ideally – discontinued for 2–3 weeks (much more for mineralocorticoid receptor antagonists) in order to perform accurately the ARR estimation. However, drug discontinuation is not always feasible in everyday clinical practice, especially in patients with severe HTN, underlying cardiovascular disease or acute target organ damage. In such cases, the treating physician has two options: (a) either to replace prior therapy with alpha-blockers as monotherapy or combined with non-dihydropyridine calcium antagonists (based on experience and clinical judgment) or (b) to perform the ARR determination while the patient continues administered antihypertensive therapy. In the latter case, the physician should be aware of the abovementioned effects of antihypertensive drugs on ARR, and evaluate the result taking into account these effects. Some studies report a minimal effect of antihypertensive drugs on ARR, thus supporting the performance of ARR without drug withdrawal [56]. However, other studies point toward a significant effect of antihypertensive drugs on ARR, thus supporting drug withdrawal before ARR determination. In a recent study, beta-blocker therapy resulted in false-positive ARR in 31 % of patients, underlining the need for drug withdrawal before screening for primary aldosteronism. The optimum time for beta-blocker withdrawal depends on the method of renin determination and is 2 weeks for direct renin concentration and 3 weeks for plasma renin activity determination [57].

In our experience, drug replacement with alpha-blockers and non-dihydropyridine calcium antagonists for 2 weeks is feasible and safe in the vast majority of cases, even in patients with severe HTN and/or history of cardiovascular disease, since the blood pressure remains practically unaffected by drug replacement and is not further elevated during this short time period. Therefore, we perform ARR after appropriate drug switching in almost all patients with dRHTN, apart from patients who are fragile or exhibit acute organ damage.

Plasma aldosterone and renin levels are greatly influenced by the posture of the patient, exhibiting lower values in the supine position and higher values in the upright position, while the corresponding values in the seating position lie in between. Supine ARR, with blood sampling in the morning after an overnight bed rest or after 1–2 h with the patient at the supine position, was for long time considered as the most accurate tool. However, many centers have adopted the seated ARR test during the last decade, with blood sampling in the morning and the patient seated for 5–15 min after walking for at least 2 h, due to its convenience. Several studies have shown the reliability of seated ARR, although with a slightly reduced power compared to the supine ARR [58, 59].

Finally, dietary sodium intake also affects ARR determination. A normal- or high-sodium diet uncovers the hormonal features of primary aldosteronism, while a low-sodium diet might mask the diagnosis of primary aldosteronism, by increasing renin levels and thus reducing ARR. Therefore, a liberal sodium diet (high or at least normal) should be recommended in all patients undergoing screening for primary aldosteronism. Of great importance, sodium intake should be checked by the measurement of 24 h urinary sodium excretion to exclude sodium depletion. Even the phase of menstrual cycle may affect renin and aldosterone levels for screening and confirming primary aldosteronism [60].

2.5.3 Expert Comment

ARR is a crude tool, unable to differentiate primary aldosteronism from low-renin hypertension. For example, a patient with low renin levels at 0.2 ng/ml/h and normal aldosterone levels at 7 ng/dl has an elevated ARR of 35, suggesting primary aldosteronism based on ARR despite normal aldosterone levels. Even more outrageous, a patient with renin levels of 0.1 ng/ml/h has an elevated ARR of 40 with aldosterone levels at 4 ng/dl, a supernormal value, which actually excludes, rather than being indicative of, primary aldosteronism. It therefore seems obvious that raised aldosterone levels are a sine qua noncriterion when screening for primary aldosteronism; otherwise, clinically unwise paths may be followed.

Assay characteristics strongly affect the screening validity of ARR in primary aldosteronism [61]. The rate of positive ARR is lower when plasma renin concentration is measured instead of plasma renin activity in treated hypertensive patients [62]. The simultaneous determination of plasma aldosterone and plasma renin concentrations using automated chemiluminescence immunoassays has been available recently, and looks like a promising and convenient alternative to traditional assays, in the effort to facilitate the screening and confirmatory process for primary aldosteronism [63].

Although most specialized centers use plasma renin activity, direct renin activity seems to prevail among general practitioners in everyday clinical practice, since its measurement is simpler and less costly and blood can be collected, transferred, and centrifuged at room temperature. It is obvious that different cutoff ARR levels apply when direct measurement of active renin is used instead of plasma renin activity.

Collectively, the aforementioned parameters confounding ARR determination underline the need for improved screening tests, which will act either complimentary or independently to ARR. Recently the N-terminal probrain natriuretic peptide (NT-proBNP) was proposed as a complimentary screening test. The confirmation of diagnosis with intravenous saline loading reached 93 % in male patients with high ARR and high NT-proBNP levels [64].

2.6 Confirmation

The confirmation of diagnosis is of paramount importance, given the high proportion of false-positive findings from screening tests that might be as high as 50 % [7]. Confirmatory tests aim to uncover the autonomous production of aldosterone, and thus establish the diagnosis of primary aldosteronism. Several tests are currently used for the confirmation of the diagnosis, and the main tests (Table 2.2) will be described in summary, along with a critical presentation of their advantages and disadvantages.

Table 2.2 Confirmatory tests for primary aldosteronism

Fludrocortisone test
Intravenous saline loading
Captopril test
Oral sodium loading

2.6.1 Oral Sodium Load

The oral sodium load is an old and cheap diagnostic test for the confirmation of diagnosis, used by the Mayo Clinic group and others. A high sodium diet (300 mmol per day) is administered to the patient for 3 days. A 24 h urine collection is performed during the third day of the test for the determination of urinary aldosterone and sodium levels. A 24 h urinary sodium value of more than 200 mEq ensures sodium loading, whereas a 24 h urinary aldosterone value of more than 12 μg confirms the diagnosis (some centers use cutoff 24 h urinary aldosterone levels of 14–17 μg to minimize false-positive tests) [65, 66].

Several factors limit the wide use of this confirmatory test. Apart from the inherent difficulties and uncertainties of accurate 24 h urinary collection, the main limitation of the test is the measurement of 24 h urinary aldosterone. Available assays often exhibit poor performance and usually measure only the 18-oxo-glucoronide fraction, a part of total aldosterone excretion that might not be excreted in chronic kidney disease. Moreover, potassium levels should be assessed daily, and appropriate supplementation is needed, in times large amounts are required.

2.6.2 Intravenous Saline Load

The intravenous saline load is the most widely used confirmatory test in Europe. In summary, the test starts at 7.00–8.30 am, and the patient has to remain in the supine position for at least 1 h; then, 2 L of normal saline are infused over a 4 h period, and serum aldosterone levels are measured before and after saline infusion. Serum aldosterone values higher than 5 ng/dl are considered diagnostic for primary aldosteronism, since saline infusion typically suppresses aldosterone levels to less than 5 ng/dl.

This test has the advantage of being performed under controlled and supervised conditions and potassium supplementation is usually not required during the test, due to its short duration (nevertheless, serum potassium levels are measured before and after the test to ensure that hypokalemia is not evident). On the other hand, the acute saline loading has its own limitations as well. First of all, safety may be compromised in patients with heart failure and/or chronic kidney disease or fragile patients who cannot tolerate an acute 2 L saline infusion. Then, the test is not very practical, since the patient needs to be in the hospital for a whole morning and should stay still in the supine position for about 6 h, experiencing the discomfort of urinating in a "bedpan." Another important limitation is the 5 ng/dl cutoff level. In our opinion, serum aldosterone below this level is definitely excluding the diagnosis of primary aldosteronism, while values between 5 and 10 ng/dl should be considered as a "gray zone," and the acute saline loading should be coupled by another confirmatory test (preferably the fludrocortisone test). Serum aldosterone levels above 10 ng/dl are definitely diagnostic of primary aldosteronism.

Recently, a modified version of the intravenous saline loading was proposed, based on the posture of the patient. Traditionally, the intravenous saline loading is performed with the patient in the supine position, potentially missing the diagnosis of posture-responsive primary aldosteronism. In a small sample of patients (24 participants), it was found that the intravenous saline loading in the seated position was significantly superior to the intravenous saline loading in the supine position, and similar to the fludrocortisone test [67]. Larger studies are needed to validate these findings, and such a larger study is currently ongoing and the results are eagerly awaited.

2.6.3 Fludrocortisone Test

The fludrocortisone test is considered the "gold standard" confirmatory test for the diagnosis of primary aldosteronism and is widely used in Australia and other specialized centers worldwide. In summary, fludrocortisone (0.1 mg four times daily) is administered for 4 days along with sodium and potassium supplementation, while patients are on a high-sodium diet. At the conclusion of the test, blood is drawn at 10 am, and the diagnosis of primary aldosteronism is confirmed when (a) serum aldosterone levels are over 6 ng/dl, (b) plasma renin activity is lower than 1 mg/ml/h, and potassium levels are within normal range [68].

This test requires close attention when performed in patients with heart failure and/or chronic kidney disease, just as with the acute saline loading. Moreover, it has to be acknowledged that it is time consuming, and requires hospitalization (recommended by many centers, including the Brisbane center with the larger experience). In our practice, hospitalization is not mandatory, provided that hypokalemia has been corrected (which is anyway a prerequisite for the proper conduction of the test along with adequate sodium intake). In our experience of more than 600 tests, no adverse events have been observed, and hospitalization was selected in a minority of cases.

Recently, a modified form of the fludrocortisone suppression test was proposed, using dexamethasone administration on the last day of the test to eliminate the potential stimulation of aldosterone by endogenous stress-induced ACTH [69]. The validity of this test needs to be confirmed in large studies from more centers, before gaining wider application.

2.6.4 Captopril Test

The captopril test is an old test, traditionally used for the diagnosis of renovascular HTN and later applied for the confirmation of primary aldosteronism. This test gained wider application after the publication of the PAPY study [33] and the support of several Italian groups and others. Captopril (25–50 mg) is administered with the patient seated for at least 1 h; serum aldosterone and plasma renin activity are measured 2 h post-captopril ingestion. The diagnosis of primary aldosteronism is confirmed when serum aldosterone is over 8.5 mg/dl (other centers use higher cutoff levels up to 15 ng/dl) or the ARR is over 30 (other centers use higher cutoff levels up to 50) [70–72]. The captopril test is cheap, very easy to perform, and devoid of risks in patients with heart failure and chronic kidney disease. However, some studies support a substantial portion of false-negative and false-positive findings [73]. Moreover, this test was reported to have a poor discriminatory ability for the diagnosis of primary aldosteronism in patients with HTN and high ARR [74], as well as in patients with 24 h urinary sodium excretion of less than 130 mEq [33], casting doubts about the use of this test as a first-line confirmatory test for the diagnosis of primary aldosteronism.

Recently, an alternative test was introduced, using valsartan or losartan instead of captopril, measuring ARR 2 h and 4 h post-valsartan ingestion, and using ARR cutoff levels of 35 or 40 [75–77]. Available data regarding the valsartan test is contradictory, and the test requires further evaluation before gaining wide application.

2.6.5 Expert Comment

The fludrocortisone suppression test is considered the "gold standard" by most experts in this field. However, head-to-head comparisons between confirmatory tests are limited, are usually post hoc and monocentric, and often are performed under different sampling conditions, and the number of participants is small [78–80]. Current data do not establish beyond any doubt that any confirmatory test is much better than another for the confirmation of the diagnosis of primary aldosteronism.

The fludrocortisone and the intravenous saline tests seem preferable, but have technical difficulties and carry potential risks, while the captopril test is devoid of these limitations but seems to underperform compared to the former tests and needs further validation in head-to-head studies with the fludrocortisone test. The choice of the confirmatory test is mainly based upon habit and the familiarity of each expert with the test and hospital amenities at each center. We prefer saline loading (intravenous and fludrocortisone) testing and perform both tests in all patients with high ARR and/or suspicion of primary aldosteronism.

Both screening and confirmatory tests, as well as disease lateralization by adrenal venous sampling depend (rely) on the accurate measurement of hormones (aldosterone, renin, cortisol). Immunoassays of aldosterone require expertise and present some problems. Mass spectrometry is much more preferred. Similarly, renin measurements have many problems, and plasma angiotensin seems preferable. Currently, automated platforms and immunometric methods are widely used in everyday clinical practice for the estimation of aldosterone and renin, in the effort to provide results more rapidly and at a lower cost.

An alternative method of aldosterone determination using high performance liquid chromatography and tandem mass spectrometry was found to be very accurate and reproducible [81], and this methodology was confirmed by other groups as well [82, 83]. The same methodology is used for angiotensin I determination [84], and might be used for the determination of angiotensin II in the near future with theoretical significant benefits. Chemiluminescence-based methods have been also introduced recently with promising results [85].

2.7 Localization

Although many forms of primary aldosteronism have been described in the literature, from the clinical point of view of primary care physicians, cardiologists, and internists should be able to make the distinction between bilateral adrenal hyperplasia that is managed medically and unilateral aldosterone-producing adenomas that are managed surgically, along with recognizing the rare cases of adrenal carcinoma and familial syndromes (Table 2.3). Other forms of primary aldosteronism such as congenital aldosteronism, primary unilateral adrenal hyperplasia, bilateral aldosterone-producing adenomas, and unilateral multinodular adrenal hyperplasia represent rare and less well-defined forms, whose description (certainly beyond the scope of this review) blurs the necessary clarity when addressing perplexed issues to nonspecialists.

2.7.1 Adrenal Venous Sampling

The most accurate and reliable test to differentiate unilateral from bilateral primary aldosteronism and to lateralize aldosterone-producing adenoma before surgery is the adrenal venous sampling. Adrenal venous sampling consists of selective blood sampling from both adrenal veins, while the inferior vena cava serves as peripheral control site. Serum aldosterone and cortisol levels are determined, in order to differentiate unilateral from bilateral disease and ensure successful cannulation of adrenal veins, respectively. Adrenal hemorrhage, adrenal vein dissection, and groin hematoma are the main adverse effects of adrenal venous sampling, and are uncommon in experienced centers (0.5–2.5 %) [86].

The successful cannulation of the adrenal veins is difficult, especially the localization of the right adrenal vein, which is more challenging [87, 88]. Successful cannulation rates as low as 44 % have been reported [89], while a large review of 47 studies found an overall success rate of 74 % [90]. Several ways have been proposed to overcome this limitation. First, the experience of the radiologist: it is obvious that the rate of successful cannulation increases with greater experience, and this can be

Table 2.3 Main forms of primary aldosteronism

1. Bilateral adrenal hyperplasia
2. Unilateral aldosterone-producing adenoma
3. Aldosterone-producing carcinoma
4. Familial hyperaldosteronism
Type I
Type II
Type III

achieved by limiting the number of interventional radiologists performing the test at each institution while increasing the number of the procedures [91, 92]. Retrospective data from the German Conn's registry revealed a 31 % successful bilateral cannulation, and more importantly, centers completing less than 20 procedures exhibited success rates between 8 and 10 %, quite disappointing [92]. Then, the imaging aid: localization of the right adrenal vein by computed tomography either before adrenal venous sampling [93] or during angiography with subsequent repositioning of the catheter in as much as 10 % of the cases [94, 95]. Finally, the hormonal aid: the intra-procedural determination of cortisol by using rapid cortisol assays provides valuable information regarding successful cannulation, and is extremely helpful in centers with relatively low success rates [96].

Along with the technical difficulties in adrenal vein cannulation, the interpretation of the findings might be tricky. Most centers use the lateralization index for the diagnosis of aldosterone-producing adenomas, which represents the ratio of aldosterone/cortisol levels in the ipsilateral/contralateral vein. Values over four are considered indicative of adenomas, values less than three are considered indicative of bilateral hyperplasia, and values between three and four represent a "gray zone" [97].

The adrenocorticotropic hormone (ACTH)-stimulating test (infusion of cosyntropin, a synthetic ACTH agent) might be extremely helpful in cases of a transient lack of cortisol secretion at the moment of blood sampling during adrenal venous sampling [98]. A potential concern with ACTH stimulation is that ACTH might stimulate the contralateral gland in patients with unilateral aldosterone-producing adenoma, perplexing the results and suggesting bilateral instead of unilateral disease [99]. However, it seems that ACTH stimulation does not affect significantly the accurate detection of adenomas, and in fact increases the selectivity success, especially in centers with low success rates of bilateral cannulation [100]. In contrast, in a recent report of the Monash group, the ACTH stimulation not only failed to improve successful cannulation rates but tended to mask lateralization [101].

An expert consensus statement on arterial vein sampling for the subtyping of primary aldosteronism has been published at 2014, in the effort to unify the way of performing the procedure and interpreting the findings of adrenal venous sampling [102]. Recently, another group of experts has formed a report addressing the same issue, with many similarities but also with some differences [97], highlighting the need for standardization of the performance and interpretation of the test.

A super-selective adrenal venous sampling has been proposed, with blood drawn from branches of the adrenal vein, in the effort to accurately sub-localize aldosterone-producing adenomas and subsequently permit for partial, rather than total adrenalectomy [103].

2.7.2 Adrenal Imaging

Computed tomography (CT) scanning has been long used for the lateralization of primary aldosteronism; however, its use has significant limitations: it cannot accurately recognize microadenomas (less than 25 % of small adenomas are detected by

CT), it cannot accurately exclude contralateral or bilateral hyperplasia, and it cannot accurately provide functional information about a nodular finding [104–109]. Magnetic resonance imaging (MRI) has the advantage of avoiding exposure to ionizing radiation, but does not seem to offer better sensitivity and specificity for the diagnosis of primary aldosteronism.

A study of more than 200 patients from Mayo Clinic revealed that accurate lateralization was achieved only in 53 % of cases, while 21.7 % of patients would have been refused an indicated operation, and 24.7 % of patients would have been unnecessarily operated [86]. In another study comparing adrenal imaging with adrenal venous sampling findings, it was reported that if the decision for adrenalectomy was based on imaging findings (CT or MRI) then: 14.6 % of patients would have been operated inappropriately, 19.1 % of patients would not have been operated inappropriately, and more dramatically, 3.9 % of patients would have been operated on the wrong side [109]. A recent systematic review of 950 patients with primary aldosteronism revealed a 37.8 % discrepancy between the findings of adrenal imaging and adrenal venous sampling [110], underlining the inability of adrenal imaging for accurate localization, and subsequently, its limited usefulness and validity in clinical practice for the lateralization of primary aldosteronism. Another recent report evaluating the localizing validity of newest imaging technology revealed that multidetector CT performed even with the latest generation multidetector CT scanners does not offer sufficient accuracy for disease lateralization and cannot replace adrenal venous sampling [111].

Recently, two new imaging techniques have been proposed for the localization of primary aldosteronism, the ^{11}C-metodimate PET/CT and the semi-quantification of NP-59 SPECT/CT with promising results [112, 113]; however, further studies in larger number of patients are needed to validate its use for disease localization in everyday clinical practice.

2.7.3 Nuclear Imaging

Nuclear scintigraphy has been used for disease lateralization for quite some time, and it is available since the 1970s. Scintigraphy with ^{131}I-6β-iodomethyl-19-norcholesterol (NP-59) offers the potential advantage of linking anatomical with functional abnormalities. However, the diagnostic accuracy of NP-59 scintigraphy is size-dependent, and this method lacks sensitivity in small adenomas (less than 1.5 cm). Therefore, nuclear scintigraphy is of limited value for small adenomas, a common finding in primary aldosteronism.

2.7.4 Expert Comment

Adrenal venous sampling is considered the method of choice for the lateralization of primary aldosteronism, but is currently unavailable in large parts of the world. Alternative localization approaches aim to overcome the main disadvantages of adrenal venous sampling, mainly the technical difficulties, its invasive nature, the necessity of highly expertise radiologists, and the "gray-zone" results that are inconclusive for differentiating between unilateral and bilateral disease. Newer imaging techniques might be of help as well as genetic testing. During the past 5 years, several somatic mutations in genes encoding potassium, sodium, and calcium ATPases have been described in more than half of aldosterone-producing adenomas [114–119]. In the case that cells with such mutations can be identified in peripheral blood and an adrenal mass is found in CT scanning, then it could be rational to assume that adrenal lateralization might be skipped in the near future in such patients. Extensive basic and clinical research is needed in this field, and many efforts are currently underway.

2.8 Management and Follow-Up

Adrenalectomy is considered the method of choice for the management of aldosterone-producing adenomas, while mineralocorticoid receptor antagonists are recommended for the management of bilateral hyperplasia.

2.8.1 Adrenalectomy

Hypertension "cure" with adrenalectomy has been reported in 17–85 % of patients [106, 120], a wide variation that might be ought to differences in studied populations (indications for adrenalectomy, patient selection, work-up algorithms). A recent review found "cure" of HTN in 42 % of patients undergoing adrenalectomy [121], meaning that the majority of patients will still require antihypertensive drugs to achieve blood pressure control [122]. Blood pressure reduction following adrenalectomy is usually observed within the first semester, but may be even more delayed in some cases. Serum potassium and ARR become normal in most patients following adrenalectomy.

Expectations for 100 % "cure" of hypertension seem naïve. First, essential HTN is expected to coexist frequently with primary aldosteronism and subsequently contribute to HTN maintenance post-adrenalectomy. Then, vascular changes induced by long-standing elevated blood pressure levels may also contribute to HTN persistence. Nevertheless, a smaller number of drugs are usually required for blood pressure control even in these patients. Very recently, another potential mechanism of HTN persistence has been described: the identification of activating autoantibodies against angiotensin II type I receptors in patients with primary aldosteronism [123–125].

Predictors of poor blood pressure response post-adrenalectomy include long-standing HTN, obesity, preoperative ARR, and advanced age, while predictors of a favorable response include younger age, short duration and absence of familial history of HTN, normal renal function, response to spironolactone, and blood pressure control with less than three antihypertensive drugs [126, 127]. A prediction scoring system based on 100 patients who underwent adrenalectomy identified body mass index >25 kg/m^2, female sex, HTN duration <6 years, and the use of less than three antihypertensive drugs as the main predictors of blood pressure response to adrenalectomy [128]. High aldosterone levels post-intravenous saline testing have been associated with better outcome following either adrenalectomy or medical therapy, as indicated [129].

The choice between open and laparoscopic adrenalectomy is mainly based on the familiarity and the experience of the surgeon. Laparoscopic adrenalectomy seems to be preferred due to lower complication rates and shorter duration of hospitalization [130]. Partial adrenalectomy has also been proposed and used, with obvious advantages, but seems to carry the risk for disease recurrence [131, 132]. Recently, a single incision laparoscopic adrenalectomy has been reported with obvious cosmetic superiority [133, 134]; however, further studies are needed to evaluate the efficacy and safety of this approach.

2.8.2 Mineralocorticoid Receptor Antagonists

Mineralocorticoid receptor antagonists are recommended for the management of bilateral hyperplasia. These drugs may also be used as alternatives to surgery for the management of aldosterone-producing adenoma in patients who are either at high risk for operation, or they do not prefer to be operated and opt for drug therapy.

The use of mineralocorticoid receptor antagonists in primary aldosteronism may follow two directions: (a) initiation with low doses (25–50 mg spironolactone) and up-titration until blood pressure reduction and potassium normalization is achieved or (b) initiation with high doses (200–400 mg spironolactone) and down-titration until finding the minimum dose of spironolactone that is adequate to maintain blood pressure control and eukalemia. Most experts prefer the second option (high doses, down-titration), because eukalemia and blood pressure control are achieved more rapidly, within a couple of weeks. The disadvantage of this approach is that it carries a higher risk of renal function deterioration and hyperkalemia, and thus a close monitoring is required.

Gynecomastia is dose related and reaches almost 50 % with high spironolactone doses (>150 mg daily), while it is much less common (5–10 %) with low doses (25–50 mg spironolactone daily) [135]. Eplerenone can be used in patients experiencing adverse effects with spironolactone. A recent randomized, double-blind trial comparing the antihypertensive effect of spironolactone and eplerenone (75–225 mg versus 100–300 mg) in hypertensive patients with evidence of primary aldosteronism revealed that spironolactone was more effective than eplerenone in blood pressure reduction, at the expense of more adverse effects (gynecomastia and female mastodynia) [136].

Aldosterone synthase inhibitors and nonsteroidal dihydropyridine-based mineralocorticoid receptor antagonists represent promising alternative medical therapies.

In a recent study, eplerenone was better than an aldosterone synthase inhibitor (LCI 699) in terms of blood pressure reduction, as well as potassium and renin normalization in patients with primary aldosteronism [137]. Nonsteroidal mineralocorticoid receptor antagonists show similar in vitro potency with spironolactone and seem devoid of the androgen- and progesterone-induced adverse effects, and clinical studies in primary aldosteronism are eagerly awaited [138].

Spontaneous remission of primary aldosteronism after long-term (>5 years) spironolactone therapy has been reported in a small portion (5 %) of patients in the German Conn's registry [139], reaching up to 50 % in other small studies [140].

2.8.3 Adrenalectomy Versus Medical Therapy

Many studies have evaluated the effects of adrenalectomy versus drug therapy with mineralocorticoid antagonists in primary aldosteronism. The majority of experts in this field consider adrenalectomy to be superior to medical therapy in patients with aldosterone-producing adenomas, with more pronounced and more rapid benefits [141, 142].

Left ventricular mass reduction was comparable with both therapeutic strategies at the end of a large follow-up period (mean, 6.4 years); however, a significant reduction in left ventricular mass at the first year was observed only in patients who underwent adrenalectomy [141]. A recent meta-analysis revealed that there was no difference in left ventricular mass reduction between patients on medical therapy or operated patients [143].

A recent large epidemiological study of more than 1700 patients reported that blood pressure was significantly reduced by surgical but not by medical therapy [144]. Observational data from the German Conn's registry of 300 patients with primary aldosteronism suggest that surgical therapy is associated with improved survival when compared to medical therapy [49]. However, the lack of large randomized studies comparing adrenalectomy with medical therapy does not permit for definite conclusions favoring adrenalectomy over the use of mineralocorticoid receptor antagonists [145].

2.9 Diagnostic and Therapeutic Algorithm

Existing guidelines and recommendations are prepared by experts and are addressed to specialists, being far too perplexed to be easily memorized by general physicians and be widely implemented in everyday clinical practice. A simple and practical algorithm is needed in order to facilitate primary care physicians, cardiologists, and internists who manage the vast majority of patients with arterial hypertension, to raise the suspicion of primary aldosteronism, and then subsequently screen and confirm the diagnosis (Fig. 2.1).

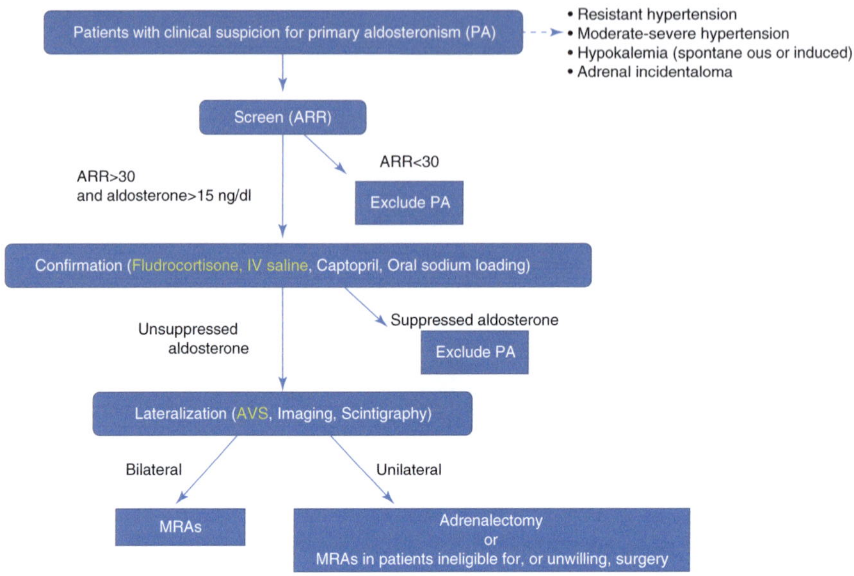

Fig. 2.1 Algorithm for the diagnosis and management of primary aldosteronism. *ARR* aldosterone to renin ratio, *AVS* adrenal venous sampling, *MRAs* mineralocorticoid receptor antagonists

2.9.1 Alternative Diagnostic Algorithms

Some groups propose skipping confirmation tests and proceeding directly to lateralization with adrenal venous sampling in selected group of patients. In general, in patients with extremely low renin, marked hypokalemia, and high aldosterone levels, some experts propose proceeding directly to lateralization and skipping confirmatory tests, based on the highly likelihood of detecting primary aldosteronism in such patients.

For example, the group of Padua proposes to proceed directly to lateralization with adrenal venous sampling in patients with pronouncedly high ARR (>100), whereas a repeat screening test should be performed in patients with high ARR (26–100) and proceed directly to lateralization in patients with confirmed high ARR in repeat testing. This approach has been adopted by the Italian Society of Hypertension recommendations for the clinical management of primary aldosteronism [146]. The group from Calgary proposes skipping confirmatory tests and proceeding directly to lateralization with adrenal venous sampling in all patients with high ARR; of note, the cutoff level is set rather low (550, with aldosterone expressed in pmol/L), in the effort to avoid missing cases of primary aldosteronism [147].

Another clinical approach regards a prediction score based on imaging findings (typical adrenal adenoma on CT), and biochemical tests (hypokalemia and normal renal function), with an acceptable predictive value for diagnosing primary aldosteronism [148]. However, other studies failed to confirm the validity of original findings, when the clinical prediction score was applied in other centers [149, 150].

The Mayo Clinic group proposed that patients younger than 40 years of age could potentially proceed to surgery skipping adrenal venous sampling, when a unilateral mass >10 mm and normal contralateral findings are observed in CT scanning, based on the rare frequency of adrenal incidentalomas in young patients [86]. Another example regards patients younger than 35 years of age with a unilateral nodule greater than 1 cm and normal CT findings of the contralateral gland. Retrospective data from the German Conn's registry demonstrates that the clinical prediction score and the age-imaging combination cannot accurately skip disease lateralization by adrenal venous sampling [149].

Measurement of peripheral 18-hydroxycortisol and 18-oxo-cortisol has been proposed as alternative to adrenal venous sampling for disease lateralization [151, 152], reporting up to 60 % discriminatory ability between unilateral and bilateral disease. Further studies are needed however to confirm these findings and establish whether these methods may limit the necessity for adrenal sampling, at least in some cases.

A recent study of 235 patients with primary aldosteronism questions the need for adrenal imaging in patients undergoing adrenal venous sampling, since when adrenal sampling was performed first, imaging could have been avoided in almost half of the cases [153].

2.9.2 Expert Comment

Although some experts propose skipping a confirmatory test in patients with high ARR (or at least some subgroups of these patients) and proceeding directly to disease localization, we believe that confirmatory testing is mandatory in all cases, mainly for two reasons: (a) the ARR is false positive in a substantial portion of patients (reaching up to 50 %), and (b) lateralization with adrenal venous sampling is costly, is difficult to perform, requires highly specialized centers, and is potentially harmful as every interventional approach. It therefore seems wise to avoid performing unnecessary and potentially harmful lateralization tests in large numbers of patients, based solely on a high ARR.

Likewise, skipping lateralization tests and proceeding directly to surgery based on imaging findings does not seem a wise approach. The findings of imaging techniques (CT, MRI) might be misleading: an adrenal nodule might be an aldosterone-producing adenoma, the prevailing nodule of bilateral hyperplasia, or an incidental nonfunctional mass, and vice versa, an aldosterone-producing adenoma might be small enough to be detected even with the newest imaging techniques.

Conclusion

Primary aldosteronism is highly prevalent in patients with dRHTN, and its detection is of paramount importance since these patients should not be candidates for interventional therapy with renal sympathetic denervation. The diagnosis of primary aldosteronism in real life is time consuming and might be tricky. The screening for primary aldosteronism (who to screen and how to screen), the confirmation of the diagnosis (four tests are currently used), and the lateralization of the disease (three tests available) remain controversial topics. Clarification of these issues is urgently needed, in order to form a simplified algorithm for the diagnosis and management of primary aldosteronism, which could be easily implemented in everyday clinical practice.

References

1. Mancia G, Fagard R, Narkiewicz K et al (2013) 2013 ESH/ESC guidelines for the management of arterial hypertension. J Hypertens 31:1281–1357
2. Faselis C, Doumas M, Papademetriou V (2011) Common secondary causes of resistant hypertension and rational for treatment. Int J Hypertens 2011:236239
3. Calhoun DA, Nishizaka MK, Zaman MA, Thakkar RB, Weissman P (2002) High prevalence of primary aldosteronism among black and white subjects with resistant hypertension. Hypertension 40:892–896
4. Eide IK, Torjesen PA, Drolsum A, Babovic A, Lilledahl NP (2004) Low-renin status in therapy-resistant hypertension: a clue to efficient treatment. J Hypertens 22:2217–2226
5. Martell N, Rodriguez-Cerrillo M, Grobee DE, Lopez-Eady MD, Fernandez-Pinilla C, Avila M, Fernandez-Cruz A, Luque M (2003) High prevalence of secondary hypertension and insulin resistance in patients with refractory hypertension. Blood Press 12:149–154
6. Umpierrez GE, Cantey P, Smiley D, Palacio A, Temponi D, Luster K, Chapman A (2007) Primary aldosteronism in diabetic subjects with resistant hypertension. Diabetes Care 30: 1699–1703
7. Douma S, Petidis K, Doumas M et al (2008) Prevalence of primary hyperaldosteronism in resistant hypertension: a retrospective observational study. Lancet 371:1921–1926
8. Florczak E, Prejbisz A, Szwench-Pietrasz E, Sliwinski P, Bielen P, Klisiewicz A, Michalowska I, Warchol E, Januszewicz M, Kala M, Witkowski A, Wiecek A, Narkiewicz K, Somers VK, Januszewicz A (2013) Clinical characteristics of patients with resistant hypertension: the RESIST-POL study. J Hum Hypertens 27:678–685
9. Papademetriou V, Tsioufis C, Doumas M (2014) Renal denervation and Symplicity HTN-3: "Dubium sapientiae initium" (doubt is the beginning of wisdom). Circ Res 115:211–214
10. Papademetriou V, Rashidi AA, Tsioufis C, Doumas M (2014) Renal nerve ablation for resistant hypertension: how did we get here, present status and future directions. Circulation 129:1440–1451
11. Doumas M, Faselis C, Papademetriou V (2011) Renal sympathetic denervation in hypertension. Curr Opin Nephrol Hypertens 20:647–653
12. Doumas M, Faselis C, Kokkinos P et al (2014) Carotid baroreceptor stimulation: a promising approach for the management of resistant hypertension and heart failure. Curr Vasc Pharmacol 12:30–37
13. Doumas M, Faselis C, Tsioufis C, Papademetriou V (2012) Carotid baroreceptor activation for the treatment of resistant hypertension and heart failure. Curr Hypertens Rep 14: 238–246
14. Doumas M, Athyros V, Papademetriou V (2015) Screening for primary aldosteronism: whom and how? J Clin Hypertens 17:547–548
15. Douma S, Petidis K, Kamparoudis A et al (2012) Surgical management of primary aldosteronism: not everything that shines is gold. Clin Exp Hypertens 34:53–56
16. Sarafidis PA, Bakris GL (2008) Resistant hypertension: an overview of evaluation and treatment. J Am Coll Cardiol 52:1749–1757
17. Calhoun DA, Jones D, Textor S et al (2008) Resistant hypertension: diagnosis, evaluation, and treatment. Circulation 117:e510–e526

18. Krum H, Schlaich M, Whitbourn R et al (2009) Catheter-based renal sympathetic denervation for resistant hypertension: a multicentre safety and proof-of-principle cohort study. Lancet 373:1275–1281
19. Symplicity HTN-2 Investigators, Esler MD, Krum H, Sobotka PA, Schlaich MP, Schmieder RE, Bohm M (2010) Renal sympathetic denervation in patients with treatment-resistant hypertension (the Symplicity HTN-2 trial): a randomised controlled trial. Lancet 376:1903–1909
20. Bhatt DL, Kandzari DE, O'Neill WW, D'Agostino R, Flack JM, Katzen BT, Leon MB, Liu M, Mauri L, Negoita M, Cohen SA, Oparil S, Rocha-Singh K, Townsend RR, Bakris GL, Symplicity HTN-3 Investigators (2014) A controlled trial of renal denervation for resistant hypertension. N Engl J Med 370:1393–1401
21. Bisognano JD, Bakris G, Nadim MK et al (2011) Baroreflex activation therapy lowers blood pressure in patients with resistant hypertension: results from the double-blind, randomized, placebo-controlled rheos pivotal trial. J Am Coll Cardiol 58:765–773
22. Nishizaka MK, Zaman MA, Calhoun DA (2003) Efficacy of low-dose spironolactone in subjects with resistant hypertension. Am J Hypertens 16:925–930
23. Conn JW (1955) Primary aldosteronism: a new clinical syndrome. J Lab Clin Med 45:3–17
24. Andersen GS, Toftdahl DB, Lund JO et al (1988) The incidence rate of phaeochromocytoma and Conn's syndrome in Denmark, 1977–1981. J Hum Hypertens 2:187–189
25. Berglund G, Andersson O, Wilhelmsen L (1976) Prevalence of primary and secondary hypertension: studies in a random population sample. Br Med J 2:554–556
26. Kaplan NM (1967) Hypokalemia in the hypertensive patient, with observations on the incidence of primary aldosteronism. Ann Intern Med 66:1079–1090
27. Sinclair AM, Isles CG, Brown I et al (1987) Secondary hypertension in a blood pressure clinic. Arch Intern Med 147:1289–1293
28. Kaplan NM (2004) The current epidemic of primary aldosteronism: causes and consequences. J Hypertens 22:863–869
29. Gordon RD, Stowasser M, Tunny TJ, Klemm SA, Rutherford JC (1994) High incidence of primary aldosteronism in 199 patients referred with hypertension. Clin Exp Pharmacol Physiol 21(4):315–318
30. Kaplan NM (2011) Primary aldosteronism: a contrarian view. Rev Endocr Metab Disord 12(1):49–52
31. Rossi GP (2004) Primary aldosteronism: a needle in a haystack or a yellow cab on Fifth Avenue? Curr Hypertens Rep 6(1):1–4
32. Funder JW, Carey RM, Fardella C, Endocrine Society et al (2008) Case detection, diagnosis, and treatment of patients with primary aldosteronism: an endocrine society clinical practice guideline. J Clin Endocrinol Metab 93:3266–3281
33. Rossi GP, Bernini G, Caliumi C et al (2006) A prospective study of the prevalence of primary aldosteronism in 1,125 hypertensive patients. J Am Coll Cardiol 48:2293–2300
34. Ito Y, Takeda R, Karashima S, Yamamoto Y, Yoneda T, Takeda Y (2011) Prevalence of primary aldosteronism among prehypertensive and stage 1 hypertensive subjects. Hypertens Res 34(1):98–102
35. Westerdahl C, Bergenfelz A, Isaksson A, Nerbrand C, Valdemarsson S (2011) Primary aldosteronism among newly diagnosed and untreated hypertensive patients in a Swedish primary care area. Scand J Prim Health Care 29(1):57–62
36. Mosso L, Carvajal C, Gonzalez A, Barraza A, Avila F, Montero J, Huete A, Gederlini A, Fardella CE (2003) Primary aldosteronism and hypertensive disease. Hypertension 42:161–165
37. Milliez P, Girerd X, Plouin PF, Blacher J, Safar ME, Mourard JJ (2005) Evidence for an increased rate of cardiovascular events in patients with primary aldosteronism. J Am Coll Cardiol 45:1243–1248
38. Born-Frontsberg E, Reincke M, Rump LC, Hahner S, Diederich S, Lorenz R, Allolio B, Seufert J, Schirpenbach C, Beuschlein F, Bidlingmaier M, Endres S, Quinkler M, Participants

of the German Conn's Registry (2009) Cardiovascular and cerebrovascular comorbidities of hypokalemic and normokalemic primary aldosteronism: results of the German Conn's Registry. J Clin Endocrinol Metab 94:1125–1130
39. Savard S, Amar L, Plouin PF, Steichen O (2013) Cardiovascular complications associated with primary aldosteronism: a controlled cross-sectional study. Hypertension 62:331–336
40. Strauch B, Petrak O, Wichterle D et al (2006) Increased arterial wall stiffness in primary aldosteronism in comparison with essential hypertension. Am J Hypertens 19:909–914
41. Lin YH, Lee HH, Liu KL et al (2011) Reversal of myocardial fibrosis in patients with unilateral hyperaldosteronism receiving adrenalectomy. Surgery 150:526–533
42. Sechi LA, Novello M, Lapenna R et al (2006) Long-term renal outcomes in patients with primary aldosteronism. JAMA 295:2638–2645
43. Nishizaka MK, Zaman MA, Green SA et al (2004) Impaired endothelium-dependent flow-mediated vasodilation in hypertensive subjects with hyperaldosteronism. Circulation 109: 2857–2861
44. Su MY, Wu VC, Yu HY et al (2012) Contrast-enhanced MRI index of diffuse myocardial fibrosis is increased in primary aldosteronism. J Magn Reson Imaging 35:1349–1355
45. Maule S, Mulatero P, Milan A et al (2006) QT interval in patients with primary aldosteronism and low-renin essential hypertension. J Hypertens 24:2459–2464
46. Mulatero P, Monticone S, Bertello C et al (2013) Long-term cardio- and cerebrovascular events in patients with primary aldosteronism. J Clin Endocrinol Metab 98:4826–4833
47. Fallo F, Veglio F, Bertello C et al (2006) Prevalence and characteristics of the metabolic syndrome in primary aldosteronism. J Clin Endocrinol Metab 91:454–459
48. Fischer E, Adolf C, Pallauf A et al (2013) Aldosterone excess impairs first phase insulin secretion in primary aldosteronism. J Clin Endocrinol Metab 98:2513–2520
49. Reincke M, Fischer E, Gerum S, Merkle K, Schulz S, Pallauf A, Quinkler M, Hanslik G, Lang K, Hahner S, Allolio B, Meisinger C, Holle R, Beuschlein F, Bidlingmaier M, Endres S (2012) Observational study mortality in treated primary aldosteronism: the German Conn's registry. Hypertension 60:618–624
50. Kearney PM, Whelton M, Reynolds K et al (2005) Global burden of hypertension: analysis of worldwide data. Lancet 365:217–223
51. Nishikawa T, Omura M, Satoh F et al (2011) Guidelines for the diagnosis and treatment of primary aldosteronism – the Japan Endocrine Society 2009. Endocr J 58:711–721
52. Monticone S, Viola A, Tizzani D, Crudo V, Burrello J, Galmozzi M, Veglio F, Mulatero P (2012) Primary aldosteronism: who should be screened? Horm Metab Res 44(3):163–169
53. Hiramatsu K, Yamada T, Yukimura Y, Komiya I, Ichikawa K, Ishihara M, Nagata H, Izumiyama T (1981) A screening test to identify aldosterone-producing adenoma by measuring plasma renin activity: results in hypertensive patients. Arch Intern Med 141:1589–1593
54. Mulatero P, Stowasser M, Loh KC, Fardella CE, Gordon RD, Mosso L, Gomez-Sanchez CE, Veglio F, Young WF Jr (2004) Increased diagnosis of primary aldosteronism, including surgically correctable forms, in centers from five continents. J Clin Endocrinol Metab 89:1045–1050
55. Luo Q, Li NF, Yao XG, Zhang DL, Abulikemu SF, Chang GJ, Zhou KM, Wang GL, Wang MH, Ouyang WJ, Cheng QY, Jia Y (2016) Potential effects of age on screening for primary aldosteronism. J Hum Hypertens 30(1):53–61
56. Mulatero P, Rabbia F, Milan A et al (2002) Drug effects on aldosterone/plasma renin activity ration in primary aldosteronism. Hypertension 40:897–902
57. Browne GA, Griffin TP, O'Shea PM, Dennedy MC (2015) β-Blocker withdrawal is preferable for accurate interpretation of the aldosterone-renin ratio in chronically treated hypertension. Clin Endocrinol (Oxf) 84:325–331 [Epub ahead of print]
58. Tiu S-C, Choi C-H, Shek C-C, Ng Y-W, Chan FKW, Ng C-M et al (2005) The use of aldosterone-renin ratio as a diagnostic test for primary hyperaldosteronism and its test characteristics under different conditions of blood sampling. J Clin Endocrinol Metab 90(1):72–78
59. Barigou M, Ah-Kang F, Orloff E, Amar J, Chamontin B, Bouhanick B (2015) Effect of postural changes on aldosterone to plasma renin ratio in patients with suspected secondary hypertension. Ann Cardiol Angeiol (Paris) 64(3):169–174

60. Ahmed AH, Gordon RD, Ward G, Wolley M, Kogovsek C, Stowasser M (2015) Should aldosterone suppression tests be conducted during a particular phase of the menstrual cycle, and if so, which phase? Results of a preliminary study. Clin Endocrinol (Oxf) 83(3): 303–307
61. Fischer E, Reuschl S, Quinkler M, Rump LC, Hahner S, Bidlingmaier M, Reincke M, Participants of the German Conn's Registry – Else Kröner-Fresenius-Hyperaldosteronism Registry (2013) Assay characteristics influence the aldosterone to renin ratio as a screening tool for primary aldosteronism: results of the German Conn's registry. Horm Metab Res 45(7):526–531
62. Lonati C, Bassani N, Gritti A, Biganzoli E, Morganti A (2014) Measurement of plasma renin concentration instead of plasma renin activity decreases the positive aldosterone-to-renin ratio tests in treated patients with essential hypertension. J Hypertens 32(3):627–634
63. Manolopoulou J, Fischer E, Dietz A, Diederich S, Holmes D, Junnila R, Grimminger P, Reincke M, Morganti A, Bidlingmaier M (2015) Clinical validation for the aldosterone-to-renin ratio and aldosterone suppression testing using simultaneous fully automated chemiluminescence immunoassays. J Hypertens 33(12):2500–2511
64. Pizzolo F, Zorzi F, Chiecchi L et al (2014) NT-proBNP, a useful tool in hypertensive patients undergoing a diagnostic evaluation for primary aldosteronism. Endocrine 45:479–486
65. Young WF (2007) Primary aldosteronism: renaissance of a syndrome. Clin Endocrinol (Oxf) 66:607–618
66. Williams JS, Williams GH, Raji A, Jeunemaitre X, Brown NJ, Hopkins PN, Conlin PR (2006) Prevalence of primary hyperaldosteronism in mild to moderate hypertension without hypokalaemia. J Hum Hypertens 20:129–136
67. Ahmed AH, Cowley D, Wolley M et al (2014) Seated saline suppression testing for the diagnosis of primary aldosteronism: a preliminary study. J Clin Endocrinol Metab 99:2745–2753
68. Stowasser M, Gordon RD, Gunasekera TG et al (2003) High rate of detection of primary aldosteronism, including surgically treatable forms, after 'non-selective' screening of hypertensive patients. J Hypertens 21:2149–2157
69. Gouli A, Kaltsas G, Tzonou A et al (2011) High prevalence of autonomous aldosterone secretion among patients with essential hypertension. Eur J Clin Invest 41:1227–1236
70. Lyons DF, Kem DC, Brown RD et al (1983) Single dose captopril as a diagnostic test for primary aldosteronism. J Clin Endocrinol Metab 57:892–896
71. Agharazii M, Douville P, Grose JH, Lebel M (2001) Captopril suppression versus salt loading in confirming primary aldosteronism. Hypertension 37:1440–1443
72. Castro OL, Yu X, Kem DC (2002) Diagnostic value of the post-captopril test in primary aldosteronism. Hypertension 39:935–938
73. Mulatero P, Bertello C, Garrone C et al (2007) Captopril test can give misleading results in patients with suspect primary aldosteronism. Hypertension 50:e26–e27
74. Westerdahl C, Bergenfelz A, Isaksson A, Valdemarsson S (2011) Captopril suppression: limitations for confirmation of primary aldosteronism. J Renin Angiotensin Aldosterone Syst 12:326–332
75. Giacchetti G, Ronconi V, Lucarelli G et al (2006) Analysis of screening and confirmatory tests in the diagnosis of primary aldosteronism: need for a standardized protocol. J Hypertens 24:737–745
76. Wu VC, Chang HW, Liu KL et al (2009) Primary aldosteronism: diagnostic accuracy of the losartan and captopril tests. Am J Hypertens 22:821–827
77. Kuo CC, Balakrishnan P, Hsein YC et al (2015) The value of losartan suppression test in the confirmatory diagnosis of primary aldosteronism in patients over 50 years old. J Renin Angiotensin Aldosterone Syst 16(3):587–598
78. Stowasser M, Gordon RD, Rutherford JC et al (2001) Diagnosis and management of primary aldosteronism. J Renin Angiotensin Aldosterone Syst 2:156–169
79. Rossi GP, Belfiore A, Bernini G, Primary Aldosteronism Prevalence in Italy Study Investigators et al (2007) Comparison of the captopril and the saline infusion test for excluding aldosterone-producing adenoma. Hypertension 50:424–431

80. Schirpenbach C, Seiler L, Maser-Gluth C et al (2006) Confirmatory testing in normokalaemic primary aldosteronism: the value of the saline infusion test and urinary aldosterone metabolites. Eur J Endocrinol 154:865–873
81. Taylor PJ, Cooper DP, Gordon RD, Stowasser M (2009) Measurement of aldosterone in human plasma by semi-automated HPLC-tandem mass spectrometry. Clin Chem 55:1155–1162
82. Hinchliffe E, Carter S, Owen LJ, Keevil BG (2013) Quantitation of aldosterone in human plasma by ultra high performance liquid chromatography tandem mass spectrometry. J Chromatogr B Analyt Technol Biomed Life Sci 913–914:19–23
83. Van Der Gugten JG, Dubland J, Liu HF, Wang A, Joseph C, Holmes DT (2012) Determination of serum aldosterone by liquid chromatography and tandem mass spectrometry: a liquid-liquid extraction method for the ABSCIEX API-5000 mass spectrometry system. J Clin Pathol 65:457–462
84. Camenzind AG, van der Gugten JG, Popp R, Holmes DT, Borchers CH (2013) Development and evaluation of an immuno-MALDI (iMALDI) assay for angiotensin I and the diagnosis of secondary hypertension. Clin Proteomics 10:20
85. Dorrian CA, Toole BJ, Alvarez-Madrazo S et al (2010) A screening procedure for primary aldosteronism based on the Diasorin Liaison automated chemiluminescent immunoassay for direct renin. Ann Clin Biochem 47:195–199
86. Young WF, Stanson AW, Thompson GB et al (2004) Role for adrenal venous sampling in primary aldosteronism. Surgery 136:1227–1235
87. Elliot P, Holmes DT (2013) Adrenal vein sampling: substantial need for technical improvement at regional referral centers. Clin Biochem 46:1399–1404
88. Pasternak JD, Epelboym I, Seiser N et al (2016) Diagnostic utility of data from adrenal venous sampling for primary aldosteronism despite failed cannulation of the right adrenal vein. Surgery 159:267–274
89. Harvey A, Kline G, Pasieka JL (2006) Adrenal venous sampling in primary hyperaldosteronism: comparison of radiographic with biochemical success and the clinical decision making with "less than ideal" testing. Surgery 140:847–853
90. Young WF, Klee GG (1988) Primary aldosteronism. Diagnostic evaluation. Endocrinol Metab Clin North Am 17:367–395
91. Harvey A, Pasieka JL, Kline G, So B (2012) Modification of the protocol for selective adrenal venous sampling results in both a significant increase in the accuracy and necessity of the procedure in the management of patients with primary hyperaldosteronism. Surgery 152:643–649
92. Vonend O, Ockenfels N, Gao X et al (2011) Adrenal venous sampling: evaluation of the German Conn's registry. Hypertension 57:990–995
93. Daunt N (2005) Adrenal vein sampling: how to make it quick, easy, and successful. Radiographics 25(suppl 1):S143–S158
94. Onozawa S, Murata S, Tajima H et al (2014) Evaluation of right adrenal vein cannulation by computed tomography angiography in 140 consecutive patients undergoing adrenal venous sampling. Eur J Endocrinol 170:601–608
95. Park SI, Rhee Y, Lim JS et al (2014) Right adrenal venography findings correlated with C-arm CT for selection during C-arm CT-assisted adrenal vein sampling in primary aldosteronism. Cardiovasc Intervent Radiol 37(6):1469–1475
96. Rossi E, Regolisti G, Perazzoli F et al (2011) Intraprocedural cortisol measurement increases adrenal vein sampling success rate in primary aldosteronism. Am J Hypertens 24:1280–1285
97. Monticone S, Viola A, Rossato D et al (2015) Adrenal vein sampling in primary aldosteronism: towards a standardised protocol. Lancet Diabetes Endocrinol 3(4):296–303
98. Kline GA, Pasieka JL, Harvey A, So B, Dias VC (2014) A marked proportional rise in IVC aldosterone following cosyntropin administration during AVS is a signal to the presence of adrenal hyperplasia in primary aldosteronism. J Hum Hypertens 28:298–302
99. Seccia TM, Miotto D, De Toni R et al (2009) Adrenocorticotropic hormone stimulation during adrenal vein sampling for identifying surgically curable subtypes of primary aldosteronism: comparison of 3 different protocols. Hypertension 53:761–766

100. Monticone S, Satoh F, Giacchetti G et al (2012) Effect of adrenocorticotropic hormone stimulation during adrenal vein sampling in primary aldosteronism. Hypertension 59:840–846
101. Teng J, Hutchinson ME, Doery JC et al (2015) Role of adrenal vein sampling in primary aldosteronism: the Monash Health experience. Intern Med J 45(11):1141–1146
102. Rossi GP, Auchus RJ, Brown M et al (2014) An expert consensus statement on use of adrenal vein sampling for the subtyping of primary aldosteronism. Hypertension 63:151–160
103. Satoh F, Morimoto R, Seiji K et al (2015) Is there a role for segmental adrenal venous sampling and adrenal sparing surgery in patients with primary aldosteronism? Eur J Endocrinol 173(4):465–477
104. Hammarstedt L, Muth A, Wangberg B et al (2010) Adrenal lesion frequency: a prospective, cross-sectional CT study in a defined region, including systematic re-evaluation. Acta Radiol 51:1149–1156
105. Rossi GP, Sacchetto A, Chiesura-Corona M et al (2001) Identification of the etiology of primary aldosteronism with adrenal vein sampling in patients with equivocal computed tomography and magnetic resonance findings: results in 104 consecutive cases. J Clin Endocrinol Metab 86:1083–1090
106. White ML, Gauger PG, Doherty GM et al (2008) The role of radiologic studies in the evaluation and management of primary hyperaldosteronism. Surgery 144:926–933
107. Zarnegar R, Bloom AI, Lee J et al (2008) Is adrenal venous sampling necessary in all patients with hyperaldosteronism before adrenalectomy? J Vasc Interv Radiol 19:66–71
108. Lin TP, Chiu AW, Chen M et al (2015) Adrenal computed tomography and NP-59 usefulness for diagnosing aldosterone-producing adenomas and idiopathic hyperaldosteronism in primary hyperaldosteronism. Urol Sci 34:1–5
109. Patel SM, Lingam RK, Beaconsfield TI et al (2007) Role of radiology in the management of primary aldosteronism. Radiographics 27:1145–1157
110. Kempers MJ, Lenders JW, van Outheusden L et al (2009) Systematic review: diagnostic procedures to differentiate unilateral from bilateral adrenal abnormality in primary aldosteronism. Ann Intern Med 151:329–337
111. Raman SP, Lessne M, Kawamoto S et al (2015) Diagnostic performance of multidetector computed tomography in distinguishing unilateral from bilateral abnormalities in primary hyperaldosteronism: comparison of multidetector computed tomography with adrenal vein sampling. J Comput Assist Tomogr 39(3):414–418
112. Burton TJ, Mackenzie IS, Balan K et al (2012) Evaluation of the sensitivity and specificity of (11)C-metomidate positron emission tomography (PET)-CT for lateralizing aldosterone secretion by Conn's adenomas. J Clin Endocrinol Metab 97:100–109
113. Lu CC, Wu VC, Wu KD et al (2014) Prognostic value of semiquantification NP-59 SPECT/CT in primary aldosteronism patients after adrenalectomy. Eur J Nucl Med Mol Imaging 41:1375–1384
114. Choi M, Scholl UI, Yue P et al (2011) K+ channel mutations in adrenal aldosterone-producing adenomas and hereditary hypertension. Science 331:768–772
115. Boulkroun S, Beuschlein F, Rossi GP et al (2012) Prevalence, clinical, and molecular correlates of KCNJ5 mutations in primary aldosteronism. Hypertension 59:592–598
116. Beuschlein F, Boulkroun S, Osswald A et al (2013) Somatic mutations in ATP1A1 and ATP2B3 lead to aldosterone-producing adenomas and secondary hypertension. Nat Genet 45:440–444
117. Scholl UI, Goh G, Stolting G et al (2013) Somatic and germline CACNA1D calcium channel mutations in aldosterone producing adenomas and primary aldosteronism. Nat Genet 45:1050–1054
118. Akerstrom T, Crona J, Delgado Verdugo A et al (2012) Comprehensive re-sequencing of adrenal aldosterone producing lesions reveal three somatic mutations near the KCNJ5 potassium channel selectivity filter. PLoS One 7:e41926
119. Kuppusamy M, Caroccia B, Stindl J et al (2014) A novel KCNJ5-insT149 somatic mutation close to, but outside, the selectivity filter causes resistant hypertension by loss of selectivity for potassium. J Clin Endocrinol Metab 99:E1765–E1773

120. Shen WT, Lim RC, Siperstein AE et al (1999) Laparoscopic vs open adrenalectomy for the treatment of primary hyperaldosteronism. Arch Surg 134:628–631
121. Viola A, Tizzani D, Monticone S et al (2013) Diagnosis and treatment of unilateral forms of primary aldosteronism. Curr Hypertens Rev 9:156–165
122. van der Linden P, Steichen O, Zinzindohoue F et al (2012) Blood pressure and medication changes following adrenalectomy for unilateral primary aldosteronism: a follow-up study. J Hypertens 30:761–769
123. Rossitto G, Regolisti G, Rossi E et al (2013) Elevation of angiotensin-II type-1-receptor autoantibodies titer in primary aldosteronism as a result of aldosterone-producing adenoma. Hypertension 61:526–533
124. Kem DC, Li H, Velarde-Miranda C et al (2014) Autoimmune mechanisms activating the angiotensin AT1 receptor in primary aldosteronism. J Clin Endocrinol Metab 99:1790–1797
125. Li H, Yu X, Cicala MV et al (2015) Prevalence of angiotensin II type 1 receptor (AT1R)-activating autoantibodies in primary aldosteronism. J Am Soc Hypertens 9:15–20
126. Sawka AM, Young WF, Thompson GB et al (2001) Primary aldosteronism: factors associated with normalization of blood pressure after surgery. Ann Intern Med 135:258–261
127. Rossi GP, Bolognesi M, Rizzoni D et al (2008) Vascular remodelling and duration of hypertension predict outcome of adrenalectomy in primary aldosteronism patients. Hypertension 51:1366–1371
128. Zarnegar R, Young WF, Lee J et al (2008) The aldosteronoma resolution score: predicting complete resolution of hypertension after adrenalectomy for aldosteronoma. Ann Surg 247:511–518
129. Weigel M, Riester A, Hanslik G et al (2015) Post-saline infusion test aldosterone levels indicate severity and outcome in primary aldosteronism. Eur J Endocrinol 172(4):443–450
130. Jacobsen NE, Campbell JB, Hobart MG (2003) Laparoscopic versus open adrenalectomy for surgical adrenal disease. Can J Urol 10:1995–1999
131. Fu B, Zhang X, Wang G-X, Lang B, Ma X, Li H-Z et al (2011) Long-term results of a prospective, randomized trial comparing retroperitoneoscopic partial versus total adrenalectomy for aldosterone producing adenoma. J Urol 185:1578–1582
132. Ishidoya S, Ito A, Sakai K et al (2005) Laparoscopic partial versus total adrenalectomy for aldosterone producing adenoma. J Urol 174:40–43
133. Shimabuku M, Sasaki A, Higa M, Kakazu M, Asato M, Shiroma H (2011) Single-incision laparoscopic adrenalectomy for primary aldosteronism: report of a case. Surg Today 41:1306–1309
134. Colon MJ, Lemasters P, Newell P, Divino C, Weber KJ, Chin EH (2011) Laparoscopic single site adrenalectomy using a conventional laparoscope and instrumentation. JSLS 15:236–238
135. Jeunemaitre X, Chatellier G, Kreft-Jais C et al (1987) Efficacy and tolerance of spironolactone in essential hypertension. Am J Cardiol 60:820–825
136. Parthasarathy HK, Ménard J, White WB et al (2011) A double-blind, randomized study comparing the antihypertensive effect of eplerenone and spironolactone in patients with hypertension and evidence of primary aldosteronism. J Hypertens 29:980–990
137. Amar L, Azizi M, Menard J, Peyrard S, Plouin PF (2013) Sequential comparison of aldosterone synthase inhibition and mineralocorticoid blockade in patients with primary aldosteronism. J Hypertens 31:624–629
138. Pitt B, Kober L, Ponikowski P et al (2013) Safety and tolerability of the novel non-steroidal mineralocorticoid receptor antagonist BAY94–8862 in patients with chronic heart failure and mild or moderate chronic kidney disease: a randomized, double-blind trial. Eur Heart J 34:2453–2463
139. Fischer E, Beuschlein F, Degenhart C et al (2012) Spontaneous remission of idiopathic aldosteronism after long-term treatment with spironolactone: results from the German Conn's Registry. Clin Endocrinol (Oxf) 76(4):473–477
140. Lucatello B, Benso A, Tabaro I et al (2013) Long-term re-evaluation of primary aldosteronism after medical treatment reveals high proportion of normal mineralocorticoid secretion. Eur J Endocrinol 168(4):525–532

141. Catena C, Colussi G, Lapenna R et al (2007) Long-term cardiac effects of adrenalectomy or mineralocorticoid antagonists in patients with primary aldosteronism. Hypertension 50: 911–918
142. Ahmed AH, Gordon RD, Sukor N et al (2011) Quality of life in patients with bilateral primary aldosteronism before and during treatment with spironolactone and/or amiloride, including a comparison with our previously published results in those with unilateral disease treated surgically. J Clin Endocrinol Metab 96:2904–2911
143. Marzano L, Colussi G, Sechi LA, Catena C (2015) Adrenalectomy is comparable with medical treatment for reduction of left ventricular mass in primary aldosteronism: meta-analysis of long-term studies. Am J Hypertens 28:312–318. doi:10.1093/ajh/hpu154
144. Miyake Y, Tanaka K, Nishikawa T et al (2014) Prognosis of primary aldosteronism in Japan: results from a nationwide epidemiological study. Endocr J 61:35–40
145. Sechi LA, Colussi GL, Novello M et al (2015) Mineralocorticoid receptor antagonists and clinical outcomes in primary aldosteronism: as good as surgery? Horm Metab Res 47:1000–1006
146. Rossi GP, Dalla CA (2014) Clinical management of primary aldosteronism: 2013 practical recommendations of the Italian Society of Hypertension (SIIA). High Blood Press Cardiovasc Prev 21(1):71–75
147. Kline GA, Pasieka JL, Harvey A, So B, Dias VC (2014) High-probability features of primary aldosteronism may obviate the need for confirmatory testing without increasing false-positive diagnoses. J Clin Hypertens 16:488–496
148. Küpers EM, Amar L, Raynaud A, Plouin PF, Steichen O (2012) A clinical prediction score to diagnose unilateral primary aldosteronism. J Clin Endocrinol Metab 97:3530–3537
149. Riester A, Fischer E, Degenhart C et al (2014) Age below 40 or a recently proposed clinical prediction score cannot bypass adrenal venous sampling in primary aldosteronism. J Clin Endocrinol Metab 99:E1035–E1039
150. Sze WC, Soh LM, Lau JH et al (2014) Diagnosing unilateral primary aldosteronism – comparison of a clinical prediction score, computed tomography and adrenal venous sampling. Clin Endocrinol (Oxf) 81:25–30
151. Mulatero P, di Cella SM, Monticone S et al (2012) 18-hydroxycorticosterone, 18-hydroxycortisol and 18-oxocortisol in the diagnosis of primary aldosteronism and its subtypes. J Clin Endocrinol Metab 97:881–889
152. Satoh F, Morimoto R, Ono Y et al (2015) Measurement of peripheral plasma 18-oxocortisol can discriminate unilateral adenoma from bilateral diseases in patients with primary aldosteronism. Hypertension 65:1096–1102
153. Asmar M, Wachtel H, Yan Y et al (2015) Reversing the established order: should adrenal venous sampling precede cross-sectional imaging in the evaluation of primary aldosteronism? J Surg Oncol 112(2):144–148

3 Pheochromocytoma/Paragangliomas

Philippe van de Borne

Abbreviations

CT	Computed tomography
HTN	Hypertension
PET	Positron emission tomography
123I-MIBG SPECT	123I-metaiodobenzylguanidine single photon emission computed tomography
18F-FDG	18F-fluorodeoxyglucose

3.1 Introduction

Pheochromocytomas are rare catecholamine-secreting tumors derived from the chromaffin cells of the embryonic neural crest arising directly from the adrenal glands, first described in 1886 by Fränkel [1]. Most cases of pheochromocytoma are sporadic in origin [2–4]. Chromaffin tumors arising from extra-adrenal autonomic paraganglia are called paragangliomas [5]. These paragangliomas derive from extra-adrenal chromaffin (noradrenaline-producing) cells that persist postnatally in the pre- or para-aortic regions in relation to sympathetic ganglia. They can occur in locations such as the carotid body, the kidney, the bladder, the retroperitoneum, as well as in the paraganglionic complex named the organ of Zuckerkandl. They consist of paired organs situated lateral to the abdominal aorta at the level of the inferior mesenteric artery. Smaller accessory paraganglia, anterior to the aorta or below the aortic bifurcation, have also been described. The Zuckerkandl organ is the largest accumulation of chromaffin cells. It regresses after birth by autophagy [6] but remains a site of origin for

P. van de Borne (✉)
Department of Cardiology, Erasme Hospital, Université Libre de Bruxelles, Brussels, Belgium
e-mail: Philippe.van.de.Borne@erasme.ulb.ac.be

C. Tsioufis et al. (eds.), *Interventional Therapies for Secondary and Essential Hypertension*, Updates in Hypertension and Cardiovascular Protection,
DOI 10.1007/978-3-319-34141-5_3

paraganglioma which occurs in association with the succinate dehydrogenase complex, subunit B (SDHB), or less frequently, subunit D (SDHD) gene mutations in more than 70 % of cases [7]. Paragangliomas of parasympathetic origin develop from non-chromaffin organs that act as chemoreceptors. They are located in glomus bodies (carotid body, aortic bodies) or are embedded in several sensory parasympathetic ganglia. Those located in the head and neck region are referred to as head and neck paragangliomas. The most common location among all parasympathetic paragangliomas is the carotid body. Next is the glomus jugulare (the jugular bulb in the jugular foramen), the glomus tympanicum or hypotympanicum (the middle ear or hypotympanum), and then the glomus vagale. Two out of three head and neck paragangliomas do not produce catecholamine. Some may however produce catecholamine and mostly dopamine. This is converted inside the tumor into 3-methoxytyramine, currently the best specific biomarker for these tumors [8–10], and known to be increased in 33 % of patients with head and neck paragangliomas [8, 9].

Malignant tumors occur in about 10 % pheochromocytomas, the others are benign [11]. Malignant pheochromocytoma/paragangliomas are defined by the presence of tumor at sites normally devoid of chromaffin cells or by local invasion by the primary tumor [12, 13]. The rate of metastatic disease is variable, with reports ranging from 1 out of 20 to almost a tenfold higher incidence [14–16]. Locoregional or metastatic recurrence occurs preferentially within 5 years of initial curative therapy but can also occur after much longer periods [16]. Tumor recurrence is more common in patients with hereditary pheochromocytoma. Extra-adrenal pheochromocytomas recur more often than in the adrenal gland [2–4]. Local lymph nodes, liver, bone, and lung are common metastatic sites [17, 18]. These malignant tumors secrete often catecholamine, in contrast to the head and neck paragangliomas, as already discussed [3, 19]. Patients with metastatic pheochromocytomas and paragangliomas have a diminished quality of life, and their overall 5-year survival rate is less than 60 % [15, 20]. Consequences of elevated catecholamine and side effects from treatments are worrisome [21, 22]. Bone metastases are painful and may induce bone fractures and hypercalcemia, as well as spinal cord compression, but seem less aggressive than non-skeletal metastases [23].

Multiple non-anatomic parameters have also been associated with metastatic disease. Pathologic features more often associated with metastatic disease include primary tumor size greater than 6 cm, necrosis, hemorrhage, and high mitotic index [24, 25]. Possible biochemical indicators of malignant disease include dopamine hypersecretion measured by methoxytyramine and markedly elevated plasma or urinary metanephrines [10, 25–27]. The most well-defined genetic risk factor for malignant disease is a mutation in the SDHB gene, which is clinically associated with an earlier onset of disease and more aggressive malignancy [3, 28, 29].

3.2 Clinical Aspects

On early diagnosis of pheochromocytomas and paragangliomas is critical, and the signs and symptoms should be recognized as soon as possible. Misdiagnosed or undiagnosed patients may present severe consequences of hypertensive crises, including heart attacks, strokes, and even death [30]. Hypertensive emergencies in patients with pheochromocytomas and paragangliomas proved lethal in 15 % [31]. The incidence of pheochromocytomas and paragangliomas in the general population is estimated to be less than 1 per 100,000 people per year [32]. The prevalence of pheochromocytomas is higher in the hypertensive population (between 0.1 and 0.6 %)[32, 33]. Patients with resistant hypertension (HTN) should thus be considered for evaluation of pheochromocytomas and paragangliomas [34]. The diagnosis takes often place in patients aged 40–50 years [32]. Importantly, however, it should be remembered that hereditary variants, such as the pheochromocytoma-paraganglioma syndrome, multiple endocrine neoplasia type 2, neurofibromatosis type 1, and Von Hippel-Lindau disease may present earlier [34]. Classically, patients experience signs of paroxysmal HTN, episodic headache, sweating, and tachycardia [35, 36]. Excessive catecholamine release account for these acute complaints, however, between these episodes blood pressure can be normal. The clinical presentation can be affected by the catecholamine-releasing profile of the tumor. Norepinephrine-secreting tumors are associated with more sustained HTN than epinephrine ones, which are more often associated with paroxysmal HTN [37, 38]. Autopsy analyses also show that many tumors remain undiagnosed [3, 13, 15], perhaps because patients can also present with a variety of nonspecific symptoms that can mimic many other conditions, such as pallor, anxiety or panic feelings, fever, and nausea or vomiting [32, 39]. Children can present with exercise-induced nausea and vomiting [40], as well as an early onset of diabetes in the absence of typical risk factors [41]. Other features are hypertensive crises caused by catecholamine surges after accidental tumor manipulation or anesthesia [32], the appearance of suspicious symptoms in patients with a family history of pheochromocytomas and paragangliomas, or incidentally discovered adrenal masses, even in the absence of symptoms [32, 42, 43].

3.3 Diagnosis

Diagnosis of pheochromocytomas and paragangliomas is based on clinical data, laboratory findings (plasma or 24-h urinary fractionated metanephrines), anatomical imaging (computed tomography and magnetic resonance imaging), and functional imaging such as 123I-metaiodobenzylguanidine single photon emission computed tomography (123I-MIBG SPECT) and 18F-fluorodeoxyglucose (18F-FDG) positron emission tomography (PET) computed tomography. 18F-FDG PET computed tomography imaging appears superior to computed tomography only and to 123I-MIBG SPECT [18, 44].

3.3.1 Laboratory Findings

Pheochromocytoma and paraganglioma tumors produce, synthesize, store, and metabolize catecholamine. Many tumors have fluctuating levels of catecholamine release, which can lead to false negatives [32]. Measurement of catecholamine in the plasma or urine is, therefore, not always the most effective approach [32, 45, 46]. Fortunately, catecholamine metabolism remains fairly constant in these tumors, leading to increased metanephrine levels [32, 45]. At the present time, there is no clear evidence favoring plasma or urine metanephrines.

Importantly, and frequently overlooked, plasma catecholamine and metanephrine levels should be drawn through an indwelling catheter after the patient has rested supine for at least 20 min in a dark and quiet room to remove any environmental impacts on stress levels. Failure to obtain blood tests under these conditions will result in false-positive elevations relative to supine reference ranges after a period of rest [47]. Moreover, patients should have fasted overnight before the blood draw [47]. Also critical is the use of appropriate age-adjusted reference ranges as this increases the sensitivity of plasma metanephrine and normetanephrine for the detection of pheochromocytomas and paragangliomas [48].

Plasma methoxytyramine measurements may also prove useful for dopamine-secreting tumors [49, 50]. Chromogranin A is often measured in pheochromocytoma and paraganglioma patients. This polypeptide is commonly secreted by chromaffin cells, together with catecholamine. Chromogranin A is a nonspecific marker of neuroendocrine tumors. However, when combined with catecholamine measurements, the sensitivity for diagnosing pheochromocytomas and paragangliomas can be close to 100 %. Chromogranin A is significantly higher in patients with certain hereditary syndromes, and the metabolite of dopamine methoxytyramine may also serve as a predictor of malignancy [10]. In most patients, especially those presenting with signs and symptoms of pheochromocytomas and paragangliomas, catecholamine and metanephrines will be elevated to levels greater than four times the upper reference limit. In these patients, diagnostic workup can immediately move forward to anatomical and functional imaging.

Other patients will disclose more equivocal results, with values between the upper reference limit and the diagnostic level, and medication interferences should be ruled out. Beta-adrenergic blockers, dopamine D2 receptor antagonists, tricyclic antidepressants, serotonin and norepinephrine reuptake inhibitors, monoamine oxidase inhibitors, sympathicomimetics, chemotherapeutic agents, opiate analgesics, neuromuscular blocking agents, and peptide and steroid hormones can cause false-positive elevations [30, 49–52]. Beverage containing caffeine can also cause elevations in catecholamine and metanephrines and should thus be avoided before repeat testing [32, 49–51]. Elevated plasma metanephrines are also common in patients with chronic kidney disease, particularly when on dialysis [53].

For patients with elevated plasma norepinephrine or normetanephrine, when medication interferences have been ruled out or if drug interferences cannot be discontinued, a clonidine suppression test should be performed, with plasma normetanephrine as the biomarker [32, 49]. Further workup for suspected pheochromocytoma and paraganglioma is required when clonidine is unable to reduce plasma normetanephrine below the upper reference limit or by 40 % of the initial value [32]. The glucagon stimulation test, also used in the past, is no longer recommended [32].

A small percentage of pheochromocytoma and paraganglioma have no abnormal hormonal activity and are often associated with SDH mutations [54, 55]. In other rare cases, pheochromocytoma and paraganglioma can also secrete other hormones, such as cortisol and adrenocorticotropic hormone (ACTH). These patients often present with Cushing's disease in addition to pheochromocytoma and paraganglioma [56–58].

3.3.2 Anatomical Imaging

As already mentioned, once the biochemical testing has been completed and is positive for elevated metanephrine/epinephrine, then imaging can be focused on the adrenal gland, because this is where the majority of tumors that secrete epinephrine are found. Computed tomography and magnetic resonance imaging are likely sufficient to detect these tumors [32]. If the pheochromocytoma is less than 3 cm, the patient is below 40 years of age, and there is no family history of pheochromocytoma, no further imaging workup is needed [59]. Should the adrenal imaging be negative, then imaging of additional body areas must be performed, namely, of the abdomen, the pelvis, the chest, and the neck. Computed tomography and magnetic resonance imaging have similar sensitivity for the detection of pheochromocytoma and paraganglioma [32]. Magnetic resonance imaging is preferred in patients in whom radiation exposure should be limited (i.e., pregnant or pediatric patients), subjects with computed tomography-contrast allergies, and perhaps in the presence of extra-adrenal tumors [32].

On computed tomography, pheochromocytoma and paraganglioma have a heterogeneous appearance, often with some cystic areas [60–63]. Attenuation values are typically greater than 10 Hounsfield units, although fatty components in some pheochromocytoma may result in an adenoma-like appearance [62]. Calcifications or hemorrhage may also be present on the computed tomography [62]. Using contrast-enhanced computed tomography, pheochromocytomas distinguish themselves from other adrenal masses because of higher intensities than 110 Hounsfield units during the arterial phase [63].

On magnetic resonance imaging, pheochromocytoma and paraganglioma typically appear as T2-bright lesions, sometimes attenuated by necrotic or cystic components [60–62]. On T1 imaging, pheochromocytoma and paraganglioma enhance similarly to the muscle but are less intense than the liver [62]. Just as with contrast-enhanced computed tomography, pheochromocytoma and paraganglioma are enhanced with gadolinium contrast agents. This can be hindered by necrotic or cystic areas [62].

Ultrasound techniques have a limited utility, unless for metastatic lesion evaluation, in the liver or in the urinary tract [62].

3.3.3 Functional Imaging

This imaging modality is important in the workup of pheochromocytoma and paraganglioma because it can detect tumors (primary or metastatic) not seen at the computed tomography or magnetic resonance, and it is able to assess their metabolic activity as well. Historically, functional imaging consisted in 123I- or 131I-MIBG scintigraphy. This is because MIBG resembles norepinephrine and enters through norepinephrine transporters in the pheochromocytoma and paraganglioma. MIBG scintigraphy has however several pitfalls: because of less intense or false-negative results in the presence of extra-adrenal tumors, when tumors are associated with succinate dehydrogenase subunit B (SDHB) mutations, as well as in the presence of head and neck paragangliomas or medications such as tricyclic antidepressants, opioids, labetalol, to name a few [59, 66, 67]. In comparison, PET is characterized by an increased sensitivity, shorter acquisition times, and higher image resolution and is now widely used for pheochromocytoma and paraganglioma characterization [59, 64]. Most frequently, the glucose analog 18F-fluorodeoxyglucose will be administered to the patient and taken up by a glucose transporter in the tumor [62, 65]. Interestingly, PET can quantify tracer uptake through standard uptake value measurements and thereby assess tumor metabolism [59]. Higher standard uptake values could prove useful to differentiate malignant from benign disease, and this is important for patients with metastatic disease or SDHB mutations [32]. The main limitation of 18F-fluorodeoxyglucose is obviously that it is not specific for pheochromocytoma and paraganglioma. It may detect hypermetabolic regions that are unrelated to the chromaffin tumor [59]. More specific tracers which enter cells via the L-type amino acid transporter system have been developed, such as 18F-fluorodopa and 18F-fluorodopamine. These tracers are however much less widely available [62, 65]. Recently, PET/CT imaging using 68Ga-labeled somatostatin was developed [68–72]. 68Ga-based PET imaging has lower spatial resolution and detection sensitivity than 18F-fluorodeoxyglucose PET imaging [73]. It is also less specific than 18F-fluorodopa and 18F-fluorodopamine. However, highly elevated tumor to background uptake ratio of the paraganglioma compensates these drawbacks. It does also not require a cyclotron to make the radiotracer and might surpass 18F-fluorodeoxyglucose PET as due to its easier production, availability, and distribution [74–76].

3.4 Treatment

3.4.1 Medical

Catecholamine-producing pheochromocytoma and paraganglioma should receive without any delay antihypertensive medications in order to alleviate symptoms and prevent complications of hypertensive crises. Preoperative management of hypertension is also mandatory since tumor manipulation during surgical treatment releases important amounts of catecholamines into the circulation. This may result in potentially life-threatening events such as myocardial ischemia or infarction, cardiac arrhythmias, and pulmonary edema. Conversely, once the tumor is removed, the patients may become severely hypotensive [77–79].

The treatment must begin with an alpha-adrenergic blocker, followed by a beta-adrenergic blocker, if needed. The reason for this is that if the treatment starts with a beta-adrenergic blocker, beta-adrenoceptor vasodilation elicited by the elevated adrenalin levels is inhibited, but it leaves alpha-adrenergic stimulation induced by the heightened catecholamine levels unopposed, with, as a result, a hypertensive crisis [32, 39, 49]. Importantly, it should be remembered that labetalol, a combined alpha- and beta-adrenoceptor antagonists, is not recommended for patients with pheochromocytoma and paraganglioma. This is because the beta-blocking activity of labetalol is by far more pronounced than its alpha-adrenoceptor blocking activity [30, 39]. Furthermore, labetalol interferes with MIBG scintigraphy [59, 66, 67].

Different alpha-adrenergic blockers can be used to treat hypertension, according to local practice and drug availability. The long-lasting alpha blocker phenoxybenzamine is frequently used in the United States [80, 81], but shorter acting alpha blockers, such as prazosin, doxazosin, and terazosin, can also be used when phenoxybenzamine is not available or hypertension is not sufficiently severe [39, 82]. Because these medications can elicit a severe orthostatic hypotension upon treatment initiation, medication should be taken at bedtime. The risk of an acute severe orthostatic hypotension, as well as the countermeasures which must be taken, should be carefully explained to the patient [39, 82]. Next, doses are progressively increased until the patient becomes normotensive or remains slightly hypertensive [30].

Phenoxybenzamine is a long-acting, noncompetitive, alpha-1- and alpha-2-adrenoceptor antagonist [81, 83, 84]. The usual starting dose is 10 mg twice daily per os and is increased until blood pressure is controlled or orthostatic hypotension arises [32, 81, 83]. Because of its noncompetitive action, alpha blockade will remain effective even when tremendous amounts of catecholamine are released in the circulation. Presynaptic alpha-2 adrenoceptor inhibition suppresses the negative feedback on norepinephrine release, with, as a result, a reflex tachycardia [38, 81]. Phenoxybenzamine passes the blood-brain barrier and induces central sedation and headaches and has long-acting properties that can lead to a prolonged postoperative hypotension. Doxazosin is a short-acting, competitive, and selective alpha-1-adrenoceptor antagonist [81, 83, 84]. Because of its competitive inhibition properties, it has a relatively short duration of action which reduces the risk of postoperative hypotension. Doxazosin may however become ineffective when plasma concentrations of catecholamine become very elevated. Doxazosin does also not induce a reflex tachycardia and, unlike phenoxybenzamine, does not induce central signs. The starting dose is usually 1 mg per os, with a recommended maximum of 16 mg a day [84, 85].

Beta blockers can be added subsequently, in order to relieve symptomatic tachyarrhythmia. The cardioselective metoprolol and atenolol, and even the noncardioselective propranolol, can be used in this indication. Labetalol should not be used, because its alpha-blocking activity is not sufficient to control blood pressure in such patients [30, 39].

Calcium channel blockers such as amlodipine, nicardipine, nifedipine, and verapamil can also be used. These agents are useful when alpha blockers are unable to achieve sufficient blood pressure reductions, when alpha blockers are not well tolerated or result in excessive hypotension because blood pressure is only mildly elevated or, conversely, when supramaximal doses of alpha blocker monotherapy are required to achieve a satisfactory blood pressure control [30, 39]. Calcium channel blockers can also be used for additional blood pressure and symptom control [30]. Patients with persistent hypertension after alpha blockers may benefit from the addition of a calcium channel blocker, rather than supramaximal doses of the alpha blocker. In addition, some patients may be unable to tolerate alpha blockers, in which case calcium channel blockers should be used. Calcium channel blockers are also valuable in the management of patients with very mild hypertension, in whom alpha blockade would cause hypotension [84].

3.4.2 Surgical

Surgical resection is the only potentially curative treatment for pheochromocytomas and paragangliomas [78]. In both patients with adrenal pheochromocytomas and extra-adrenal paragangliomas, laparoscopic surgery can be successfully performed with similar outcomes to open surgery. Thus, when feasible, laparoscopy is the preferred technique [32, 86–94]. Laparoscopy may still be used for tumors >6 cm, although these are frequently converted intraoperatively to open procedures [86, 93]. Open resection is preferable to ensure complete removal of multiple, metastatic, or recurrent tumors, although laparoscopic tumor removal can also be tried by experienced surgeons [20, 84, 94]. Robotic assistance or robotic procedures are alternative solutions with similar success rates, lower morbidity, less postoperative pain, and shorter hospitalization [95]. In patients with bilateral tumors or a high risk of bilateral tumors, cortex-sparing surgery may be sufficient if the tumor is small enough, in order to reduce the need for steroid replacement [32, 84, 96–102]. For patients with adrenal pheochromocytomas, full adrenalectomies should be performed in the absence of a genetic background, if patients are at a low risk of bilateral disease, or if they disclose larger tumors. Operative mortality is very low if the experienced surgical team is accompanied by an anesthesiologist capable to suppress the intraoperative hypertensive crises and administer fluid replacement to prevent any postoperative hypotension for the reasons already mentioned [32]. Surgery is a curative treatment for primary, recurrent, or limited metastatic tumors. In patients with extensive metastatic disease, surgery can also be used as a debulking technique to alleviate symptoms and complications from tumor size; however, long-term benefits are often elusive [15, 45, 84, 103].

3.4.3 Palliative Therapy

Surgical removal of a pheochromocytoma and abdominal paraganglioma can be difficult due to their anatomical locations [98]. Moreover, paragangliomas can appear in unusual and surgically inaccessible locations which will not allow complete tumor resection or may result in tumor spillage [104]. Some of these tumors can benefit of radiofrequency ablation. This has been reported in small series of patients for liver and bone metastases [84, 105–108]. Radiofrequency ablation releases catecholamine during the procedure, and an experienced anesthesiologist is required during the procedure to prevent hypertensive crises [105]. External palliative beam radiation can be used for symptom relief, bone lesion treatment, and nonremovable head and neck paraganglioma [15, 20]. For patients with positive MIBG scintigraphy, 131I-MIBG treatment therapy is another palliative treatment modality. Beta particles emission by the radioactive compound taken into tumor cells lead to their destruction [32]. Novel therapies targeting somatostatin receptors are currently also under investigation [84]. Last, some chemotherapy regimens may prolong patient survival and improve quality of life. Traditional chemotherapy with cyclophosphamide, vincristine, and dacarbazine is an effective treatment for widespread metastatic disease [15, 20]. The tyrosine kinase inhibitor sunitinib is currently investigated in this indication [84].

3.5 Follow-Up

For patients with small tumors, surgical resection can be curative, although hypertension may persist [32, 84, 109]. In the absence of genetic background, with complete tumor removal, rates of metastases and recurrence can be very low. In a large study of patients who underwent successful removals of pheochromocytoma and paraganglioma, only 14 % developed recurrent or metastatic disease [109]. The risk of recurrence with cortical-sparing adrenalectomies was small (approximately 7 %), as long as the whole tumor is removed [98]. Repeat subtotal adrenalectomies can be successfully performed if tumors recur [84, 96, 97]. Patients with hereditary pheochromocytoma and extra-adrenal pheochromocytoma recur more often and require a closer follow-up [2–4]. Increased rates of adrenal recurrence have also been demonstrated in laparoscopic interventions, in contrast to open procedure [98]. There is also an increased risk of recurrence in younger patients and in case of larger tumors [34, 84, 110]. Surgical removal is the first-line treatment if there is a recurrence. Because there is no clear method for distinguishing benign from malignant tumors, patients should always undergo close clinical follow-up after surgery, at least annually, regardless of the pathological features of the tumor [32, 84, 109]. Current guidelines suggest that all patients with a pheochromocytoma should be followed during at least 10 years after surgery [111]. In case of an extra-adrenal tumor or genetic pheochromocytoma, the patient should be followed lifelong [84].

References

1. Fränkel F (1886) Ein Fall von doppelseitigem, völlig latent verlaufenen Nebennierentumor und gleichzeitiger Nephritis mit Veränderungen am Circulationsapparat und Retinitis. Arch Pathol Anat Physiol Klin Med 103:244–263
2. Gimenez-Roqueplo AP, Burnichon N, Amar L, Favier J, Jeunemaitre X, Plouin PF (2008) Recent advances in the genetics of pheochromocytoma and functional paraganglioma. Clin Exp Pharmacol Physiol 35(4):376–379

3. Neumann HP, Pawlu C, Peczowska M, Bausch B, McWhinney SR, Muresan M et al (2004) Distinct clinical features of paraganglioma syndromes associated with SDHB and SDHD gene mutations. JAMA 292(8):943–951
4. Kaltsas GA, Papadogias D, Grossman AB (2004) The clinical presentation (symptoms and signs) of sporadic and familial chromaffin cell tumours (phaeochromocytomas and paragangliomas). Front Horm Res 31:61–75
5. DeLellis RA (2004) Pathology and genetics of tumours of endocrine organs. IARC Press, Lyon
6. Schober A, Parlato R, Huber K, Kinscherf R, Hartleben B, Huber TB, Schutz G, Unsicker K (2013) Cell loss and autophagy in the extra-adrenal chromaffin organ of Zuckerkandl are regulated by glucocorticoid signalling. J Neuroendocrinol 25(1):34–47
7. Lodish MB, Adams KT, Huynh TT, Prodanov T, Ling A, Chen C, Shusterman S, Jimenez C, Merino M, Hughes M et al (2010) Succinate dehydrogenase gene mutations are strongly associated with paraganglioma of the organ of Zuckerkandl. Endocr Relat Cancer 17(3):581–588
8. van Duinen N, Steenvoorden D, Kema IP, Jansen JC, Vriends AH, Bayley JP, Smit JW, Romijn JA, Corssmit EP (2010) Increased urinary excretion of 3-methoxytyramine in patients with head-and-neck paragangliomas. J Clin Endocrinol Metab 95(1):209–214
9. van Duinen N, Corssmit EP, de Jong WH, Brookman D, Kema IP, Romijn JA (2013) Plasma levels of free metanephrines and 3-methoxytyramine indicate a higher number of biochemically active HNPGL than 24-h urinary excretion rates of catecholamines and metabolites. Eur J Endocrinol/Eur Federation of Endocrine Soc 169:377–382
10. Eisenhofer G, Lenders JW, Siegert G, Bornstein SR, Friberg P, Milosevic D, Mannelli M, Linehan WM, Adams K, Timmers HJ et al (2012) Plasma methoxytyramine: a novel biomarker of metastatic pheochromocytoma and paraganglioma in relation to established risk factors of tumour size, location and SDHB mutation status. Eur J Cancer 48(11):1739–1749
11. Brouwers FM, Elkahloun AG, Munson PJ et al (2006) Gene expression profiling of benign and malignant pheochromocytoma. Ann N Y Acad Sci 1073:541–556
12. O'Riordain DS, Young WF Jr et al (1996) Clinical spectrum and outcome of functional extraadrenal paraganglioma. World J Surg 20:916–921, discussion 922
13. Wangberg B, Muth A, Khorram-Manesh A et al (2006) Malignant pheochromocytoma in a population-based study: survival and clinical results. Ann N Y Acad Sci 1073:512–516
14. Zarnegar R, Kebebew E, Duh QY, Clark OH (2006) Malignant pheochromocytoma. Surg Oncol Clin N Am 15:555–571
15. Adjalle R, Plouin PF, Pacak K, Lehnert H (2009) Treatment of malignant pheochromocytoma. Horm Metab Res 41:687–696
16. Pacak K, Eisenhofer G, Ahlman H et al (2007) Pheochromocytoma: recommendations for clinical practice from the First International Symposium October 2005. Nat Clin Pract Endocrinol Metab 3:92–102
17. Loh KC, Fitzgerald PA, Matthay KK et al (1997) The treatment of malignant pheochromocytoma with iodine-131 metaiodobenzylguanidine (131I-MIBG): a comprehensive review of 116 reported patients. J Endocrinol Invest 20:648–658
18. Bravo EL (1994) Evolving concepts in the pathophysiology, diagnosis and treatment of pheochromocytoma. Endocr Rev 15:356–368
19. Schwaber MK, Glasscock ME, Nissen AJ et al (1984) Diagnosis and management of catecholamine secreting glomus tumors. Laryngoscope 94:1008–1015
20. Jimenez C, Rohren E, Habra MA et al (2013) Current and future treatments for malignant pheochromocytoma and sympathetic paraganglioma. Curr Oncol Rep 15:356–371
21. Plouin PF, Fitzgerald P, Rich T et al (2012) Metastatic pheochromocytoma and paraganglioma: focus on therapeutics. Horm Metab Res 44:390–399
22. van Hulsteijn LT, Louisse A, Havekes B et al (2013) Quality of life is decreased in patients with paragangliomas. Eur J Endocrinol 168:689–697
23. Ayala-Ramirez M, Palmer JL, Hofmann MC et al (2013) Bone metastases and skeletal-related events in patients with malignant pheochromocytoma and sympathetic paraganglioma. J Clin Endocrinol Metab 98:1492–1497

24. Strong VE, Kennedy T, Al-Ahmadie H et al (2008) Prognostic indicators of malignancy in adrenal pheochromocytomas: clinical, histopathologic, and cell cycle/apoptosis gene expression analysis. Surgery 143:759–768
25. Park J, Song C, Park M et al (2011) Predictive characteristics of malignant pheochromocytoma. Korean J Urol 52:241–246
26. John H, Ziegler WH, Hauri D, Jaeger P (1999) Pheochromocytomas: can malignant potential be predicted? Urology 53:679–683
27. Khorram-Manesh A, Ahlman H, Nilsson O et al (2005) Long-term outcome of a large series of patients surgically treated for pheochromocytoma. J Intern Med 258:55–66
28. Amar L, Baudin E, Burnichon N et al (2007) Succinate dehydrogenase B gene mutations predict survival in patients with malignant pheochromocytomas or paragangliomas. J Clin Endocrinol Metabol 92:3822–3828
29. King KS, Prodanov T, Kantorovich V et al (2011) Metastatic pheochromocytoma/paraganglioma related to primary tumor development in childhood or adolescence: significant link to SDHB mutations. J Clin Oncol 29:4137–4142
30. Pacak K (2007) Preoperative management of the pheochromocytoma patient. J Clin Endocrinol Metab 92:4069–4079
31. Whitelaw B, Prague JK, Mustafa O et al (2014) Pheochromocytoma crisis. Clin Endocrinol (Oxf) 80(1):13–22
32. Lenders JW, Eisenhofer G, Mannelli M, Pacak K (2005) Phaeochromocytoma. Lancet 366:665–675
33. Beard CM, Sheps SG, Kurland LT, Carney JA, Lie JT (1983) Occurrence of pheochromocytoma in Rochester, Minnesota, 1950 through 1979. Mayo Clin Proc 58:802–804
34. Maher ER, Eng C (2002) The pressure rises: update on the genetics of pheochromocytoma. Hum Mol Genet 11:2347–2354
35. Stein PP, Black HR (1991) A simplified diagnostic approach to pheochromocytoma. A review of the literature and report of one institution's experience. Medicine (Baltimore) 70:46–66
36. Bravo EL (1991) Pheochromocytoma: new concepts and future trends. Kidney Int 40:544–556
37. Bravo EL, Tagle R (2003) Pheochromocytoma: state-of-the-art and future prospects. Endocr Rev 24:539–553
38. Langer SZ (1980) Presynaptic regulation of the release of catecholamines. Pharmacol Rev 32:337–362
39. Mazza A, Armigliato M, Marzola MC et al (2014) Anti-hypertensive treatment in pheochromocytoma and paraganglioma: current management and therapeutic features. Endocrine 45(3):469–478
40. King KS, Darmani NA, Hughes MS et al (2010) Exercise-induced nausea and vomiting: another sign and symptom of pheochromocytoma and paraganglioma. Endocrine 37:403–407
41. La Batide-Alanore A, Chatellier G, Plouin PF (2003) Diabetes as a marker of pheochromocytoma in hypertensive patients. J Hypertens 21:1703–1707 [PubMed: 129234030]
42. Arnaldi G, Boscaro M (2012) Adrenal incidentaloma. Best Pract Res Clin Endocrinol Metab 26:405–419
43. Mannelli M, Lenders JWM, Pacak K et al (2012) Subclinical phaeochromocytoma. Best Pract Res Clin Endocrinol Metab 26:507–515
44. Timmers HJ, Kozupa A, Chen CC et al (2007) Superiority of fluorodeoxyglucose positron emission tomography to other functional imaging techniques in the evaluation of metastatic SDHB-associated pheochromocytoma and paraganglioma. J Clin Oncol 25:2262–2269
45. Chen H, Sippel RS, O'Dorisio MS et al (2010) The North American Neuroendocrine Tumor Society consensus guideline for the diagnosis and management of neuroendocrine tumors: pheochromocytoma, paraganglioma, and medullary thyroid cancer. Pancreas 39:775–783
46. Lenders JWM, Pacak K, Walther MM et al (2002) Biochemical diagnosis of pheochromocytoma: which test is best? JAMA 287:1427–1434

47. Därr R, Pamporaki C, Peitzsch M et al (2014) Biochemical diagnosis of phaeochromocytoma using plasma free normetanephrine, metanephrine and methoxytyramine: importance of supine sampling under fasting conditions. Clin Endocrinol (Oxf) 80(4):478–486
48. Eisenhofer G, Lattke P, Herberg M et al (2013) Reference intervals for plasma free metanephrines with an age adjustment for normetanephrine for optimized laboratory testing of phaeochromocytoma. Ann Clin Biochem 50:62–69
49. Eisenhofer G, Goldstein DS, Sullivan P et al (2005) Biochemical and clinical manifestations of dopamine-producing paragangliomas: utility of plasma methoxytyramine. J Clin Endocrinol Metab 90:2068–2075
50. Poirier É, Thauvette D, Hogue JC (2013) Management of exclusively dopamine-secreting abdominal pheochromocytomas. J Am Coll Surg 216:340–346
51. Eisenhofer G, Siegert G, Kotzerke J et al (2008) Current progress and future challenges in the biochemical diagnosis and treatment of pheochromocytomas and paragangliomas. Horm Metab Res 40:329–337
52. Neary NM, King KS, Pacak K (2011) Drugs and pheochromocytoma–don't be fooled by every elevated metanephrine. N Engl J Med 364:2268–2270
53. Niculescu DA, Ismail G, Poiana C (2014) Plasma free metanephrine and normetanephrine levels are increased in patients with chronic kidney disease. Endocr Pract 20(2):139–144
54. Timmers HJLM, Pacak K, Huynh TT et al (2008) Biochemically silent abdominal paragangliomas in patients with mutations in the succinate dehydrogenase subunit B gene. J Clin Endocrinol Metab 93:4826–4832
55. Timmers HJLM, Gimenez-Roqueplo AP, Mannelli M et al (2009) Clinical aspects of SDHx-related pheochromocytoma and paraganglioma. Endocr Relat Cancer 16:391–400
56. Nijhoff MF, Dekkers OM, Vleming LJ et al (2009) ACTH-producing pheochromocytoma: clinical considerations and concise review of the literature. Eur J Intern Med 20:682–685
57. Kumar M, Kumar V, Talukdar B et al (2010) Cushing syndrome in an infant due to cortisol secreting adrenal pheochromocytoma: a rare association. J Pediatr Endocrinol Metab 23:621–625
58. Berenyi MR, Singh G, Gloster ES et al (1977) ACTH-producing pheochromocytoma. Arch Pathol Lab Med 101:31–35
59. Taïeb D, Timmers HJ, Hindié E et al (2012) EANM 2012 guidelines for radionuclide imaging of phaeochromocytoma and paraganglioma. Eur J Nucl Med Mol Imaging 39:1977–1995
60. Bhatia KSS, Ismail MM, Sahdev A et al (2008) 123I-metaiodobenzylguanidine (MIBG) scintigraphy for the detection of adrenal and extra-adrenal phaeochromocytomas: CT and MRI correlation. Clin Endocrinol (Oxf) 69:181–188
61. Havekes B, King K, Lai EW et al (2010) New imaging approaches to phaeochromocytomas and paragangliomas. Clin Endocrinol (Oxf) 72:137–145
62. Leung K, Stamm M, Raja A et al (2013) Pheochromocytoma: the range of appearances on ultrasound, CT, MRI, and functional imaging. AJR Am J Roentgenol 200:370–378
63. Northcutt BG, Raman SP, Long C et al (2013) MDCT of adrenal masses: Can dual-phase enhancement patterns be used to differentiate adenoma and pheochromocytoma? AJR Am J Roentgenol 201:834–839
64. Hartung-Knemeyer V, Rosenbaum-Krumme S, Buchbender C et al (2012) Malignant pheochromocytoma imaging with [124I]mIBG PET/MR. J Clin Endocrinol Metab 97:3833–3834
65. Chen CC, Carrasquillo JA (2012) Molecular imaging of adrenal neoplasms. J Surg Oncol 106:532–542
66. Fonte JS, Robles JF, Chen CC et al (2012) False-negative 123I-MIBG SPECT is most commonly found in SDHB-related pheochromocytoma or paraganglioma with high frequency to develop metastatic disease. Endocr Relat Cancer 19:83–93
67. Apeldoorn L, Voerman HJ, Hoefnagel CA (1995) Interference of MIBG uptake by medication: a case report. Neth J Med 46:239–243
68. Maurice JB, Troke R, Win Z, Ramachandran R, Al-Nahhas A, Naji M, Dhillo W, Meeran K, Goldstone AP, Martin NM et al (2012) A comparison of the performance of (68)

Ga-DOTATATE PET/CT an (123)I-MIBG SPECT in the diagnosis and follow-up of pheochromocytoma and paraganglioma. Eur J Nucl Med Mol Imaging 39(8):1266–1270
69. Naji M, Al-Nahhas A (2012) (68)Ga-labelled peptides in the management of neuroectodermal tumours. Eur J Nucl Med Mol Imaging 39 Suppl 1:S61–S67
70. Kroiss A, Putzer D, Frech A, Decristoforo C, Uprimny C, Gasser RW, Shulkin BL, Url C, Widmann G, Prommegger R et al (2013) A retrospective comparison between (68)Ga-DOTATOC PET/CT and (18)F-DOPA PET/CT in patients with extra-adrenal paraganglioma. Eur J Nucl Med Mol Imaging 40(12):1800–1808
71. Sharma P, Thakar A, Suman KCS, Dhull VS, Singh H, Naswa N, Reddy RM, Karunanithi S, Kumar R, Malhotra A et al (2013) 68Ga-DOTANOC PET/CT for baseline evaluation of patients with head and neck paraganglioma. J Nucl Med 54(6):841–847
72. Janssen I, Blanchet EM, Adams K, Chen CC, Millo C, Herscovitch P, Taieb D, Kebebew E, Lehnert H, Fojo AT et al (2015) Superiority of [68Ga]- DOTATATE PET/CT to other functional imaging modalities in the localization of SDHB-associated metastatic pheochromocytoma and paraganglioma. Clin Cancer Res 21(17):3888–3895
73. Sanchez-Crespo A (2013) Comparison of Gallium-68 and Fluorine-18 imaging characteristics in positron emission tomography. Appl Radiat Isot 76:55–62
74. Taieb D, Timmers HJ, Hindie E, Guillet BA, Neumann HP, Walz MK, Opocher G, de Herder WW, Boedeker CC, de Krijger RR et al (2012) EANM2012 guidelines for radionuclide imaging of pheochromocytoma and paraganglioma. Eur J Nucl Med Mol Imaging 39(12):1977–1995
75. Castinetti F, Kroiss A, Kumar R, Pacak K, Taieb D (2015) 15 YEARS OF PARAGANGLIOMA: imaging and imaging-based treatment of pheochromocytoma and paraganglioma. Endocr Relat Cancer 22(4):T135–T145
76. Hofman MS, Lau WF, Hicks RJ (2015) Somatostatin receptor imaging with (68)Ga DOTATATE PET/CT: clinical utility, normal patterns, pearls, and pitfalls in interpretation. Radiographics 35(2):500–516
77. Kinney MA, Warner ME, vanHeerden JA et al (2000) Perianesthetic risks and outcomes of pheochromocytoma and paraganglioma resection. Anesth Analg 91:1118–1123
78. Zhu Y, He HC, Su TW et al (2010) Selective alpha1-adrenoceptor antagonist (controlled release tablets) in preoperative management of pheochromocytoma. Endocrine 38:254–259
79. Prys-Roberts C (2000) Phaeochromocytoma–recent progress in its management. Br J Anaesth 85:44–57
80. Hamilton CA, Reid JL, Sumner DJ (1983) Acute effects of phenoxybenzamine on alpha-adrenoceptor responses in vivo and in vitro: relation of in vivo pressor responses to the number of specific adrenoceptor binding sites. J Cardiovasc Pharmacol 5:868–873
81. van der Horst-Schrivers AN, Kerstens MN, Wolffenbuttel BH (2006) Preoperative pharmacological management of pheochromocytoma. Neth J Med 64:290–295
82. van der Zee PA, de Boer A (2014) Pheochromocytoma: a review on preoperative treatment with phenoxybenzamine or doxazosin. Neth J Med 72(4):190–201
83. Domi R, Laho H (2012) Management of pheochromocytoma: old ideas and new drugs. Niger J Clin Pract 15:253–257
84. Martucci VL, Pacak K (2014) Pheochromocytoma and paraganglioma: diagnosis, genetics, management, and treatment. Curr Probl Cancer 38(1):7–41
85. Prys-Roberts C, Farndon JR (2002) Efficacy and safety of doxazosin for perioperative management of patients with pheochromocytoma. World J Surg 26:1037–1042
86. Conzo G, Musella M, Corcione F et al (2013) Laparoscopic adrenalectomy, a safe procedure for pheochromocytoma. A retrospective review of clinical series. Int J Surg 11:152–156
87. Cheah WK, Clark OH, Horn JK et al (2002) Laparoscopic adrenalectomy for pheochromocytoma. World J Surg 26:1048–1051
88. Goers TA, Abdo M, Moley JF et al (2013) Outcomes of resection of extra-adrenal pheochromocytomas/paragangliomas in the laparoscopic era: a comparison with adrenal pheochromocytoma. Surg Endosc 27:428–433
89. Henry JF, Defechereux T, Raffaelli M et al (2000) Complications of laparoscopic adrenalectomy: results of 169 consecutive procedures. World J Surg 24:1342–1346

90. Hwang JJ, Shoaf G, Uchio EM et al (2004) Laparoscopic management of extra-adrenal pheochromocytoma. J Urol 171:72–76
91. Janetschek G, Finkenstedt G, Gasser R et al (1998) Laparascopic surgery for pheochromocytoma: adrenalectomy, partial resection excision of paragangliomas. J Urol 160:330–334
92. Sprung J, O'Hara JF, Gill IS et al (2000) Anesthetic aspects of laparoscopic and open adrenalectomy for pheochromocytoma. Urology 55:339–343
93. Vargas HI, Kavoussi LR, Bartlett DL et al (1997) Laparoscopic adrenalectomy: a new standard of care. Urology 49:673–678
94. Walz MK, Peitgen K, Neumann HPH et al (2002) Endoscopic treatment of solitary, bilateral, multiple, and recurrent pheochromocytomas and paragangliomas. World J Surg 26:1005–1012
95. Aliyev S, Karabulut K, Agcaoglu O et al (2013) Robotic versus laparoscopic adrenalectomy for pheochromocytoma. Ann Surg Oncol 20(13):4190–4194. doi:10.1245/s10434-013-3134-z
96. Brauckhoff M, Gimm O, Brauckhoff K et al (2004) Repeat adrenocortical-sparing adrenalectomy for recurrent hereditary pheochromocytoma. Surg Today 34:251–255
97. Fallon SC, Feig D, Lopez ME et al (2013) The utility of cortical-sparing adrenalectomy in pheochromocytomas associated with genetic syndromes. J Pediatr Surg 48:1422–1425
98. Grubbs EG, Rich TA, Ng C et al (2013) Long-term outcomes of surgical treatment for hereditary pheochromocytoma. J Am Coll Surg 216:280–289
99. Neumann HPH, Reincke M, Bender BU et al (1999) Preserved adrenocortical function after laparoscopic bilateral adrenal sparing surgery for hereditary pheochromocytoma. J Clin Endocrinol Metab 84:2608–2610
100. Volkin D, Yerram N, Ahmed F et al (2012) Partial adrenalectomy minimizes the need for long-term hormone replacement in pediatric patients with pheochromocytoma and von Hippel-Lindau syndrome. J Pediatr Surg 47:2077–2082
101. Walther MM, Herring J, Choyke PL et al (2000) Laparascopic partial adrenalectomy in patients with hereditary forms of pheochromocytoma. J Urol 164:14–17
102. Yip L, Lee JE, Shapiro SE et al (2004) Surgical management of hereditary pheochromocytoma. J Am Coll Surg 198:525–534
103. Ellis RJ, Patel D, Prodanov T et al (2013) Response after surgical resection of metastatic pheochromocytoma and paraganglioma: can postoperative biochemical remission be predicted? J Am Coll Surg 217:489–496
104. Goldstein RE, O'Neill JA, Holcomb GW, Morgan WM, Neblett WW, Oates JA et al (1999) Clinical experience over 48 years with pheochromocytoma. Ann Surg 229(6):755–764
105. Mamlouk MD, van Sonnenberg E, Stringfellow G et al (2009) Radiofrequency ablation and biopsy of metastatic pheochromocytoma: emphasizing safety issues and dangers. J Vasc Interv Radiol 20:670–673
106. McBride JF, Atwell TD, Charboneau WJ et al (2011) Minimally invasive treatment of metastatic pheochromocytoma and paraganglioma: efficacy and safety of radiofrequency ablation and cryoablation therapy. J Vasc Interv Radiol 22:1263–1270
107. Pacak K, Fojo T, Goldstein DS et al (2001) Radiofrequency ablation: a novel approach for treatment of metastatic pheochromocytoma. J Natl Cancer Inst 93:648–649
108. Venkatesan AM, Locklin J, Lai EW et al (2009) Radiofrequency ablation of metastatic pheochromocytoma. J Vasc Interv Radiol 20:1483–1490
109. Plouin PF, Chatellier G, Fofol I et al (1997) Tumor recurrence and hypertension persistence after successful pheochromocytoma operation. Hypertension 29:1133–1139
110. Bryant J, Farmer J, Kessler LJ (2003) Pheochromocytoma: the expanding genetic differential diagnosis. J Natl Cancer Inst 95(1):1196–1204
111. Erickson D, Kudva YC, Ebersold MJ, Thompson GB, Grant CS, van Heerden JA et al (2001) Benign paragangliomas: clinical presentation and treatment outcomes in 236 patients. J Clin Endocrinol Metab 86(11):5210–5216

Coarctation of the Aorta

4

Maria Boutsikou, Anselm Uebing, and Michael A. Gatzoulis

Abbreviations

CoA	Coarctation of the aorta
CT	Computed tomography
ECG	Electrocardiography
LV	Left ventricular
MRI	Magnetic resonance imaging

Coarctation of the aorta (CoA) is a congenital malformation of the aorta, first described by Morgagni in 1760 [1]. The overall incidence of CoA is 5–8 % of all congenital heart disease, and the condition is 1.7 times more frequent in white males than white females [2]. Aortic coarctation can present as a localised discrete stenosis of the aortic isthmus, but segmental tubular hypoplasia of the aortic arch is also commonly associated. The usual site of CoA is distal to the left subclavian artery.

The aetiology of CoA has not yet been clearly identified. Potential pathogenic mechanisms include abnormalities of blood flow in the aorta during fetal life or excessive distribution of aberrant ductal tissue around the aortic isthmus [3, 4]. An increase in collagen production with reduced smooth muscle content has also been found in the CoA segment [5, 6].

M. Boutsikou, MD, MSc, PhD (✉)
Adult Congenital Heart Centre and Centre for Pulmonary Hypertension, Royal Brompton Hospital, Sydney Street, London SW3 6NP, UK
e-mail: M.Boutsikou@rbht.nhs.uk

A. Uebing, MD, PhD • M.A. Gatzoulis, MD, PhD, FACC, FESC
Adult Congenital Heart Centre and Centre for Pulmonary Hypertension, Royal Brompton Hospital, and the National Heart & Lung Institute, Imperial College, Sydney Street, London SW3 6NP, UK

National Heart & Lung Institute, Imperial College, Sydney Street, London SW3 6NP, UK

C. Tsioufis et al. (eds.), *Interventional Therapies for Secondary and Essential Hypertension*, Updates in Hypertension and Cardiovascular Protection,
DOI 10.1007/978-3-319-34141-5_4

Aortic coarctation may occur as an isolated lesion but may also coexist with other cardiac lesions, most commonly with a bicuspid aortic valve (in up to 50 % of the cases), ventricular septal defects or mitral valve abnormalities. It can also be part of complex congenital anomalies such as transposition of the great arteries, Taussig–Bing anomaly, double-inlet left ventricle or hypoplastic left heart syndrome. It is also commonly found in genetic syndromes such as Turner, Williams and Noonan [7].

4.1 Clinical Presentation and Diagnosis

Early diagnosis of CoA is of paramount importance. Diagnosis in fetal life may be based on indirect signs such as ventricular disproportion (right ventricular dilatation) and great vessel disproportion (pulmonary artery dilatation). Direct imaging of the coarctation site with fetal echocardiography is challenging [8].

Postnatal presentation may vary according to the severity of CoA. In cases with prenatal suspicion of CoA, neonates should be kept under close monitoring with echocardiography after delivery. Once the diagnosis of significant CoA with duct-dependent perfusion of the descending aorta is confirmed, administration of prostaglandins is maintained from birth until repair [8].

Neonates with severe CoA present with signs and symptoms of heart failure or even cardiogenic shock after duct closure. Untreated high-grade CoA that presents with signs of heart failure and complicated cases have a mortality rate of up to 90 % during the first year of life [7, 8].

Diagnosis of CoA in adulthood is often incidental. Adult patients usually present with upper limb hypertension. The femoral pulses are weak and delayed or absent. A continuous systolic–diastolic murmur between the scapulae is typical for significant CoA with blood flow through collateral vessels. Auscultation may also reveal a suprasternal thrill and a systolic ejection murmur in the aortic area in cases with concomitant aortic valve disease.

Some of the patients present with leg fatigue and claudication. Other typical symptoms in adults with untreated CoA may include headache, epistaxis, dizziness and cold feet. Complications include intracranial aneurysms, intracranial haemorrhage, left ventricular (LV) failure, infective endocarditis, aortic rupture/dissection and premature coronary artery disease [9, 10].

The eletrocardiography (ECG) may show signs of LV hypertrophy and dilatation.

Chest X-ray in adults may show a normal cardiac contour. Double contouring of the descending aorta known as the '3 sign' beneath the aortic notch is characteristic and represents narrowing of the aorta at the level of CoA and dilatation of the aorta before and after CoA. Rib notching caused by the intercostal collateral arteries can be visible in older patients with severe CoA (Fig. 4.1).

Echocardiography is essential to image and evaluate the severity of CoA. The site of CoA is best visualised from the suprasternal view. Colour Doppler demonstrates turbulent flow at the CoA site, while spectral Doppler provides information

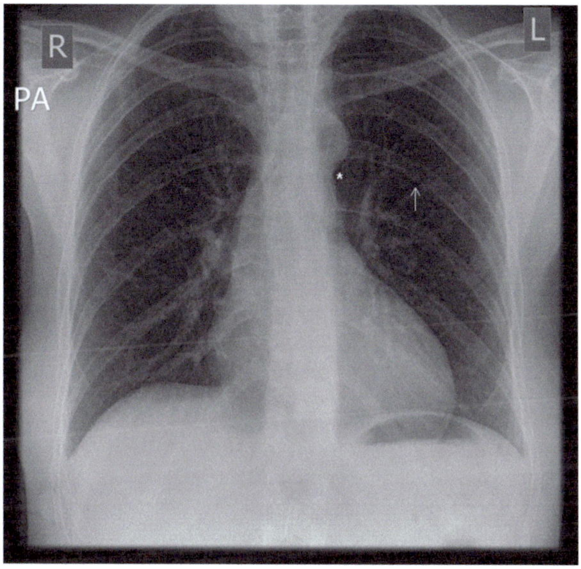

Fig. 4.1 Chest X-ray of a patient with CoA. The typical findings of the '3 sign' beneath the aortic notch (marked by *asterisk*) and the rib notching (*arrow*) are visible

on the severity of stenosis. Through continuous wave Doppler, the maximum velocity and the peak and mean pressure gradients across the CoA site can be estimated using the modified Bernoulli equation. Continuous wave Doppler typically shows continuous forward flow through the CoA site with continuous high-velocity flow during diastole ('sawtooth flow pattern', Fig. 4.2). Echocardiography also provides valuable information on LV size, systolic and diastolic function and hypertrophy and associated lesions.

The exact anatomy of the entire aorta in the adolescent and adult is best assessed by cardiac magnetic resonance imaging (MRI) and computed tomography (CT) (Fig. 4.3). MRI also provides information on the size and function of the LV and the structure and function of the aortic valve. Using phase contrast flow imaging, the blood flow and the pressure gradients through the coarctation site can also be estimated [11].

Three-dimensional reconstructions with CT or MRI angiography detect complications from CoA treatment such as residual stenosis, pseudoaneurysm formation or dissection. Since CT requires radiation exposure, MRI is the preferable imaging modality in cases where repeat imaging is required. However, CT is superior in patients with previously implanted CoA stents as it is less susceptible to artefacts caused by the stent material. CT is also the preferred three-dimensional imaging modality of the aorta for patients with pacemaker devices and patients with previous clipping of intracranial aneurysms. It is also superior to cardiac MRI in cases where the coronary anatomy shall also be studied.

Cardiac catheterisation with pressure measurement and angiography determines the pressure gradient across the CoA site and delineates the anatomy of the aorta and its branches. The coronary anatomy and LV function and pressures can also be assessed.

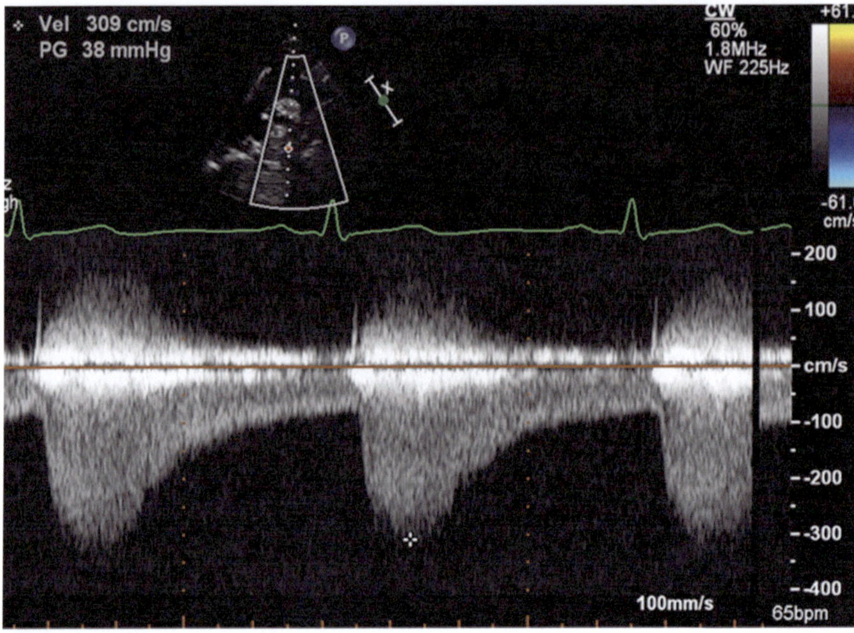

Fig. 4.2 'Sawtooth flow pattern' on continuous wave Doppler in a patient with native CoA

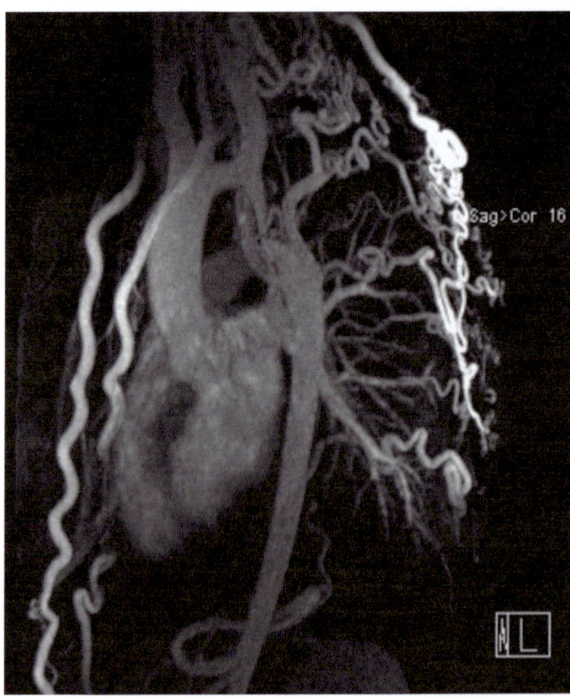

Fig. 4.3 MR angiography in a case of severe CoA distal to the left common carotid artery. Extensive collateral arteries are present

4.2 Indications for Intervention

The most recent ESC recommendations for management of CoA are presented in Table 4.1 [12, 13]. Interventional therapy is indicated:

- In all patients with non-invasive pressure difference >20 mmHg between upper and lower limbs
- In patients with upper limb hypertension (>140/90 mmHg), abnormal blood pressure response during exercise of LV hypertrophy regardless of symptoms

4.3 Therapy

Without treatment, the outcome for CoA patients is poor. Data on the natural history of patients with CoA who survived beyond infancy showed a mean age of death of 34 years and 75 % mortality at the age of 43 years. Death was from congestive heart failure, aortic dissection or rupture, endocarditis and intracranial bleeding [15].

The treatment of CoA is either surgical or interventional. The type of treatment depends on patient's age at the time of diagnosis, the severity of stenosis, complexity of the anatomy, clinical presentation and concomitant cardiac lesions.

Medical therapy and monitoring alone is preserved for patients with mild coarctation and no significant systemic hypertension. The 2008 ACC/AHA guidelines for the management of adult patients with congenital heart disease recommended the use of b-blockers, angiotensin-converting enzymc inhibitors and angiotensin receptor blockers as first-line treatment of systemic hypertension in this group taking into consideration the presence of any concomitant anomalies such as aortic root dilatation or aortic valve regurgitation [16] (Table 4.2).

Table 4.1 ESC guidelines on time for intervention in adult patients with CoA

Recommendations	Class[a]	Level[b]
In all patients with non-invasive pressure difference >20 mmHg between upper and lower limbs regardless of symptoms but with upper limb hypertension (>140/90 mmHg in adults), abnormal blood pressure response during exercise or significant LV hypertrophy, an intervention is indicated	I	C
Independent of the pressure gradient, hypertensive patients with >50 % aortic narrowing relative to the aortic diameter at the diaphragm level (on MRI, CT or invasive angiography) should be considered for intervention	IIa	C
Independent of the pressure gradient and the presence of hypertension with >50 % aortic narrowing relative to the aortic diameter at the diaphragm level (on MRI, CT or invasive angiography) may be considered for intervention	IIb	C

[a] class of recommendation
[b] level of evidence

Table 4.2 AHA guidelines for catheter intervention in paediatric patients with CoA [14]

Recommendations for transcatheter balloon angioplasty of coarctation/re-coarctation of the aorta		
Transcatheter systolic coarctation gradient of > 20 mmHg and suitable anatomy, irrespective of patient age	I	C
Transcatheter systolic coarctation gradient of < 20 mmHg in the presence of significant collateral vessels and suitable angiographic anatomy, irrespective of patient age, as well as in patients with univentricular heart or with significant ventricular dysfunction	I	C
As a palliative measure to stabilise a patient when extenuating circumstances are present, such as severely depressed ventricular function, severe mitral regurgitation, low cardiac output or systemic disease affected by the cardiac condition	IIa	C
Beyond 4–6 months of age when associated with a transcatheter systolic coarctation gradient > 20 mmHg and suitable anatomy	IIb	C
Native or recurrent coarctation of the aorta in patients with complex coarctation anatomy or systemic conditions such as connective tissue disease or Turner syndrome but should be scrutinised on a case-by-case basis	IIb	C
Recommendations for stent placement in native coarctation and re-coarctation of the aorta		
Recurrent coarctation patients of sufficient size for safe stent placement, in whom the stent can be expanded to an adult size, and who have a transcatheter systolic coarctation gradient >20 mmHg	I	B
1. Transcatheter systolic coarctation gradient of >20 mmHg Transcatheter systolic coarctation gradient of <20 mmHg but with systemic hypertension associated with an anatomic narrowing that explains the hypertension Long-segment coarctation with a transcatheter systolic coarctation gradient >20 mmHg 2. When balloon angioplasty has failed, as long as a stent that can be expanded to an adult size can be implanted	IIa	B C B B
1. In infants and neonates when complex aortic arch obstruction exists despite surgical or catheter-mediated attempts to relieve this obstruction and when further surgery is regarded as high risk 2. Transcoarctation gradient of <20 mmHg but with an elevated LV end-diastolic pressure and an anatomic narrowing Transcoarctation gradient of <20 mmHg but in whom significant aortic collaterals exist, which results in an underestimation of coarctation	IIb	C C C

4.4 Surgical Treatment

Numerous surgical techniques have been developed for the treatment of aortic coarctation (Fig. 4.4). The choice of the surgical technique depends on the patient's age and the anatomy of the aorta and CoA site.

Surgery is performed as early as possible balancing the prognostic benefit of early surgery versus the age-related risks for procedural complications. The optimal age for elective surgical repair is likely between 2 and 5 years of age [7]. The risk of persistent systemic hypertension increases with age at CoA repair. The prevalence of systemic hypertension in patients with repaired CoA ranges from 25 to 68 % [17]. Surgical repair in adulthood is characterised by an increased mortality risk due to degenerative changes in aortic wall, coronary artery disease and end-organ damage due to long-standing hypertension.

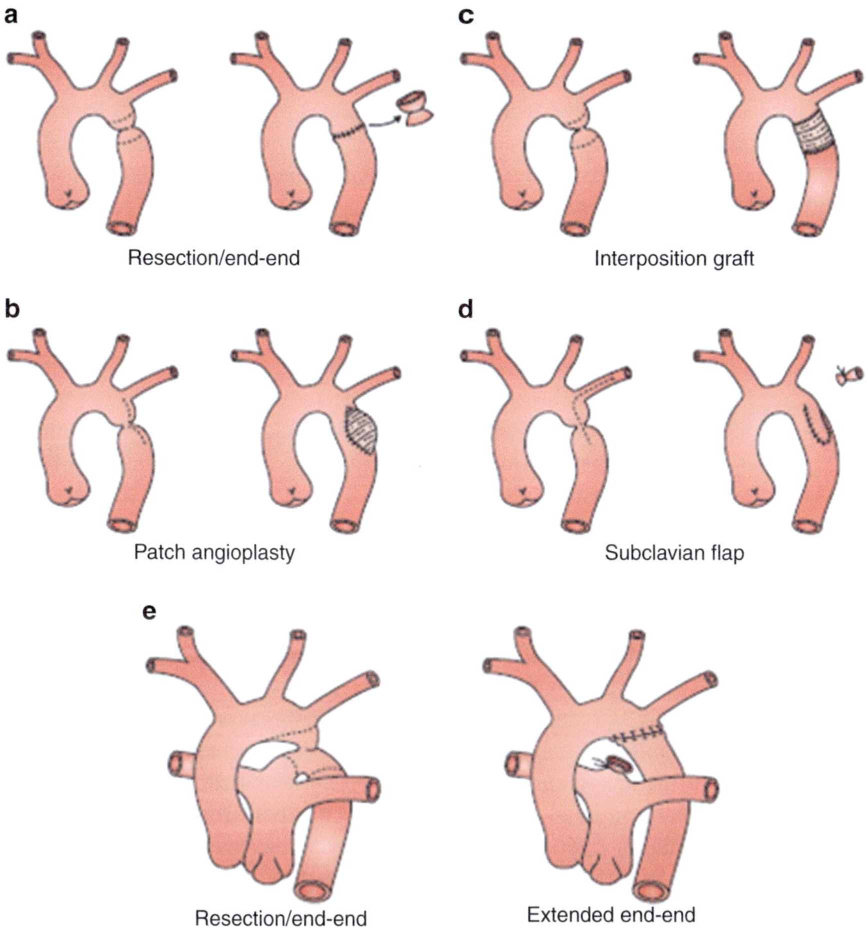

Fig. 4.4 (**a–e**) Different types of surgical interventions in CoA (From Ref. [7])

The first successful surgical repair of CoA was carried out by Crafoord in 1944 and included resection of the stenotic aortic segment and end-to-end anastomosis of the aorta [18]. This procedure remains the gold standard treatment in infants and young children with circumscriptive stenosis. The advantage of this procedure is that it offers excision of the abnormal aortic and ductal tissue. However, there is a risk of restenosis at the site of circumferential suture which is as high as 20 %.

Coarctation repair with an aortoplasty patch was introduced in 1957 by Vossschulte [19] and included augmentation of the coarctation segment with a prosthetic patch. This type of repair offered lower rates of re-coarctation compared to end-to-end anastomosis technique, but is commonly complicated by aneurysm formation [20, 21]. It is therefore avoided nowadays.

The subclavian flap repair is an alternative surgical procedure used in infants with CoA. This technique was first described by Waldhausen and Nahrwold in 1966 [22]. The subclavian artery is divided and ligated followed by a longitudinal incision of the proximal part of the vessel. An incision on the aortic wall is performed at the site of coarctation with ligation and division of the duct. The opened proximal end of the subclavian artery forms a flap which is folded down reconnected with the aortic edges to form a patch that enlarges the aorta. The advantage of this procedure is that autologous tissue is used for the repair which allows growth of the aorta. However, the left subclavian artery is sacrificed with potential implications on growth of the left arm and the potential for subclavian steal, left arm weakness and claudication [23, 24].

CoA repair with resection and replacement of interposition graft is an appropriate technique for adult patients with long-segment coarctation or re-coarctation. Other surgical procedures include placement of bypass tube graft more appropriate in patients with fragile aortic tissue or in long-segment coarctation. In very complex cases coarctation repair may include the placement of an extra-anatomic bypass graft from ascending to descending aorta (Fig. 4.4).

4.5 Transcatheter Therapies

Lock and colleagues were the first to describe balloon angioplasty as an interventional alternative to conventional surgery in 1982 [25]. It was initially recommended for re-coarctation only, to reduce the number of repeat operations, but its subsequent use for native coarctation remains controversial. The development of re-coarctation and aneurysm formation remains a particular concern of balloon angioplasty of native CoA especially in infants and young children. Apart from critically ill neonates with CoA, balloon angioplasty is often avoided in this age group as complications involving the femoral artery are a concern [26–28].

Intravascular stent angioplasty for CoA was initially introduced in 1993 [29, 30] and is by many considered the preferred treatment option for adolescent and adult patients with native or recurrent CoA [31]. It is also occasionally used in infants who cannot undergo surgery as a bridging therapy towards later surgical repair.

CoA stenting is effective and safe in adults and older children with good early and midterm reduction in upper limb blood pressure (Fig. 4.5), pressure gradients across the coarctation segment and low rates of aneurysm formation or dissection [32, 33].

Covered stents for the treatment of CoA were initially introduced in 2001 [34]. The fabric around the stent shall provide protection from bleeding due to aortic rupture. A recent study comparing bare versus covered stents showed similarly high success rates for both types of stents. It also showed a low incidence of pseudoaneurysms after covered stenting during follow-up [35].

Recently, the results of the Coarctation of the Aorta Stent Trial (COAST), a study aimed to assess the safety and efficacy of Cheatham-Platinum stents (CP stents) in children and adults with native or recurrent CoA, were published. During the 2-year follow-up, no deaths, serious adverse events or surgical intervention were reported. All patients experienced satisfactory post-procedural results with low rates of

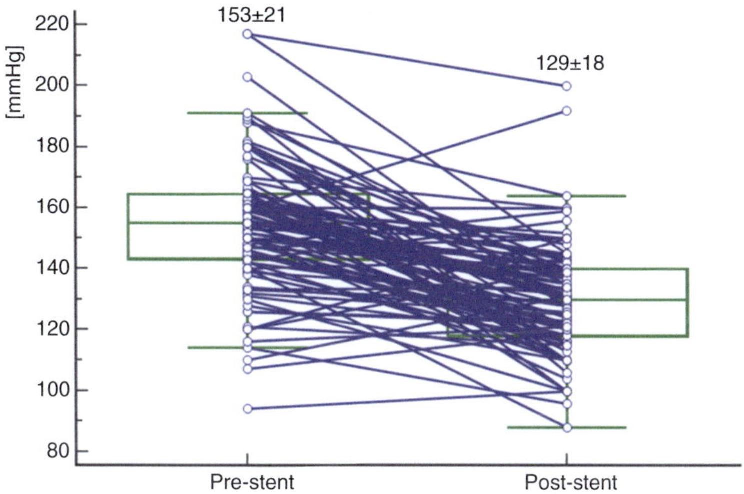

Fig. 4.5 Pre- and immediate post-procedural data from the Royal Brompton Hospital cohort of 147 CoA patients undergoing stenting between 2004 and 2015. A significant reduction in ascending aortic blood pressure is documented

complications including aneurysms and stent fracture with loss of stent integrity, stent embolisation, aortic wall injury or re-obstruction. Re-interventions that occurred during the 2-year follow-up period were for stent re-dilatation in order to account for the patients' somatic growth [33].

The CoA stent placement procedure requires very accurate measurements of the coarctation area and very careful choice of balloons and stents to be delivered. The procedure is usually performed under general anaesthesia. Once peak-to-peak systolic pressures have been obtained across the coarctation segment, a detailed angiogram is performed [36]. The stent and balloon are selected according to the size of the aorta adjacent to the CoA site. The balloon/stent system is advanced over a wire that is placed across the coarctation segment usually from the femoral. The stent has been placed by balloon inflation. A final angiogram and pressure measurement in the ascending and descending aorta is performed to exclude damage to the aortic wall, confirm appropriate stent placement and document the residual gradient. Stent implantation is considered successful if a residual gradient < 10 mmHg and improvement in vessel calibre > 80 % of the normal adjacent aortic arch are achieved [34] (Fig. 4.6).

4.6 Repair of Thoracic Pseudoaneurysms Late After Coarctation Repair

Especially patients with Dacron patch repair of aortic coarctation are at risk to develop often large para-CoA pseudoaneurysms. These patients are at high risk to operate. Furthermore, extensive aneurysms are usually not amenable to conventional stent technology.

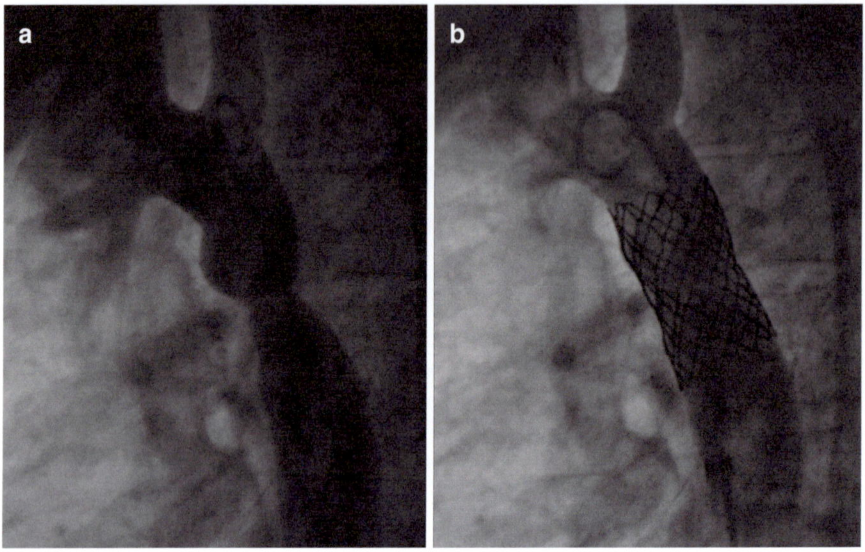

Fig. 4.6 (**a**, **b**) Angiographic images of a patient with native CoA undergoing stenting

New generation stent grafts have therefore recently been used to cover such large aneurysms. Depending on the anatomy of the aorta, preparative vascular surgery to the head and neck vessels is needed to create an appropriate implantation zone to allow safe and successful stent deployment without compromising blood flow to these vessels. Early reports on the use of this approach and technology are promising [37] (Fig. 4.7).

4.7 Long-Term Outcomes

Long-term survival after CoA repair remains lower than in the general population. This is mainly due to the long-term effects of persistent systemic hypertension [38]. Data on a historic single centre cohort of patients who underwent operative repair of CoA between 1946 and 1981 reported a long survival rate of 72 % at 30 years follow-up [39]. For patients operated before the age of 14, 20-year survival rate was 91 % and significantly better compared to the patients operated after the age of 14. The most common mode of death was coronary artery disease, accounting for 37 % of late deaths, and systolic hypertension was predictive of late death [39]. Not surprisingly patients with other cardiac defects in addition to CoA have worse outcomes [40]. More recent reports have reported improved survival rates following CoA repair with an actuarial survival of 89 % at 60 years of age [41].

Aortic valve disease is the most common associated defect requiring surgical management in patients with repaired CoA. A bicuspid aortic valve is present in up

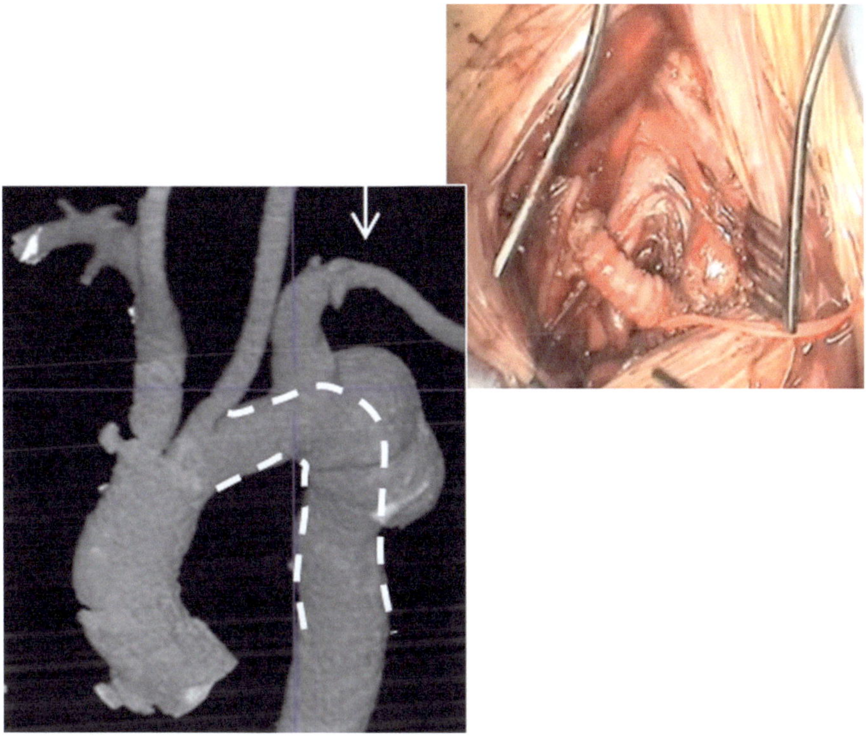

Fig. 4.7 CT aortogram of a large para-coarctation pseudoaneurysm late after CoA repair with a Dacron patch involving the origin of the left subclavian artery. Carotid to left subclavian bypass grafting (right panel) was performed to prepare the aortic arch for implantation of a stent graft (area of intended implantation zone marked by dotted lines) [37]

to 50 % of patients with CoA and is often associated with dilatation of the ascending aorta [42].

4.8 Medical Management of Systemic Arterial Hypertension

The prevalence of persistent systemic hypertension after successful CoA repair ranges from 25 to 68 % [17, 43]. There is consensus that systemic hypertension is the most important single outcome variable in patients with repaired CoA and that lifelong meticulous blood control is paramount to achieve optimal long-term outcome in this patient group.

An adverse aortic arch anatomy with residual obstruction can be an important contributor for upper limb hypertension. The causes for systemic hypertension in the absence of an anatomical obstruction following CoA repair are not fully understood. There is evidence of reset of the baroreceptors in the aortic arch and carotid arteries in the presence of abnormal arterial compliance resulting in sympathetic hyper-activation [44]. There is also evidence for impaired aortic elasticity even in patients with timely and ideal CoA repair [45–49].

4.9 Surgical Versus Percutaneous Treatment

The optimal surgical or interventional treatment of a patient with CoA has to be decided on depending on age at presentation, clinical status and anatomy. Treatment must be individualised weighing the risk and benefits for each patient. There is no universally accepted, uniform treatment algorithm available for how to best repair CoA.

In most centres surgical repair is preferred for the infant or young child with native coarctation. Balloon dilatation or even stenting in this age group is only used in the young child that is compromised and considered too unwell for surgery.

The risk for aneurysm formation and re-coarctation and the risk for vascular complications are the concern with balloon angioplasty in neonates and infants.

Surgery is also preferred in patient with complex aortic arch anatomy including those with transverse arch hypoplasia.

Balloon angioplasty is usually the treatment of choice in the younger child with recurrent coarctation after previous repair. Aneurysm formation is less of a concern in this patient group.

Stent placement in small children is a concern due to the relatively large sheath sizes and the problem of somatic growth and the inability to enlarge small stents to dimensions appropriate for an adolescent or adult. Endovascular stenting of CoA, however, has become a widely used and accepted treatment option for older children, adolescents and adults with native or recurrent CoA. Lower intra-procedural complication rates, good short and intermediate follow-up results, shorter hospitalisation stay and the avoidance of surgical trauma and thoracotomy/sternotomy which follow an open surgery are among the advantages of endovascular stent repair.

Data on the direct comparison of surgical and interventional treatment of CoA is limited and observational. Carr collected comparative data on angioplasty/stenting (633 patients) and surgery (213 patients) in adolescent and adult CoA patients. Although the reported morbidity was similar between the studied methods, the rate of re-intervention was higher after endovascular therapy. Post-procedure freedom from hypertension was similar between groups [50].

Forbes et al. published the results of a multicentre observational study comparing the safety and efficacy of surgical repair (72 patients), stent (217 patients) and balloon angioplasty (67 patients) as treatment of native CoA acutely and at follow-up. All three treatment modalities showed a significant improvement in systolic blood pressure and pre- versus post-procedure gradient. The rate of acute complications was lower after stent implantation compared to balloon angioplasty or surgery. However, planned re-intervention was more likely in the group of stented patients. Stent implantation and surgery achieved a superior haemodynamic result than balloon angioplasty [51].

In a recent systematic review, Padua et al. attempted to analyse the effectiveness and safety of stent placement compared with open surgery in patients with CoA. The authors conclude that there is insufficient evidence to prove which the best treatment for CoA is and suggest the need for further prospective randomised controlled clinical trials with an emphasis on outcomes such as quality of life and long-term survival [52].

4.10 Follow-Up

Patients with repaired CoA require lifelong surveillance. Current guidelines recommend at least annual follow-up for these patients [16]. It is important to identify complications such as restenosis, aortic aneurysm formation and systolic arterial hypertension promptly. Thorough clinical examination and echocardiography are first-line diagnostic tools for follow-up. Advanced imaging such as cardiac MRI and CT is the preferred imaging modality for more comprehensive evaluation of these patients [53].

References

1. Perloff JK (1994) The clinical recognition of congenital heart disease, 4th edn. WB Saunders, Philadelphia
2. Samanek M, Slavik Z, Zborilova B et al (1989) Prevalence, treatment, and outcome of heart disease in live-born children: a prospective analysis of 91,823 live-born children. Pediatr Cardiol 10(4):205–11
3. Rudolph AM, Spitznas U, Heymann MA (1972) Hemodynamic considerations in development of narrowing of aorta. Am J Cardiol 30:514–25
4. Russell GA, Berry PJ, Watterson K, Dhasmana JP, Wisheart JD (1991) Patterns of ductal tissue in coarctation of the aorta in the first three months of life. J Thorac Cardiovasc Surg 102: 596–601
5. Sehested J, Baandrup U, Mikkelsen E (1982) Different reactivity and structure of the prestenotic and post-stenotic aorta in human coarctation: implications for baroreceptor function. Circulation 65:1060–5
6. Xu CP, Zarins CK, Bassiouny HS, Briggs WH, Reardon C, Glagov S (2000) Differential transmural distribution of gene expression for collagen types I and III proximal to aortic coarctation in the rabbit. J Vasc Res 37:170–82
7. Kaemmerer H (2011) Aortic coarctation and interrupted aortic arch. In: Diagnosis and management of adult congenital heart disease, 2nd edn. Elselvier Saunders, Philadelphia
8. Rosenthal E (2005) Coarctation of the aorta from fetus to adult: curable condition or life long disease process? Heart 91:1495–502
9. Connelly MS, Webb GD, Somerville J et al (1998) Canadian consensus conference on adult congenital heart disease 1996. Can J Cardiol 14:395–452
10. Curtis SL, Bradley M, Wilde P et al (2012) Results of screening for intracranial aneurysms in patients with coarctation of the aorta. AJNR Am J Neuroradiol 33(6):1182–6
11. Shepherd B, Abbas A, McParland P et al (2015) MRI in adult patients with aortic coarctation: diagnosis and follow-up. Clin Radiol 70(4):433–45
12. Erbel Erbel R, Aboyans V, Boileau C, Bossone E, Di Bartolomeo R, Eggebrecht H, Evangelista A, Falk V, Frank H, Gaemperli O, Grabenwo¨ ger M, Haverich A, Iung B, Manolis AJ, Meijboom F, Nienaber CA, Roffi M, Rousseau H, Sechtem U, Sirnes PA, Von Allmen RS,

Vrints CJM (2014) 2014 ESC Guidelines on the diagnosis and treatment of aortic diseases. Eur Heart J 35:2873–926
13. Baumgartner H, Bonhoeffer P, De Groot N, de Haan F, Deanfield JE, Galie N, Gatzoulis MA, Gohlke-Baerwolf C, Kaemmerer H, Kilner P, Meijboom F, Mulder BJM, Oechslin E, Oliver JM, Serraf A, Szatmari A, Thaulow A, Vouhe PR, Walma E (2010) ESC Guidelines for the management of grown-up congenital heart disease. Eur Heart J 31:2915–57
14. Feltes TF, Bacha E, Beekman RH 3rd et al.; on behalf of the American Heart Association Congenital Cardiac Defects Committee of the Council on Cardiovascular Disease in the Young, Council on Clinical Cardiology, and Council on Cardiovascular Radiology and Intervention (2011) Indications for cardiac catheterization and intervention in paediatric cardiac disease: a scientific statement from the American Heart Association. Circulation 123:2607–2652
15. Campbell M (1970) Natural history of coarctation of the aorta. Br Heart J 32:633–40
16. Warnes CA, Williams RG, Bashore TM et al (2008) ACC/AHA 2008 guidelines for the management of adults with congenital heart disease: a report of the American College of Cardiology/American heart association Task Force on Practice guidelines (Writing Committee to Develop Guidelines on the Management of Adults With Congenital Heart Disease). Developed in Collaboration with the American Society of Echocardiography, Heart Rhythm Society, International Society for Adult Congenital Heart Disease, Society for Cardiovascular Angiography and Interventions, and Society of Thoracic Surgeons. J Am Coll Cardiol 52(23):e143–263
17. Canniffe C, Ou P, Walsh K et al (2013) Hypertension after repair of aortic coarctation: a systematic review. Int J Cardiol 167(6):2456–61
18. Crafoord C, Nylin G (1945) Congenital coarctation of the aorta and its surgical treatment. J Thorac Surg 14:347–61
19. Vossschulte K (1957) Isthmusplastik zur Behandlung der Aortenisthmusstenose. Thoraxchirurgie 4(5):443–50
20. Backer CL, Paape K, Zales VR, Weigel TJ, Mavroudis C (1995) Coarctation of the aorta. Repair with polytetrafluoroethylene patch aortoplasty. Circulation 92:II132–6
21. Walhout RJ, Lekkerkerker JC, Oron GH, Hitchcock FJ, Meijboom EJ, Bennink GB (2003) Comparison of polytetrafluoroethylene patch aortoplasty and end-to-end anastomosis for coarctation of the aorta. J Thorac Cardiovasc Surg 126:521–8
22. Waldhausen JA, Nahrwold DL (1966) Repair of coarctation of the aorta with a subclavian flap. J Thorac Cardiovasc Surg 51(4):532–3
23. Meier MA, Lucchese FA, Jazbik W, Nesralla IA, Mendonça JT (1986) A new technique for repair of aortic coarctation. Subclavian flap aortoplasty with preservation of arterial blood flow to the left arm. J Thorac Cardiovasc Surg 92(6):1005–12
24. Adams EE, Davidson WR Jr, Swallow NA et al (2013) Long-term results of the subclavian flap repair for coarctation of the aorta in infants. World J Pediatr Congenit Heart Surg 4(1):13–8
25. Lock JE, Bass JL, Amplatz K, Fuhrman BP, Castaneda-Zuniga W (1983) Balloon dilation angioplasty of aortic coarctations in infants and children. Circulation 68:109–16
26. Tynan M, Finley JP, Fontes V, Hess J, Kan J (1990) Balloon angioplasty for the treatment of native coarctation: results of Valvuloplasty and Angioplasty of Congenital Anomalies Registry. Am J Cardiol 65:790–2
27. Mendelsohn AM, Lloyd TR, Crowley DC, Sandhu SK, Kocis KC, Beekman RH (1994) Late follow-up of balloon angioplasty in children with a native coarctation of the aorta. Am J Cardiol 74:696–700
28. Fawzy ME, Fathala A, Osman A, Badr A, Mostafa MA, Mohamed G, Dunn B (2008) Twenty-two years of follow-up results of balloon angioplasty for discreet native coarctation of the aorta in adolescents and adults. Am Heart J 156:910–7
29. O'Laughlin MP, Perry SB, Lock JE, Mullins CE (1991) Use of endovascular stents in congenital heart disease. Circulation 83(6):1923–39
30. Redington AN, Booth P, Shore DF et al (1990) Primary balloon dilatation of coarctation of the aorta in neonates. Br Heart J 64:277–81

31. Morrow WR, Palmaz JC, Tio FO, Ehler WJ, VanDellen AF, Mullins CE (1993) Re-expansion of balloon-expandable stents after growth. J Am Coll Cardiol 22(7):2007–13
32. Holzer R, Qureshi S, Ghasemi A, Vincent J, Sievert H, Gruenstein D, Weber H, Alday L, Peirone A, Zellers T, Cheatham J, Slack M, Rome J (2010) Stenting of aortic coarctation: acute, intermediate, and long-term results of a prospective multi-institutional registry–Congenital Cardiovascular Interventional Study Consortium (CCISC). Catheter Cardiovasc Interv 76:553–63
33. Meadows J, Minahan M, McElhinney DB, McEnaney K, Ringel R (2015) Intermediate outcomes in the prospective, multicenter coarctation of the aorta stent trial (COAST). Circulation 131:1656–64
34. Cheatham JP (2001) Stenting of coarctation of the aorta. Catheter Cardiovasc Interv 54(1):112–25
35. Sohrabi B, Jamshidi P, Yaghoubi A, Habibzadeh A, Hashemi- Aghdam Y, Moin A, Kazemi B, Ghaffari S, Abdolahzadeh Baghayi MR, Mahmoody K (2014) Comparison between covered and bare Cheatham-Platinum stents for endovascular treatment of patients with native post-ductal aortic coarctation: immediate and intermediate-term results. JACC Cardiovasc Interv 7:416–23
36. Forbes TJ, Moore P, Pedra CA, Zahn EM, Nykanen D, Amin Z et al (2007) Intermediate follow-up following intravascular stenting for treatment of coarctation of the aorta. Catheter Cardiovasc Interv 70(4):569–77
37. Perera AH, Rudarakanchana N, Hamady M, Kashef E, Mireskandari M, Uebing A, Cheshire NJ, Bicknell CD (2014) New-generation stent grafts for endovascular management of thoracic pseudoaneurysms after aortic coarctation repair. J Vasc Surg 60:330–336
38. Brown ML, Burkhart HM, Connolly HM et al (2010) Late outcomes of reintervention on the descending aorta after repair of aortic coarctation. Circulation 122(11 Suppl):S81–4
39. Cohen M, Fuster V, Steele PM et al (1989) Coarctation of the aorta. Long-term follow-up and prediction of outcome after surgical correction. Circulation 80(4):840–5
40. Ungerleider RM, Pasquali SK, Welke KF et al (2013) Contemporary patterns of surgery and outcomes for aortic coarctation: an analysis of the Society of Thoracic Surgeons Congenital Heart Surgery Database. J Thorac Cardiovasc Surg 145(1):150–7 [discussion: 157–8]
41. Choudhary P, Canniffe C, Jackson DJ, Tanous D, Walsh K, Celermajer DS (2015) Late outcomes in adults with coarctation of the aorta. Heart 101(15):1190–5
42. Warnes CA (2003) Bicuspid aortic valve and coarctation: two villains part of a diffuse problem. Heart 89:965–6
43. Hager A, Kanz S, Kaemmerer H, Schreiber C, Hess J (2007) Coarctation Long-term Assessment (COALA): significance of arterial hypertension in a cohort of 404 patients up to 27 years after surgical repair of isolated coarctation of the aorta, even in the absence of restenosis and prosthetic material. J Thorac Cardiovasc Surg 134(3):738–45
44. Johnson D, Perrault H, Vobecky SJ et al (2001) Resetting of the cardiopulmonary baroreflex 10 years after surgical repair of coarctation of the aorta. Heart 85:318–25
45. Gardiner HM, Celermajer DS, Sorensen KE et al (1994) Arterial reactivity is significantly impaired in normotensive young adults after successful repair of aortic coarctation in childhood. Circulation 89:1745–50
46. de Divitiis M, Pilla C, Kattenhorn M et al (2001) Vascular dysfunction after repair of coarctation of the aorta: impact of early surgery. Circulation 104(Suppl I):I165–70
47. Guenthard J, Wyler F (1995) Exercise-induced hypertension in the arms due to impaired arterial reactivity after successful coarctation resection. Am J Cardiol 75:814–7
48. Pfammatter J-P, Berdat P, Carrel T (2004) Impaired poststenotic aortic pulsatility after hemodynamically ideal coarctation repair in children. Pediatr Cardiol 25:495–9
49. Brili S, Dernellis J, Aggeli C et al (1998) Aortic elastic properties in patients with repaired coarctation of aorta. Am J Cardiol 82:1140–3
50. Carr JA (2006) The results of catheter-based therapy compared with surgical repair of adult aortic coarctation. J Am Coll Cardiol 47(6):1101–7

51. Forbes TJ, Kim DW, Du W, Turner DR, Holzer R, Amin Z et al (2011) Comparison of surgical, stent, and balloon angioplasty treatment of native coarctation of the aorta: an observational study by the CCISC (Congenital Cardiovascular Interventional Study Consortium). J Am Coll Cardiol 58(25):2664–74
52. Pádua LMS, Garcia LC, Rubira CJ, de Oliveira Carvalho PE (2012) Stent placement versus surgery for coarctation of the thoracic aorta. Cochrane Database Syst Rev (5):CD008204. doi:10.1002/14651858.CD008204.pub2
53. Nguyen L, Cook SC (2015) Coarctation of the aorta: strategies for improving outcomes. Cardiol Clin 33:521–30

Part II

Adjunctive Therapies

Sleep Apnea

5

Gianfranco Parati, Carolina Lombardi,
and Juan Eugenio Ochoa

Abbreviations

ABPM	Ambulatory blood pressure monitoring
AHI	Apnea–hypopnea index
baPWV	Brachial–ankle pulse wave velocity
BMI	Body mass index
BP	Blood pressure
cfPWV	Carotid–femoral pulse wave velocity
CPAP	Continuous positive air pressure
CRP	C-reactive protein
CV	Cardiovascular
eNOS	Endothelial nitric oxide synthase
ERS	European Respiratory Society
ESH	European Society of Hypertension
FMD	Flow-mediated dilation
HTN	Hypertension
ICAM-1	Intercellular adhesion molecule-1
MSNA	Muscle sympathetic nerve activity
NO	Nitric oxide
NOS	Nitric oxide synthase

G. Parati (✉)
Department of Medicine and Surgery, University of Milano-Bicocca, Milan, Italy

Department of Cardiovascular, Neural and Metabolic Sciences, St. Luke Hospital, IRCCS
Istituto Auxologico Italiano and University of Milan-Bicocca, Piazza Brescia 20, Milan, Italy
e-mail: gianfranco.parati@unimib.it

C. Lombardi • J.E. Ochoa
Department of Cardiovascular, Neural and Metabolic Sciences, St. Luke Hospital, IRCCS
Istituto Auxologico Italiano and University of Milan-Bicocca, Piazza Brescia 20, Milan, Italy

C. Tsioufis et al. (eds.), *Interventional Therapies for Secondary and Essential Hypertension*, Updates in Hypertension and Cardiovascular Protection,
DOI 10.1007/978-3-319-34141-5_5

OSA	Obstructive sleep apnea
OSAS	Obstructive sleep apnea syndrome
TNF-alpha	Tumor necrosis factor-alpha
VCAM-1	Vascular cell adhesion molecule-1

5.1 Introduction

Obstructive sleep apnea syndrome (OSAS) is associated with an increased prevalence of hypertension (HTN) and is currently recognized as a cause of secondary HTN [1], with the severity of OSAS being directly correlated with the degree of blood pressure (BP) elevation, with its resistance to antihypertensive treatment and with the presence of alterations in day-to-night BP changes [2–4]. The adverse cardiovascular (CV) prognosis associated with these alterations underlines the importance of OSAS-related hypertension and the need of implementing specific treatment strategies (that is, continuous positive airway pressure (CPAP)) in order to promote BP control and optimize CV protection. The present chapter will review the evidence supporting the association of OSAS with often resistant arterial HTN and the proposed mechanisms for this association. It will also address the role of ambulatory blood pressure monitoring (ABPM) in the confirmation of HTN in subjects with OSAS and whether the proper identification and management of OSAS in subjects with resistant HTN will improve BP control. Particular emphasis will be put on the role of CPAP ventilation for the treatment of OSAS, which is known to be effective in reducing the sympathetic nervous system overdrive, a major contributing mechanism for OSAS-related HTN.

5.2 OSAS and BP Levels

OSAS, combining nighttime occurring intermittent obstruction of upper airways with daytime somnolence, is not only a recognized cause of secondary HTN [1] but is associated with a high prevalence of severe and resistant BP elevation [2–4]. OSAS is defined as the presence of recurrent obstructive breathing events generated by complete upper airway obstruction during sleep or of sleep hypoventilation syndrome, accompanied by daytime symptoms [5]. Alterations in breathing patterns in OSAS may importantly influence many regulatory mechanisms involved in BP control. OSA events occurring during night (i.e., obstructive apnea and hyperventilation episodes alternating during sleep) have been shown to be accompanied by acute changes in autonomic CV control and in hemodynamic regulation, which in turn induce marked increases in BP levels during nighttime [6]. Indeed, HTN related to OSAS is predominantly nocturnal in its early stages and frequently accompanied by a non-dipper profile of BP (i.e., nocturnal BP fall <10 % compared to daytime BP levels) [7, 8]. Nonetheless, the increase in BP levels in OSAS subjects is not limited to the nighttime hours, during which OSA episodes occur, but is often sustained also during the daytime. Indeed, case–control studies using 24-h ABPM have provided evidence that, compared to matched control subjects, OSAS patients show significantly higher ambulatory BP levels not only during the nighttime sleep but also during daytime wakefulness [9–11].

5.3 Epidemiological Evidence of the Association Between OSAS and Hypertension

The association between OSAS and HTN has been extensively confirmed across a number of studies of different natures either in the general population or in cohorts of OSAS patients [2, 12–15]. Overall, these studies have indicated a variable frequency of HTN in subjects with OSAS that may range from 35 to 80 % [7, 16]. Conversely, when properly investigated, OSAS has been shown to be present in up to 40 % of hypertensive subjects [17]. Whether the association between OSAS and HTN is explained by the presence of other CV risk factors other than OSAS itself, this is still a matter of debate. For instance, OSAS is often associated with obesity, which in turn is considered to explain about 65–75 % of cases of essential HTN [18, 19]. Indeed, some studies have indicated that much of the relationship between OSAS and HTN may be explained by the associated obesity [20]. Conversely, other reports have indicated that the association between obesity and HTN may be explained by the presence of OSAS in a substantial number of subjects. In addition to body mass index (BMI), other factors such as sex and age have been shown to significantly influence the relationship between OSAS and elevated BP levels [21]. Evidence for this has been provided both from cross-sectional [12] and longitudinal studies [20, 22] showing that OSAS is more strongly associated with resistant HTN in young to middle-aged adults (<50 years of age) [21]. This association is more frequently observed in men than in women [23]. It is thus clear that disentangling the independent contribution of OSAS, obesity, and other CV risk factors to elevation in BP levels is rather difficult. Despite this difficulty, several longitudinal studies have supported the association between OSAS and HTN independently of other potential contributing factors such as BMI, also indicating that OSAS is not only associated with an increased risk of prevalent HTN but may also be an independent and significant predictor of future development of HTN in particular if not properly treated [3, 15, 20, 24] (Fig. 5.1).

In particular, in the Wisconsin Sleep Cohort Study, a dose–response relationship between sleep-disordered breathing at baseline and the development of HTN after 4 years of follow-up was reported independently of baseline BP levels, BMI, neck and waist circumference, age, sex, and other potential confounders, suggesting that sleep-disordered breathing is likely to be an independent risk factor for HTN and resultant CV morbidity in the general population [3].

However, in spite of such suggestion, there is still some controversy regarding the specific role of OSAS in the development of HTN. This is because of the variable role played by several confounders, the large heterogeneity of the available studies populations in terms of ethnicity, age, BMI and metabolic risk factors and the

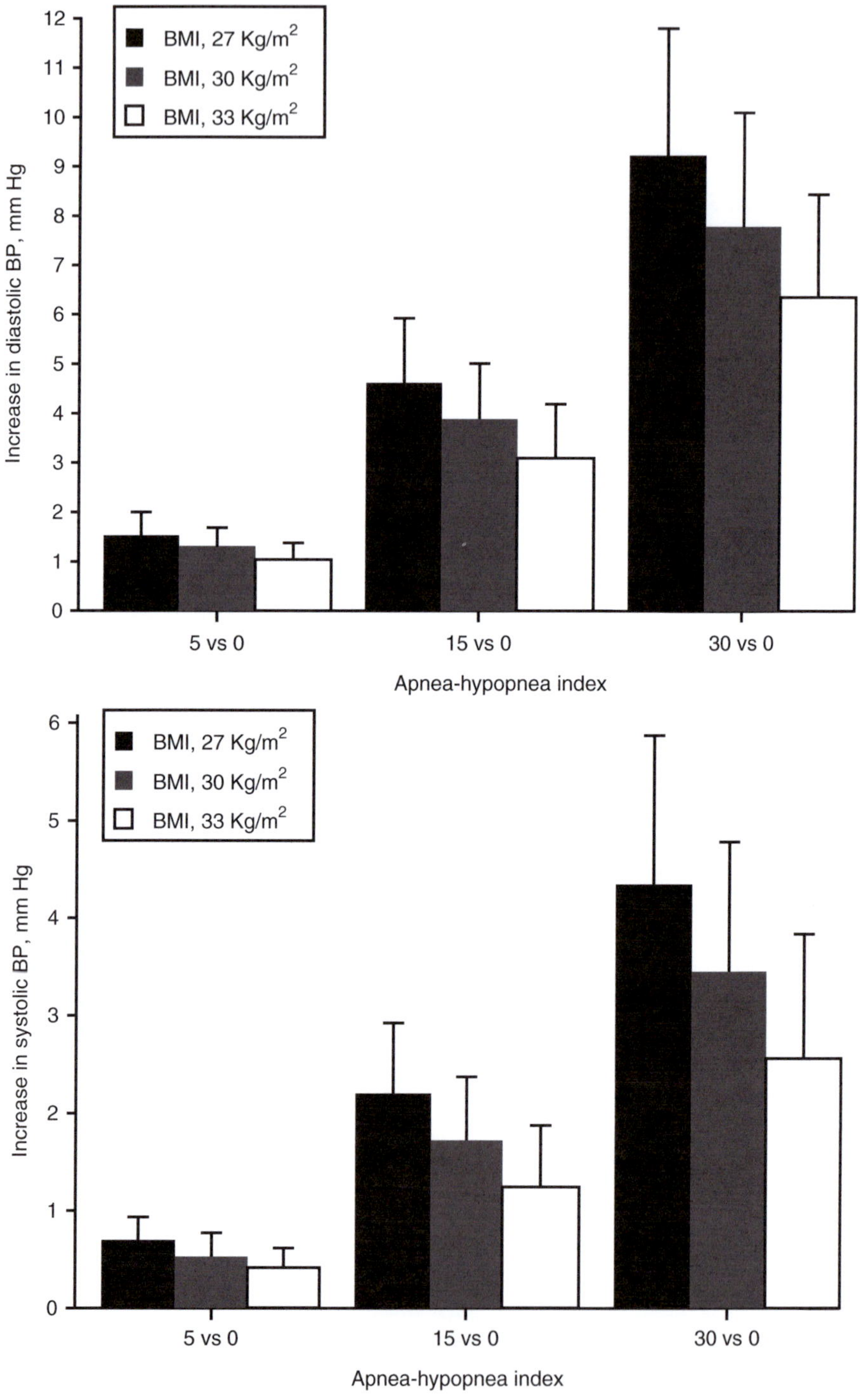

Fig. 5.1 Predicted increase in systolic blood pressure (SBP) and in diastolic blood pressure (DBP) associated with sleep-disordered breathing at three body mass index (BMI) categories in the Wisconsin Sleep Cohort Study (Modified from young et al. [15] by permission)

variable methodologies used to ascertain the presence of OSAS (i.e., in-laboratory polysomnography, in-home polysomnography, in-home polygraphy), combined with variable follow-up periods and different definitions of hypertension.

Most available longitudinal studies suffer from an inherent weakness, i.e., the lack of relevant history on subjects' sleep breathing patterns prior to the start of the study. Thus, it is possible that subjects who had HTN at baseline and were thus excluded from the study were those rapidly developing HTN because of previous exposure to sleep apnea, while normotensive subjects who had obstructive sleep apnea (OSA) at baseline were less responsive to the apneic events and therefore less likely to develop HTN at follow-up. The percentage of subjects who had HTN at baseline in these studies is indeed of substantial size.

Change in body weight over time, another important confounder for incident HTN, was not taken into account in most of available prospective studies, and majority of participants in these studies had mild OSA, with less than 13 % of patients having moderate-to-severe OSA.

A relatively short follow-up period of OSA cohorts predominantly comprising patients with mild OSA may thus importantly contribute to explain discrepant findings reported so far.

More recently, the results of a prospective cohort study of 1889 participants without HTN at baseline more convincingly showed a risk of incident hypertension to be directly related to the severity of OSA [25]. In addition, this study showed that OSA treatment with CPAP therapy was associated with a lower risk of hypertension (Fig. 5.2).

Several studies have identified OSAS as an important risk factor for resistant HTN also showing a dose–response relationship between OSAS severity and the degree of BP elevation [2, 26, 27]. It has also been shown that HTN occurring in individuals with OSAS is more likely to be severe, resistant to treatment and associated with alterations in day-to-night BP changes (i.e., nocturnal HTN and non-dipping profile of BP on 24-h ABPM) [2, 26, 27]. Conversely, an extremely high prevalence of OSA of about 80 % has been reported among adult patients with drug-resistant HTN [23]. It has also been shown that rates of BP control decrease as the severity of sleep-related breathing disorder increases [2]. Although all the above evidence supports a potential role of OSAS in the pathogenesis of HTN and drug-resistant HTN, there is still only partial understanding of the pathophysiological mechanisms by which OSAS promotes arterial HTN.

5.4 Proposed Mechanisms for OSAS-Related Hypertension

Evidence from experimental and clinical studies has indicated that the pathogenesis of OSAS-related HTN is likely to be multifactorial, involving alterations in several regulatory systems: activation of the sympathetic nervous system in the frame of complex alterations in autonomic CV modulation involving both arterial baro- and chemoreflexes, activation of renin–angiotensin–aldosterone system, endothelial dysfunction, systemic and vascular inflammation, oxidative stress, metabolic abnormalities, increased arterial stiffness and alterations in cardiac function and structure.

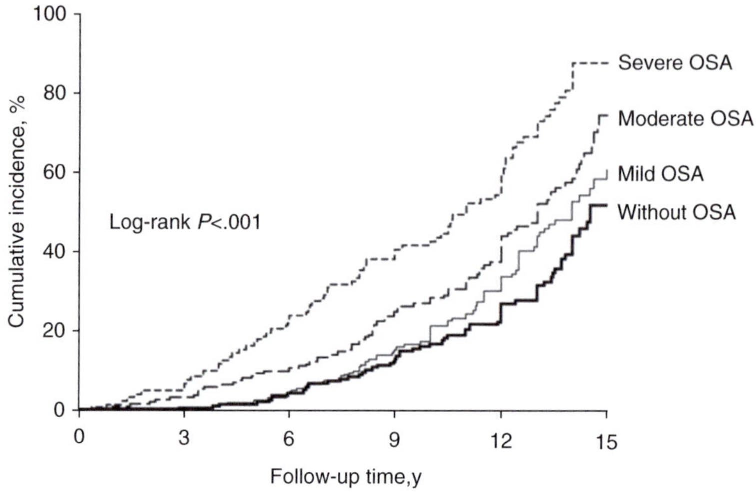

No. at risk

Severe OSA	199	184	141	119	62	37
Moderate OSA	258	222	202	162	114	67
Mild OSA	298	289	260	194	127	59
Without OSA	310	306	269	211	152	72

Fig. 5.2 Risk of incident hypertension and severity of OSA. OSA indicates obstructive sleep apnea. Severity of OSA was defined by the apnea–hypopnea index (AHI) as mild OSA (AHI, 5.0–14.9), moderate OSA (AHI, 15.0–29.9), and severe OSA (AHI, ≥30.0). *P* value reflects an overall log-rank χ^2 test, providing an overall survival difference among the four study groups (Taken from Marin et al. [25] by permission)

Sympathetic Nervous System Activation Activation of the sympathetic nervous system is considered a major pathophysiological mechanism underlying the alterations in BP regulation reported in OSAS (Fig. 5.3). This has been consistently demonstrated by several studies implementing direct techniques for assessment of sympathetic nervous system activity (i.e., recording of efferent postganglionic muscle sympathetic nerve activity via microneurography (MSNA) and assessment of norepinephrine plasma levels) in which an increase in central sympathetic drive was positively correlated with increases in BP levels independently of other contributing factors. The sympathetic activation in OSAS is largely explained by stimulation of the peripheral and central chemoreflexes, triggered by the reductions in arterial oxygen content and by hypercapnia, respectively. Moreover, sleep fragmentation, related to repeated arousals after each apnea/hypopnea event, might play an additional role in this context. The resultant increases in sympathetic drive to the heart and peripheral vasculature lead to important increases in heart rate and vascular tone which in turn are responsible for the marked increases in BP levels during resumption of ventilation after each apnoeic episode [28] (Fig. 5.4a).

This increase in central sympathetic drive has also been shown to be associated with alterations in circadian BP variation (i.e., absence of nocturnal BP fall or

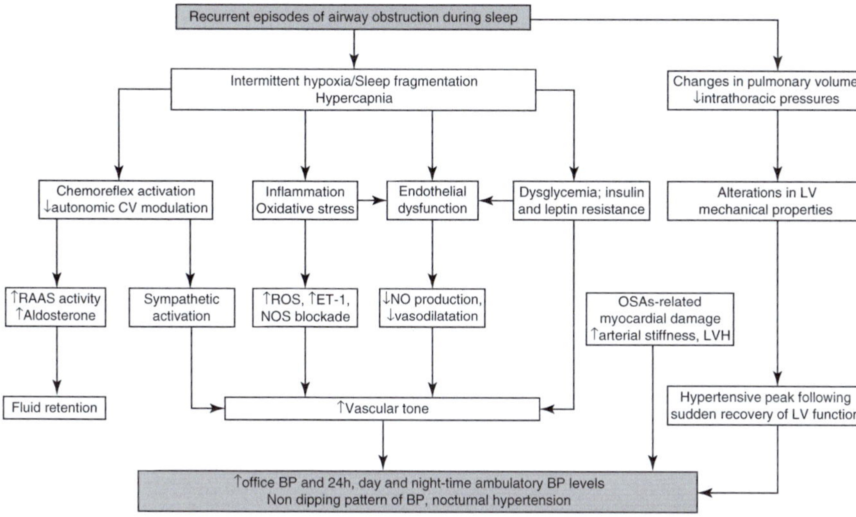

Fig. 5.3 Mechanisms by which OSAS contributes to resistant hypertension. *CV* cardiovascular, *LV* left ventricular, *RAAS* renin–angiotensin–aldosterone system, *ROS* reactive oxygen species, *ET-1* endothelin-1, *NOS* nitric oxide synthase, *NO* nitric oxide, *LVH* left ventricular hypertrophy, *BP* blood pressure

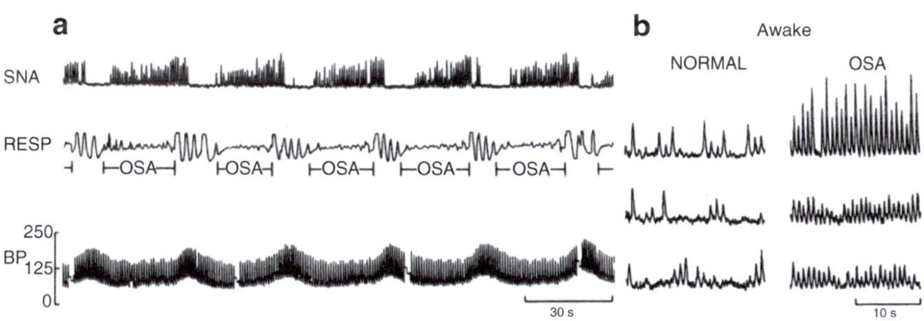

Fig. 5.4 (**a**) Recordings of sympathetic nerve activity (*SNA*), respiration (*RESP*), and blood pressure (*BP*) during 3 min of stage II sleep, showing incessant oscillations in BP and SNA in response to the repetitive OSAs. These oscillations occurred continuously during sleep, throughout all sleep stages. (**b**) Recordings of SNA during wakefulness in patients with OSAS and matched controls showing high levels of SNA in patients with OSA (Taken from reference Somers et al. [28] by permission)

increase in BP at night), and nocturnal HTN is frequently observed in OSAS patients [29]. In addition, several studies using MSNA recordings have indicated that the sympathetic activation in OSAS subjects is not only limited to nighttime but may persist even after resuming normal breathing pattern during daytime wakefulness, despite normal arterial oxygen saturation and carbon dioxide levels [28, 30] (Fig. 5.4b). Remarkably, in several studies long-term implementation of CPAP resulted in marked reductions in sympathetic nerve traffic [28] and BP levels [31] both during nighttime and daytime wakefulness [32], further supporting the pathogenetic role of the sympathetic activation in explaining BP elevation in OSAS.

Alterations in Integrated Autonomic CV Modulation In normal physiological conditions, control of BP levels is achieved through a complex combination between central and reflex neural influences, leading to a continuous modulation of efferent sympathetic and parasympathetic nerve activity and the associated activity of neurohormonal systems primarily regulated by the hypothalamus. In OSAS, the sustained chemoreflex activation, the related adrenergic overactivity, and the resulting HTN may blunt and/or reset arterial and cardiopulmonary reflexes which in turn may lead to chemoreflex potentiation [33, 34]. In addition, dysfunction of neural reflexogenic areas (i.e., baroreflex impairment) may lead to a reduced sympathoinhibition and to impaired cardiac parasympathetic modulation [35, 36] further contributing to adrenergic overdrive and rise in BP levels (Fig. 5.3).In particular, the observation of a reduced spontaneous cardiac baroreflex sensitivity (as assessed by the sequence method), and the absence of 24-h baroreflex modulation (i.e., blunted increase in baroreflex sensitivity during sleep compared with its values during wakefulness) in OSAS patients [35], has provided indirect support to the concept that baroreflex dysfunction and not only chemoreceptor stimulation by hypoxia may contribute to the acute and long-term sympathetic activation in OSAS patients (Fig. 5.5). The depressed cardiac baroreflex sensitivity during sleep may thus in turn contribute to the pathophysiology of HTN in OSAS patients.

This concept has been further supported by the results of interventional studies in OSAS patients showing a significant improvement in baroreflex sensitivity after long-term implementation of CPAP treatment [37–39]. Other independent studies, applying spectral analysis to estimate variability of MSNA, BP, and heart rate, have provided additional evidence on the impaired autonomic CV modulation in OSA based on the demonstration of significant increases in heart rate and sympathetic drive, but also of a reduced heart rate variability and a marked increase in BP variability (more than double the variance in healthy controls) [40] (Fig. 5.6).

Further evidence that sleep-related breathing disorders may induce alterations in autonomic CV modulation has been provided by a study in untreated subjects with OSA of different severities indicating that excessive daytime sleepiness is accompanied by lower baroreflex sensitivity and significantly higher low-to-high-frequency power ratio of heart rate variability (which is believed to be a marker of sympathetic activity) during the different stages of nocturnal sleep as compared not only to control subjects but also to OSA patients without daytime somnolence [41] (Fig. 5.7).

Activation of Renin–Angiotensin–Aldosterone System (Increase in Aldosterone Levels) The frequent association of OSAS with hyperaldosteronism reported in patients with resistant HTN has led to suggest that both these factors may interact on a pathophysiological basis contributing to BP elevation [42–44]. Although evidence is

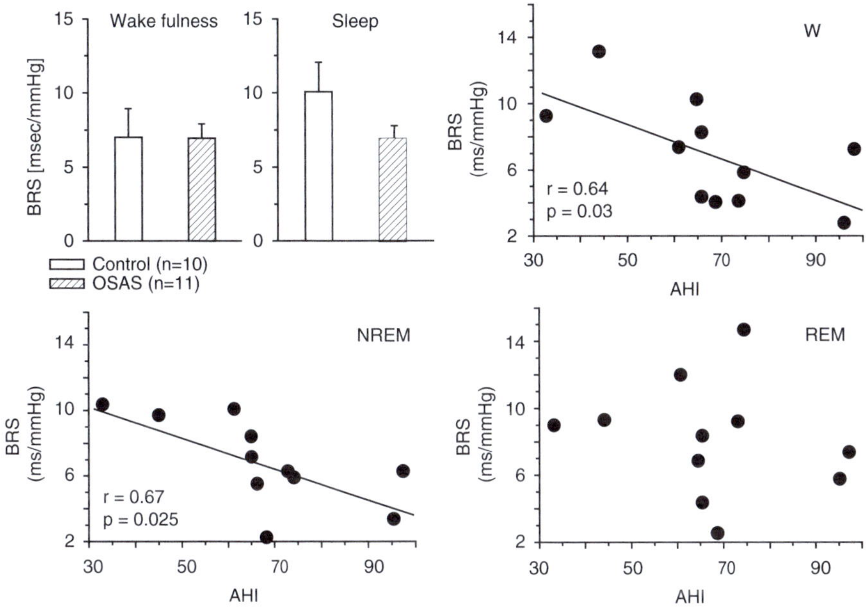

Fig. 5.5 Relationship between spontaneous baroreflex sensitivity (*BRS*) and the severity of obstructive sleep apnea syndrome, as quantified by the apnea–hypopnea index (*AHI*). Data are shown as individual values in 11 patients separately for a period of wakefulness (*W*), a period of non-rapid eye movement (*NREM*) sleep, and a period of rapid eye movement (*REM*) sleep (Taken from Parati et al. [35] by permission)

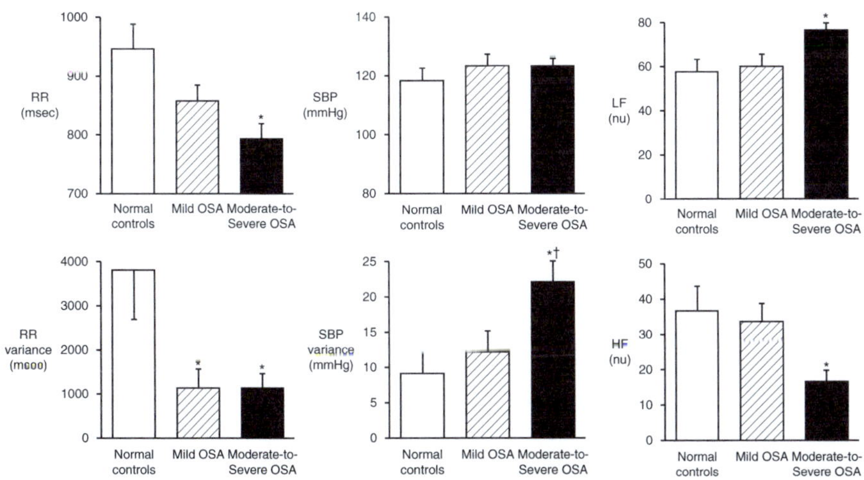

Fig. 5.6 RR interval and systolic blood pressure (*SBP*) mean values and their variances and normalized low-frequency (*LF*) and high-frequency (*HF*) spectral components of RR interval in control subjects, patients with mild OSA, and patients with moderate-to-severe OSA $*P<0.05$ versus control subjects. $\dagger P<0.05$ versus mild OSA. Data are mean ± SEM (Modified from Ref. [40] by permission)

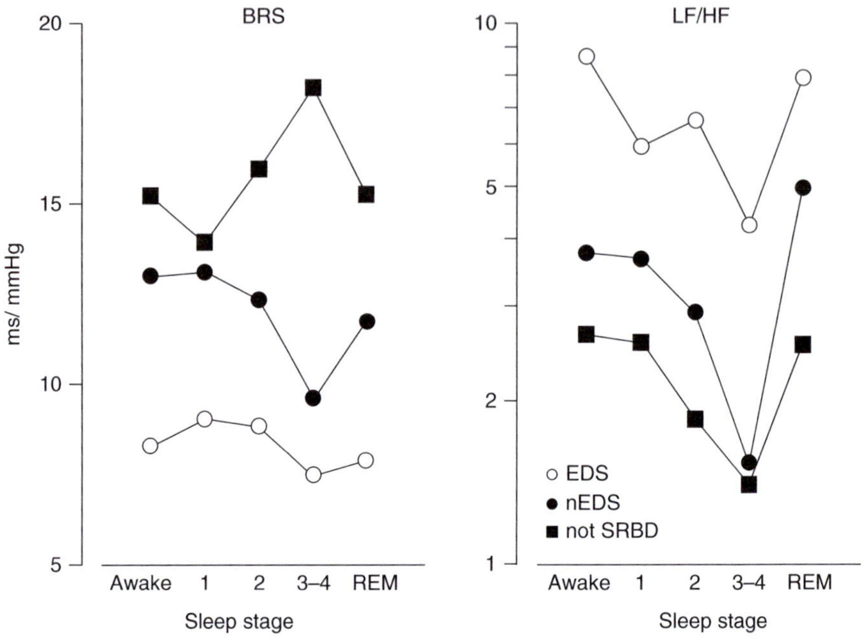

Fig. 5.7 Trends of baroreflex sensitivity (*BRS*), and of the ratio between low- and high-frequency powers of RRI (*LF/HF*), in healthy controls without sleep-related breathing disorders (*SRBD*, *square symbols*), in patients with OSA and excessive daytime sleepiness (*EDS*, *open circles*), and in patients with OSA not affected by EDS (*nEDS*, *solid circles*) (Taken from Lombardi et al. [41] by permission)

still needed to determine the causality of this association, it has been hypothesized that OSAS may contribute to the pathogenesis of resistant HTN by stimulating aldosterone secretion [45] (Fig. 5.3). Evidence supporting this concept has been provided by several studies showing positive and significant correlations between plasma aldosterone concentrations and OSAS severity in patients with resistant HTN, but not in normotensive subjects nor in treated hypertensives with controlled BP [46, 596]. It is likely that aldosterone excess by promoting fluid accumulation in the neck, and thus increasing upper airway resistance, may increase the severity of OSA and the related increase in BP levels [17, 47]. Indirect evidence favoring this concept has been provided by interventional studies in subjects with OSAS and resistant HTN where addition of spironolactone to current antihypertensive treatment resulted in significant reductions in the severity of OSA (i.e., reductions in apnea–hypopnea index and the number of central and obstructive events) on top of its BP-lowering effects [48]. Additional evidence is still needed, however, to consistently determine a causal association between aldosterone excess in OSAS and resistant hypertension.

Endothelial Dysfunction The intermittent hypoxia, the associated neural and humoral alterations, and repeated BP surges during OSA episodes may contribute to impairment in endothelial function. In turn, the inhibition of nitric oxide (NO) production, decreased vasodilatation, and increased vasoconstriction associated with endothelial dysfunction may substantially contribute to BP elevation (Fig. 5.3). Several studies assessing brachial artery endothelium-dependent flow-mediated dilation (FMD, an indirect marker of endothelial NO-mediated reactivity) and forearm blood flow responses to different stimuli (i.e., infusion of acetylcholine, sodium nitroprusside, nitroglycerin) have shown that compared to healthy controls, patients with OSAS often exhibit an impairment of resistance-vessel endothelium-dependent vasodilation [49, 50]. Even when accounting for important confounding factors such as body weight, brachial artery FMD has been shown to be significantly lower in normal-weight OSAS patients than in OSAS-free controls [51]. Additional evidence that OSAS may importantly influence both indices of macrovascular and microvascular endothelial function was provided by a recent study showing abnormal myocardial perfusion, attenuated brachial artery reactivity, and reduced cutaneous perfusion response in OSAS patients compared to healthy controls [52]. Remarkably, several interventional studies have shown substantial improvements in different indices of endothelial function following implementation of regular CPAP use in subjects with hypertension and OSAS [50–52] which indirectly supports a role for endothelial dysfunction in the pathogenesis of arterial hypertension in OSAS.

Vascular Inflammation and Oxidative Stress Repetitive episodes of hypoxia/reoxygenation during transient cessation of breathing in OSA may also reduce NO availability, promoting vascular endothelial inflammation and elevated oxidative stress [49, 50, 53–55] (Fig. 5.3). When compared to OSAS-free controls and regardless of the presence of obesity, OSAS patients have been shown to present a reduced expression of endothelial NO synthase (eNOS) and phosphorylated eNOS (proteins that regulate basal NO production and activity) as well as an increased expression of nitrotyrosine (a marker of oxidative stress) and of nuclear factor-K B (NFkB) (a marker of inflammation) [51]. Most importantly, after 1 month of regular treatment with CPAP, flow-mediated dilation, expression of eNOS, and phosphorylated eNOS were significantly increased, whereas expression of nitrotyrosine and nuclear factor-K B was decreased [51]. It has also been proposed that intermittent hypoxia/hypercapnia associated with OSAS may contribute to the pathogenesis of hypertension by increasing endothelin-1 production. This has been supported by experimental studies in rats showing significant increases in plasma levels of endothelin-1 (a potent vasoconstrictor) and higher BP levels in rats exposed to intermittent hypoxia (i.e., cycles of hypoxia/hypercapnia of 8 h a day during 11 days) compared to those breathing normoxic air [56].

Data from several studies have indicated that selective activation of inflammatory pathways may be an additional important molecular mechanism for the pathogenesis of arterial HTN in OSAS. This has been supported by translational studies showing a selective activation of the pro-inflammatory transcription factor NFkB in HeLa cells of OSAS patients exposed to intermittent hypoxia/reoxygenation cycles [57].

In addition, compared to healthy controls, subjects with OSAS showed significantly higher levels of circulating pro-inflammatory cytokines (i.e., tumor necrosis factor-alpha (TNF-alpha) and the adaptive factor erythropoietin) as well as higher levels of circulating neutrophils. Interestingly, levels of TNF-alpha were normalized after 6 weeks of continuous treatment with CPAP [57]. Other studies have shown that compared to healthy controls, serum levels of inflammatory markers (i.e., C-reactive protein, CRP) are significantly higher in OSAS patients and independently associated with OSAS severity [58]. Interestingly, interventional studies have shown significant reductions in serum levels of CRP and interleukin-6 following implementation of regular CPAP treatment [59]. Finally, evidence has also been provided that OSAS may induce activation of adhesion molecules participating in inflammation. This has been supported by case–control studies showing significantly higher levels of intercellular adhesion molecule-1 (ICAM-1), vascular cell adhesion molecule-1 (VCAM-1), and L-selectin in OSA patients compared to healthy controls [60].

Arterial Stiffness An increased arterial stiffness is a recognized risk factor contributing to the pathogenesis of arterial HTN [61–63]. A recent systematic review of relevant studies has indicated an independent effect of OSAS on arterial stiffness, which in turn may contribute to elevation in BP levels and to resistant HTN [64] (Fig. 5.3). A number of studies have consistently reported significantly higher values of carotid–femoral pulse wave velocity (cfPWV) (which is considered the "gold standard" measure of aortic stiffness), in patients with OSAS compared to healthy controls [64, 65]. Of note, the increase in cfPWV has been shown to be directly related to the severity of OSAS and to be even higher in subjects with OSAS and associated HTN or in the presence of other CV risk factors [66]. In Asian populations, several studies implementing brachial–ankle PWV (baPWV) have also reported significant associations between OSAS and increased arterial stiffness [67]. Even when comparisons have been performed between individuals with or without OSAS entirely free from other CV risk factors, an independent effect of OSAS on arterial stiffening has been reported [68]. Remarkably, in randomized interventional studies, effective treatment of OSAS with CPAP has been associated with significant decreases in arterial stiffness [69, 70]. In one of such studies, CPAP was also associated with significant reductions in sympathetic nerve activity and in ambulatory BP and with significant improvements in arterial baroreflex sensitivity [69].

Metabolic Factors In addition to the hemodynamic changes, OSAS has been frequently associated with metabolic alterations (i.e., alterations in glucose metabolism, insulin resistance, and leptin resistance) which in turn may contribute to the pathogenesis of arterial hypertension (Fig. 5.3). Although alterations in glucose metabolism are thought to be the consequence of other conditions associated with OSAS (i.e., an increased BMI, metabolic syndrome, and/or type 2 diabetes) rather than being OSAS outcomes, evidence has been provided that OSAS, independently of the presence of other confounding factors, is associated with alterations in glucose metabolism which may indeed favor development of type 2 diabetes [71]. In addition, interventional studies have shown the efficacy of regular CPAP treatment in improving the abnormalities in glucose metabolism in OSAS patients [71]. Compared to healthy controls, OSAS patients have also been shown to have a higher degree of insulin and leptin resistance [72–74] even after accounting for body fat content [75]. Although the above-mentioned metabolic alterations should theoretically contribute to the pathogenesis of HTN in OSAS, their relative contribution to BP elevation independent of other concomitant factors still needs to be further explored.

5.5 Prognostic Relevance of OSAS-Related Hypertension

Evidence from several studies has supported an independent association between OSAS and CV disease [76]. OSAS, particularly if severe, has been linked to fatal and nonfatal CV events [77–81], to development and progression of congestive heart failure [79], and with all-cause mortality [82, 83]. However, because the link between OSAS and CV disease may be related to age, obesity, and visceral adiposity, in some of these studies, the associations have lost strength when adjusting for these factors. When it comes to subclinical organ damage, evidence has also been provided that OSAS is independently associated with cardiac (i.e., LV hypertrophy and dysfunction) [70, 84, 85], vascular (i.e., increased carotid intima-media thickness, increased arterial stiffness) [64], renal organ damage (i.e., increased urinary albumin excretion) [86, 87], and endothelial dysfunction (i.e., blunted endothelium-dependent dilatation) [64]. Evidence has also been provided that resistant HTN which is more frequent among OSAS patients considerably increases the risk for CV complications including myocardial infarction, stroke, congestive heart failure, and chronic kidney disease [88–90]. In consideration of the increased CV risk associated with OSAS and resistant HTN, current guidelines for the management of arterial HTN include OSAS among the modifiable causes to be considered in the diagnostic approach to resistant HTN, in order to properly manage both of these conditions [1, 91, 92]. It should be mentioned, however, that no studies have specifically addressed how and to which extent the addition of HTN to OSAS may increase the risk of CV disease independent of other CV risk factors that are often clustered in the context of OSAS. Although OSAS and resistant hypertension have been shown to be independent predictors of CV prognosis, evidence is still needed to determine the actual prognostic relevance of their interaction independently of other concomitant CV risk factors.

Not only the presence of resistant HTN but also the higher frequency of alterations in day-to-night BP profiles and nocturnal HTN contributed to the elevated CV risk of OSAS patients. As mentioned above, nocturnal sympathetic activation during OSAS episodes importantly contributes to increases in BP during sleep, thus attenuating the physiologic nocturnal dipping of BP (i.e., on average by 10–20 % of daytime BP values) or even increasing nocturnal BP levels (rising pattern of nighttime BP). It is thus not surprising the high frequency of non-dipping profile of BP (i.e., nocturnal BP fall <10 % compared to daytime BP levels) reported in OSA patients independently of the presence of HTN [93]. Remarkably, the degree of impairment in nocturnal BP fall has been found to be related to the severity of OSAS [94]. On the other hand, an increased prevalence of alterations in day-to-night BP profiles and nocturnal HTN has been reported in subjects with resistant HTN regardless of the presence of OSAS [90, 95, 96]. It is thus expected that alterations in day-to-night BP changes might be even more pronounced in subjects with OSAS and resistant HTN. From a prognostic point of view, identification of nocturnal HTN and alterations in day-to-night BP changes in subjects with OSAS-related HTN is of utmost relevance on the background of the evidence showing the superior prognostic value of nocturnal BP compared to awake or 24-h BP means in predicting CV morbidity and mortality [97–102], the development of CV events [97, 98, 103–105] as well as overall mortality [97–99, 104, 106, 107]. Identification of "non-dipping" pattern of BP in OSAS patients is also important if we consider that subjects in whom nocturnal decrease in BP is blunted have been reported to have a higher prevalence of subclinical organ damage [108, 109] and an increased risk of CV events [110] and mortality [102], which is even higher in patients in whom BP increases rather than decreases at night (so-called risers or inverted dippers). Despite the very high prevalence of nocturnal HTN and alterations in day-to-night BP changes in OSAS patients, these are often undiagnosed (thus representing a form of so-called masked resistant hypertension), mainly because BP measurements are prevalently measured during daytime at the moment of the clinical visit. Given their relevant prognostic value, alterations in circadian BP should be properly investigated in patients with OSAS-resistant HTN through the use of 24-h ABPM in order to guide antihypertensive treatment toward their normalization and optimization of CV protection.

5.6 Diagnostic Approach to OSAS-Related Resistant Hypertension

Confirming the diagnosis of OSAS in subjects with HTN and in particular in those with resistant HTN is relevant in order to implement specific treatment strategies (i.e., CPAP, weight reduction). This might allow achievement of BP control reducing the elevated CV risk of these subjects. Polysomnography is currently considered the standard technique for diagnosis of OSAS and requires simultaneous monitoring of several CV and respiratory variables during night sleep (i.e., sleep, air flow, respiratory effort, oxygen saturation, and brain activity through electroencephalogram). Based on the number of apneas and hypopneas lasting >10 s during each hour of recording, the severity of the disease is graded using the apnea–hypopnea index (AHI) [111]. Whether polysomnography should be employed systematically in individuals with resistant HTN is still a matter of debate in the absence of cost-effectiveness studies supporting this suggestion. According to a recent position paper of the European Respiratory Society (ERS)/European

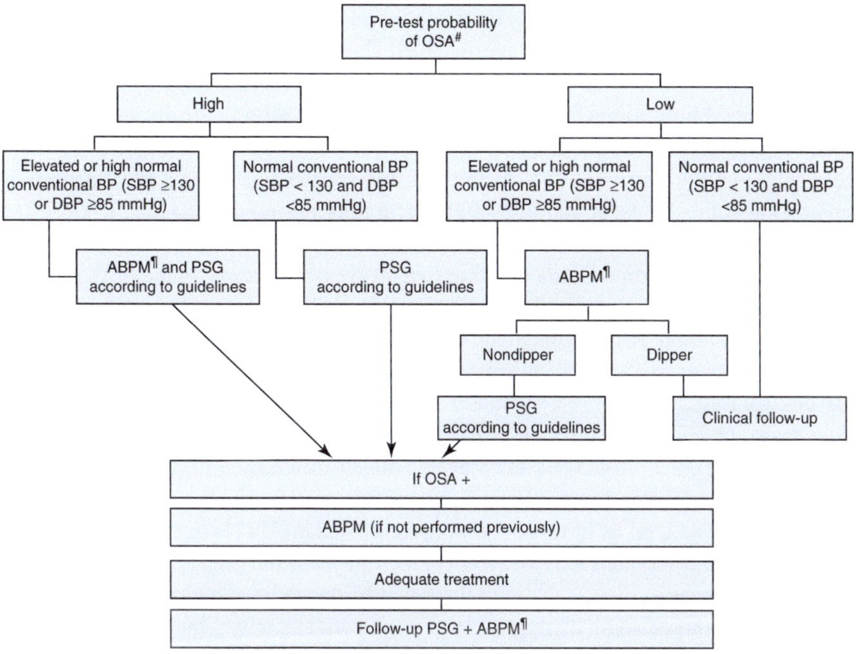

Fig. 5.8 Proposed algorithm for the diagnostic management of patients with hypertension associated with obstructive sleep apnea (*OSA*). *BP* blood pressure, *SBP* systolic BP, *DBP* diastolic BP, *ABPM* ambulatory blood pressure monitoring, *PSG* polysomnography. # according to clinical evaluation and questionnaires, e.g., Epworth and Berlin; ¶ hypertension guidelines recommend the use of home BP monitoring in most hypertensive patients (Reproduced by permission from Parati et al. [112])

Society of Hypertension (ESH) [112], polysomnography should be performed in all subjects with a high pretest probability of OSA based on structured questionnaires (e.g., Epworth and Berlin questionnaires).

Considering the extremely high frequency of alterations in ambulatory BP profiles during nighttime in subjects with resistant HTN and OSAS, the task force of the ERS/ESH also recommends performing ABPM in order to identify alterations in day-to-night BP changes in subjects with resistant HTN in order to guide the decision to perform polysomnography in subjects with otherwise a low probability of OSA based on questionnaires. Indeed, in subjects with a low pretest probability of OSAS, polysomnography is only recommended in those who present alterations in day-to-night BP changes (i.e., non-dipping pattern of BP). See Fig. 5.8.

It is worth mentioning that before starting the instrumental tests to discard OSAS, a first step in the diagnostic approach of the patient with suspected OSAS-related hypertension consists in confirming whether resistance to antihypertensive treatment is true, or corresponds to false resistance. Current guidelines for the management of arterial hypertension define resistant hypertension as the persistence of BP values above the BP goal (i.e., ≥140/90 mmHg for office systolic/diastolic BP) despite the concomitant use of three optimally dosed antihypertensive medications from different classes at near-maximal doses, one of which should ideally be a diuretic [91, 92]. However, this definition is based on office BP measurements which have acknowledged limitations in assessing BP control including the inherent inaccuracy of the technique, the observer's bias and digit preference, a variable interference by the "white-coat effect," and the inability of this approach to collect information on BP during subjects' usual activities and over a long period of time [113]. Thus, for confirmation of true resistant HTN, out-of-office BP-measuring techniques such as ambulatory and/or home BP monitoring (which are not affected by the limitations of office BP) should be performed in addition to office BP measurements. Based on the measures obtained with these methods, a substantial and sometimes larger than expected number of subjects initially diagnosed with resistant hypertension or with BP control based on OBP may actually correspond to false resistant HTN or white-coat resistant HTN (i.e., elevated OBP but normal out-of-office BP values) or to masked HTN (i.e., normal OBP but elevated out-of-office BP values) [90, 114, 115].

From a prognostic point of view, identification of OSAS patients with true resistant HTN as well as of those with masked resistant HTN (treated patients with normal OBP and elevated ABP or HBP) [116, 117] is of the highest relevance on the background of the evidence showing these conditions to be associated with a higher prevalence of target organ damage [118, 119], as well as with a higher risk of future CV and renal events when compared to those with true BP control [105, 120, 121] which ultimately translates in greater healthcare costs [27, 122, 123]. The most recent ESH/ESC arterial HTN guidelines have included OSAS among the causes responsible for true resistant HTN [92].

5.7 Effects of Different Therapeutic Strategies on OSAS-Related Resistant Hypertension

5.7.1 Effects of Lifestyle Changes and Weight Loss on OSAS-Related Hypertension

Obesity is the single most important cause of OSAS and elevation in BP levels. It is thus expected that weight loss might reduce the severity of OSAS and BP levels. Indeed, in subjects who achieve significant reductions in body weight either through dietary [124], pharmacological [125], or surgical [126] measures, considerable reductions of various indices of OSA severity (i.e., AHI) and in BP levels have been reported. In particular, bariatric surgery has been shown to be a highly effective measure to achieve OSAS improvement and BP control as supported by a large meta-analysis of 136 randomized controlled trials [127]. It has to be emphasized that BP was normalized in 61.7 % of patients and normalized or better controlled in 78.5 %. OSA was cured in 85.7 % of patients and was cured or improved in 83.6 % of patients [127]. However, despite its efficacy, bariatric surgery is reserved for selected patient groups, i.e., type 2 diabetes mellitus, patients with severe obesity (BMI >35 kg/m^2), and moderately obese patients (BMI 30–35 kg/m^2) who are inadequately controlled by conventional medical and behavioral therapies to reduce body weight.

5.7.2 Effects of CPAP Treatment on OSAS-Related Hypertension

Nasal CPAP is currently considered the optimal treatment for OSA [128]. When properly implemented, CPAP not only provides relative instant relief of clinical symptoms [129] and reduction in the severity of OSA (i.e., AHI) but also improves many of the acute and chronic pathophysiological alterations induced by OSAS, such as arterial baroreflex impairment and sympathetic activation, systemic inflammation, endothelial dysfunction, RAAS activation, arterial stiffness, and metabolic alterations (insulin resistance).

Of note, CPAP use has been shown to induce marked and acute reductions in MSNA not only during nighttime sleep but also during daytime wakefulness if maintained in the long term [28] (Fig. 5.9). As mentioned above, several studies have indeed also shown the effectiveness of CPAP in improving baroreflex impairment [69], systemic inflammation [51, 57, 59], endothelial dysfunction [50–52], RAAS activation [130], arterial stiffness [69, 70], and metabolic alterations [71].

Although improvements in these pathophysiological alterations should theoretically translate into substantial BP reductions, most interventional trials in OSAS and subsequent meta-analyses have indicated that although CPAP has a significant effect on BP levels, the overall effect on 24-h, daytime, and nighttime systolic and diastolic ambulatory BP levels is rather small (in the order of 1–3 mmHg only) [131–133]. In spite of this, the effects of CPAP on BP levels have been shown to be variable as a function of patients' compliance with nocturnal CPAP, of the number of CPAP hours during nighttime, and of the implementation of ambulatory BP monitoring to assess its effects. In some subgroups of patients, in particular those with more severe OSAS [134], or with resistant HTN [135], substantial effects of CPAP on BP levels have been reported. Indeed, effective CPAP treatment in patients with moderate-to-severe OSAS has been shown to induce important reductions both in day- and nighttime BP levels [134]. This has also been the case of subjects with resistant HTN in whom regular CPAP implementation has resulted in marked reductions in ambulatory BP levels not only during nighttime but also during daytime wakefulness [135]. In a study addressing the effects of 1-year treatment with CPAP, whereas no effects on BP levels were observed in patients with BP controlled at baseline, marked and significant reductions in BP levels were observed in subjects with resistant HTN [136].

A critical aspect when assessing the clinical effects of CPAP is to guarantee patients' adherence to therapy. Given the mechanical nature of CPAP (i.e., facial interface mask and the pressure required to prevent airway collapse), this therapeutic intervention is not always well accepted by patients specially those free of OSA-related symptoms. Indeed, compliance with CPAP has been shown to be directly related to the severity of OSAS [137]. On the other hand, several studies have indicated that in order to observe an effect of CPAP on BP, CPAP treatment should

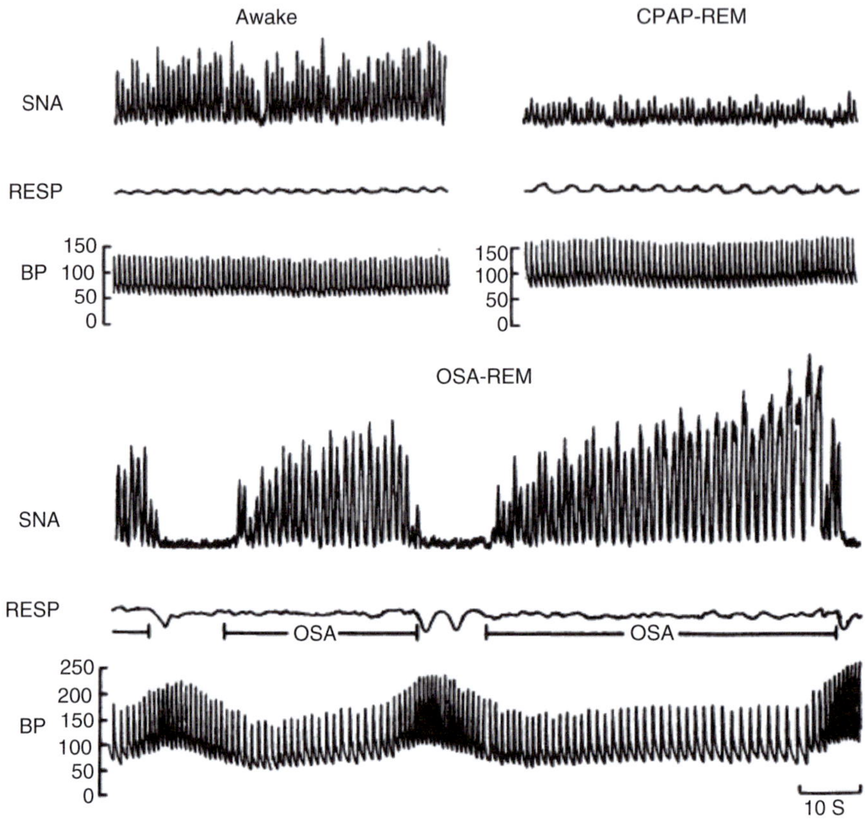

Fig. 5.9 Elimination of apneas by continuous positive airway pressure (*CPAP*) reduces muscle sympathetic nerve activity (*SNA*) and prevents blood pressure (*BP*) surge during rapid eye movement (*REM*) sleep (Taken from Somers et al. [28] by permission)

be implemented for enough time and for a sufficient number of hours per night, and its effects on BP levels ideally assessed by means of ABPM. Proof of this has been provided by several studies in OSAS in which the benefits of CPAP have been evident only in subjects with confirmed resistant HTN (i.e., persistent elevation of both in-office and out-of-office BP levels), in whom CPAP has been implemented for at least 3 months and for more than 5.8 h per night [138]. A positive effect of CPAP has also been reported in non-sleepy hypertensive patients with OSA, among whom the most significant reductions in BP have been observed in those patients using CPAP for more than 5.6 h per night [137]. Further studies are still needed, however, focusing on early start of CPAP treatment before HTN organ damage develops and makes HTN control more difficult, in order to better determine whether CPAP implementation in OSAS patients with HTN is indeed associated with better BP control rates and/or with reduction in the number of antihypertensive medications needed in order to achieve BP control.

A recent meta-analysis of a randomized control trial (RCT) [139] addressing the effect of CPAP on BP in patients with OSA and HTN evaluated seven randomized controlled trials reporting 24-h ambulatory BP data. Overall, CPAP was associated with significant reductions in 24-h ambulatory systolic BP (−2.32 mmHg; 95 % confidence interval [CI], −3.65 to −1.00) and diastolic BP (−1.98 mmHg; 95 % CI, −2.82 to −1.14). CPAP led to more significant improvement in nocturnal systolic BP than that in daytime systolic BP. Subgroup analysis showed that patients with resistant HTN or receiving antihypertensive drugs benefited most from CPAP. Meta-regression indicated that CPAP compliance, age, and baseline systolic BP were positively correlated with decrease in 24-h diastolic BP, but not with reduction in 24-h systolic BP.

A recent study addressing the effect of CPAP treatment on BP in patients with OSA and resistant HTN reported that CPAP treatment for 12 weeks compared with untreated OSA patients as controls resulted in a significant decrease in 24-h mean BP (3.1 mmHg [95 % CI, 0.6–5.6]; $P=0.02$) and 24-h DBP (3.2 mmHg [95 % CI, 1.0–5.4]; $P=0.005$), but not in 24-h systolic BP (3.1 mmHg [95 % CI, −0.6–6.7]; $P=0.10$). Moreover, the percentage of patients displaying a nocturnal BP dipping pattern at the 12-week follow-up was greater in the CPAP group than in the control group (35.9 vs. 21.6 %; adjusted odds ratio [OR], 2.4 [95 % CI, 1.2–5.1]; $P=0.02$) [140].

Another study evaluated the effect of CPAP on BP in patients with resistant HTN and OSA in the frame of a randomized controlled clinical trial with blinded assessment of outcomes in 117 patients with moderate/severe OSA, defined by apnea–hypopnea index ≥15 apneic events per hour. Subjects were randomized to 6-month CPAP treatment (57 patients) or no therapy (60 patients), while maintaining antihypertensive treatment. Clinic and 24-h ambulatory BPs were obtained before and after 6-month treatment. Primary outcomes were changes in clinic and ambulatory BPs and in nocturnal BP fall patterns. On intention-to-treat analysis, there was no significant difference in any BP change, neither in nocturnal BP fall, between CPAP and control groups. The best effect of CPAP was on nighttime systolic BP in per-protocol analysis, with a tendentially although nonsignificantly greater reduction of 4.7 mmHg (95 % confidence interval, −11.3 to +3.1 mmHg; $P=0.24$) and an increase in nocturnal BP fall of 2.2 % (95 % confidence interval, −1.6 to +5.8 %; $P=0.25$), in comparison with control group. The conclusion of this study is that CPAP treatment had no significant effect on clinic and ambulatory BPs in patients with resistant HTN and moderate/severe OSA, although a beneficial effect on nighttime systolic BP and on nocturnal BP fall might exist in patients with uncontrolled ambulatory BP levels [141].

Overall, also in the light of these recent trials, the reported poor efficacy of CPAP in reducing BP levels in OSA patients with HTN may depend on a combination of different factors, including poor patients' compliance with nocturnal CPAP use, too short treatment duration, inaccurate CPAP calibration, failure to use 24-h ABPM to evaluate CPAP effects on BP, and, most importantly, delayed use of CPAP in the clinical history of OSA patients when HTN may have become more resistant to treatment due to appearance of organ damage.

5.7.3 Effects of Renal Sympathetic Denervation in OSAS-Related Resistant Hypertension

Sympathetic activation in OSAS determines an increase in sympathetic drive to the heart, the peripheral vasculature and the kidneys. In relation to the latter, the sympathetic nerves arriving to the renal district have been identified as a major contributing factor to the pathophysiology of HTN both in experimental models and in human studies [142]. This has been the basis for the development of interventional strategies aimed at modulating renal sympathetic nerve activity through radiofrequency catheter-based renal sympathetic denervation (RDN) [143]. In subjects with uncontrolled HTN, RDN has been shown to induce significant reductions in renal sympathetic efferent nerve activity, in whole-body sympathetic nerve activity and norepinephrine spillover, as well as substantial and sustained reductions in BP levels [144]. Small interventional studies in OSAS patients who were refractory to lifestyle modifications, weight loss, pharmacological treatment, and CPAP have also suggested that RDN may represent an effective strategy for the management of resistant HTN associated with OSA, inducing significant and sustained changes in BP levels at 3 and 6 months of follow-up [145]. Remarkably, the changes in BP levels reported in this study have also been accompanied by improvements in OSAS severity as indicated by the significant reductions in AHI at 3 and 6 months after denervation [145]. Renal sympathetic denervation might thus represent a potentially useful option for the management of resistant HTN in OSAS patients, who are refractory to lifestyle modifications, weight loss, pharmacological treatment and CPAP. Nonetheless, given the very small sample size of this paper, adequately powered longitudinal studies are needed to confirm these anecdotal findings and to assess the long-term impact of RDN on HTN control, as well as its benefits in terms of organ damage and incidence of CV morbid-mortality in subjects with OSAS.

5.8 Do Different Antihypertensive Drug Classes Have Different Effects on OSAS-Related Hypertension?

Different antihypertensive drug classes might have a differential effect on the pathophysiological mechanisms involved in the pathogenesis of OSAS-related HTN. However, the few studies that have comparatively assessed the BP-lowering effects of different drug classes in OSAS have been of small size, and their statistical power was limited to derive consistent conclusions. In a randomized study assessing the effects of different classes of antihypertensive drugs (i.e., beta-blockers, calcium antagonists, angiotensin-converting enzyme inhibitors, angiotensin receptor blockers, and thiazide diuretics) on office and ambulatory BP levels in patients with HTN and OSAS, no significant differences between drug classes were observed in their ability to reduce office and daytime ambulatory BP levels. However, treatment with β-blockers was more effective in reducing nighttime ambulatory BP than administration of other compounds, probably through their effects on sympathetic activation. In general, however, no consistent evidence has been provided supporting a superior antihypertensive efficacy of any antihypertensive drug in OSA patients [146]. Long-term effects of treatment with different antihypertensive agents on hypertension severity in OSAS have not been systematically addressed in clinical trials, however. Evidence is therefore still needed in order to identify preferred compounds for an adequate BP control in this group of high-risk patients.

Recent studies in resistant HTN have suggested that spironolactone should be considered in all patients with uncontrolled HTN on three or more antihypertensive agents [147]. In some studies, addition of spironolactone in doses of 25–50 mg a day to the current antihypertensive treatment in resistant hypertensive patients was shown to reduce the severity of OSAS on top of its BP-lowering effects [48]. This is in line with the concept that aldosterone-mediated chronic fluid retention may influence severity of OSA.

Conclusions

Consistent evidence has supported the association between OSAS and HTN [2, 4, 12–15] showing a dose–response relationship between OSAS severity and the degree of BP elevation [2, 26, 27]. It has also been shown that HTN occurring in individuals with OSAS is more likely to be severe, resistant to treatment, and associated with alterations in day-to-night BP changes [2, 26, 27]. The pathogenesis of OSAS-related HTN is likely to be multifactorial, involving alterations in several regulatory systems. However, the mechanisms by which OSAS promotes arterial HTN still need to be better understood. Although OSAS and drug-resistant HTN are independent predictors of CV morbid-mortality, evidence from longitudinal studies is still needed to determine the actual prognostic relevance of OSAS-related HTN. In a subject with resistant HTN and suspected OSAS, ABPM should be performed whenever possible for confirmation of resistant HTN, for identification of alterations in day-to-night BP changes and in order to define the need of performing additional diagnostic procedures (i.e., polysomnography) and/or implementing more aggressive pharmacological or interventional strategies for the management of resistant HTN. In turn, identification of OSAS and proper implementation of specific treatment strategies for its treatment (i.e., CPAP) in subjects with resistant HTN might favor achievement of BP control optimizing CV protection. Evidence from additional longitudinal interventional studies in OSAS controlling for potential confounders (i.e., visceral obesity, increased BMI) is still needed, however, not only to determine the prognostic relevance of the interaction between OSAS and HTN but also for determining whether treating OSAS in resistant HTN confers significant benefits in terms of CV protection.

References

1. Mancia G, De Backer G, Dominiczak A, Cifkova R, Fagard R, Germano G et al (2007) 2007 Guidelines for the Management of Arterial Hypertension: the Task Force for the Management of Arterial Hypertension of the European Society of Hypertension (ESH) and of the European Society of Cardiology (ESC). J Hypertens 25(6):1105–1187. Epub 2007/06/15

2. Grote L, Hedner J, Peter JH (2000) Sleep-related breathing disorder is an independent risk factor for uncontrolled hypertension. J Hypertens 18(6):679–685. Epub 2000/06/29
3. Peppard PE, Young T, Palta M, Skatrud J (2000) Prospective study of the association between sleep-disordered breathing and hypertension. N Engl J Med 342(19):1378–1384. Epub 2000/05/11
4. Nieto FJ, Young TB, Lind BK, Shahar E, Samet JM, Redline S et al (2000) Association of sleep-disordered breathing, sleep apnea, and hypertension in a large community-based study. Sleep Heart Health Study. JAMA 283(14):1829–1836. Epub 2000/04/19
5. Medicine AAoS (2005) International classification of sleep disorders: diagnostic and coding manual, 2nd edn. American Academy of Sleep Medicine, Westchester
6. Coccagna G, Mantovani M, Brignani F, Parchi C, Lugaresi E (1972) Continuous recording of the pulmonary and systemic arterial pressure during sleep in syndromes of hypersomnia with periodic breathing. Bull Physiopathol Respir 8(5):1159–1172. Epub 1972/09/01
7. Baguet JP, Hammer L, Levy P, Pierre H, Rossini E, Mouret S et al (2005) Night-time and diastolic hypertension are common and underestimated conditions in newly diagnosed apnoeic patients. J Hypertens 23(3):521–527. Epub 2005/02/18
8. Hla KM, Young T, Finn L, Peppard PE, Szklo-Coxe M, Stubbs M (2008) Longitudinal association of sleep-disordered breathing and nondipping of nocturnal blood pressure in the Wisconsin Sleep Cohort Study. Sleep 31(6):795–800. Epub 2008/06/14
9. Lavie P, Herer P, Hoffstein V (2000) Obstructive sleep apnoea syndrome as a risk factor for hypertension: population study. BMJ 320(7233):479–482. Epub 2000/03/04
10. Davies CW, Crosby JH, Mullins RL, Barbour C, Davies RJ, Stradling JR (2000) Case–control study of 24 hour ambulatory blood pressure in patients with obstructive sleep apnoea and normal matched control subjects. Thorax 55(9):736–740. Epub 2000/08/19
11. Pankow W, Nabe B, Lies A, Becker H, Kohler U, Kohl FV et al (1997) Influence of sleep apnea on 24-hour blood pressure. Chest 112(5):1253–1258. Epub 1997/11/21
12. Bixler EO, Vgontzas AN, Lin HM, Ten Have T, Leiby BE, Vela-Bueno A et al (2000) Association of hypertension and sleep-disordered breathing. Arch Intern Med 160(15):2289–2295. Epub 2000/08/06
13. Duran J, Esnaola S, Rubio R, Iztueta A (2001) Obstructive sleep apnea-hypopnea and related clinical features in a population-based sample of subjects aged 30 to 70 yr. Am J Respir Crit Care Med 163(3 Pt 1):685–689. Epub 2001/03/20
14. Tanigawa T, Tachibana N, Yamagishi K, Muraki I, Kudo M, Ohira T et al (2004) Relationship between sleep-disordered breathing and blood pressure levels in community-based samples of Japanese men. Hypertens Res: Off J Jap Soc Hypertens 27(7):479–484. Epub 2004/08/11
15. Young T, Peppard P, Palta M, Hla KM, Finn L, Morgan B et al (1997) Population-based study of sleep-disordered breathing as a risk factor for hypertension. Arch Intern Med 157(15):1746–1752. Epub 1997/08/11
16. Kiely JL, McNicholas WT (2000) Cardiovascular risk factors in patients with obstructive sleep apnoea syndrome. Eur Res J Off J Eur Soc Clini Res Physiol 16(1):128–133. Epub 2000/08/10
17. Calhoun DA (2010) Obstructive sleep apnea and hypertension. Curr Hypertens Rep 12(3):189–195. Epub 2010/04/29
18. Garrison RJ, Kannel WB, Stokes J 3rd, Castelli WP (1987) Incidence and precursors of hypertension in young adults: the Framingham Offspring Study. Prev Med 16(2):235–251. Epub 1987/03/01
19. Bramlage P, Pittrow D, Wittchen HU, Kirch W, Boehler S, Lehnert H et al (2004) Hypertension in overweight and obese primary care patients is highly prevalent and poorly controlled. Am J Hypertens 17(10):904–910. Epub 2004/10/16
20. O'Connor GT, Caffo B, Newman AB, Quan SF, Rapoport DM, Redline S et al (2009) Prospective study of sleep-disordered breathing and hypertension: the Sleep Heart Health Study. Am J Respir Crit Care Med 179(12):1159–1164. Epub 2009/03/07
21. Kapa S, Sert Kuniyoshi FH, Somers VK (2008) Sleep apnea and hypertension: interactions and implications for management. Hypertension 51(3):605–608. Epub 2008/01/30

22. Haas DC, Foster GL, Nieto FJ, Redline S, Resnick HE, Robbins JA et al (2005) Age-dependent associations between sleep-disordered breathing and hypertension: importance of discriminating between systolic/diastolic hypertension and isolated systolic hypertension in the Sleep Heart Health Study. Circulation 111(5):614–621. Epub 2005/02/09
23. Logan AG, Perlikowski SM, Mente A, Tisler A, Tkacova R, Niroumand M et al (2001) High prevalence of unrecognized sleep apnoea in drug-resistant hypertension. J Hypertens 19(12):2271–2277. Epub 2001/11/29
24. Cano-Pumarega I, Duran-Cantolla J, Aizpuru F, Miranda-Serrano E, Rubio R, Martinez-Null C et al (2011) Obstructive sleep apnea and systemic hypertension: longitudinal study in the general population: the Vitoria Sleep Cohort. Am J Respir Crit Care Med 184(11):1299–1304. Epub 2011/08/27
25. Marin JM, Agusti A, Villar I, Forner M, Nieto D, Carrizo SJ et al (2012) Association between treated and untreated obstructive sleep apnea and risk of hypertension. JAMA 307(20):2169–2176. Epub 2012/05/24
26. Somers VK, White DP, Amin R, Abraham WT, Costa F, Culebras A et al (2008) Sleep apnea and cardiovascular disease: an American Heart Association/american College Of Cardiology Foundation Scientific Statement from the American Heart Association Council for High Blood Pressure Research Professional Education Committee, Council on Clinical Cardiology, Stroke Council, and Council on Cardiovascular Nursing. In collaboration with the National Heart, Lung, and Blood Institute National Center on Sleep Disorders Research (National Institutes of Health). Circulation 118(10):1080–1111. Epub 2008/08/30
27. Calhoun DA, Jones D, Textor S, Goff DC, Murphy TP, Toto RD (2008) Resistant hypertension: diagnosis, evaluation, and treatment. A scientific statement from the American Heart Association Professional Education Committee of the Council for High Blood Pressure Research. Hypertension 51(6):1403–1419. Epub 2008/04/09
28. Somers VK, Dyken ME, Clary MP, Abboud FM (1995) Sympathetic neural mechanisms in obstructive sleep apnea. J Clin Invest 96(4):1897–1904. Epub 1995/10/01
29. Portaluppi F, Provini F, Cortelli P, Plazzi G, Bertozzi N, Manfredini R et al (1997) Undiagnosed sleep-disordered breathing among male nondippers with essential hypertension. J Hypertens 15(11):1227–1233. Epub 1997/12/31
30. Narkiewicz K, van de Borne PJ, Cooley RL, Dyken ME, Somers VK (1998) Sympathetic activity in obese subjects with and without obstructive sleep apnea. Circulation 98(8):772–776. Epub 1998/09/04
31. Ali NJ, Davies RJ, Fleetham JA, Stradling JR (1992) The acute effects of continuous positive airway pressure and oxygen administration on blood pressure during obstructive sleep apnea. Chest 101(6):1526–1532. Epub 1992/06/01
32. Narkiewicz K, Kato M, Phillips BG, Pesek CA, Davison DE, Somers VK (1999) Nocturnal continuous positive airway pressure decreases daytime sympathetic traffic in obstructive sleep apnea. Circulation 100(23):2332–2335. Epub 1999/12/11
33. Hedner JA, Wilcox I, Laks L, Grunstein RR, Sullivan CE (1992) A specific and potent pressor effect of hypoxia in patients with sleep apnea. Am Rev Respir Dis 146(5 Pt 1):1240–1245. Epub 1992/11/01
34. Narkiewicz K, van de Borne PJ, Pesek CA, Dyken ME, Montano N, Somers VK (1999) Selective potentiation of peripheral chemoreflex sensitivity in obstructive sleep apnea. Circulation 99(9):1183–1189. Epub 1999/03/09
35. Parati G, Di Rienzo M, Bonsignore MR, Insalaco G, Marrone O, Castiglioni P et al (1997) Autonomic cardiac regulation in obstructive sleep apnea syndrome: evidence from spontaneous baroreflex analysis during sleep. J Hypertens 15(12 Pt 2):1621–1626. Epub 1998/03/06
36. Narkiewicz K, Pesek CA, Kato M, Phillips BG, Davison DE, Somers VK (1998) Baroreflex control of sympathetic nerve activity and heart rate in obstructive sleep apnea. Hypertension 32(6):1039–1043. Epub 1998/12/18
37. Noda A, Nakata S, Koike Y, Miyata S, Kitaichi K, Nishizawa T et al (2007) Continuous positive airway pressure improves daytime baroreflex sensitivity and nitric oxide production

in patients with moderate to severe obstructive sleep apnea syndrome. Hypertens Res: Off J Jap Soc Hypertens 30(8):669–676. Epub 2007/10/06

38. Ryan S, Ward S, Heneghan C, McNicholas WT (2007) Predictors of decreased spontaneous baroreflex sensitivity in obstructive sleep apnea syndrome. Chest 131(4):1100–1107. Epub 2007/04/12
39. Bonsignore MR, Parati G, Insalaco G, Marrone O, Castiglioni P, Romano S et al (2002) Continuous positive airway pressure treatment improves baroreflex control of heart rate during sleep in severe obstructive sleep apnea syndrome. Am J Respir Crit Care Med 166(3):279–286. Epub 2002/08/03
40. Narkiewicz K, Montano N, Cogliati C, van de Borne PJ, Dyken ME, Somers VK (1998) Altered cardiovascular variability in obstructive sleep apnea. Circulation 98(11):1071–1077. Epub 1998/09/16
41. Lombardi C, Parati G, Cortelli P, Provini F, Vetrugno R, Plazzi G et al (2008) Daytime sleepiness and neural cardiac modulation in sleep-related breathing disorders. J Sleep Res 17(3):263–270. Epub 2008/05/28
42. Gonzaga CC, Gaddam KK, Ahmed MI, Pimenta E, Thomas SJ, Harding SM et al (2010) Severity of obstructive sleep apnea is related to aldosterone status in subjects with resistant hypertension. J Clini Sleep Med JCSM Official Pub Am Ac Sleep Med 6(4):363–368. Epub 2010/08/24
43. Pimenta E, Calhoun DA, Oparil S (2009) Sleep apnea, aldosterone, and resistant hypertension. Prog Cardiovasc Dis 51(5):371–380. Epub 2009/03/03
44. Goodfriend TL, Calhoun DA (2004) Resistant hypertension, obesity, sleep apnea, and aldosterone: theory and therapy. Hypertension 43(3):518–524. Epub 2004/01/21
45. Calhoun DA, Nishizaka MK, Zaman MA, Harding SM (2004) Aldosterone excretion among subjects with resistant hypertension and symptoms of sleep apnea. Chest 125(1):112–117. Epub 2004/01/14
46. Pratt-Ubunama MN, Nishizaka MK, Boedefeld RL, Cofield SS, Harding SM, Calhoun DA (2007) Plasma aldosterone is related to severity of obstructive sleep apnea in subjects with resistant hypertension. Chest 131(2):453–459. Epub 2007/02/14
47. Dudenbostel T, Calhoun DA (2012) Resistant hypertension, obstructive sleep apnoea and aldosterone. J Hum Hypertens 26(5):281–287. Epub 2011/06/10
48. Gaddam K, Pimenta E, Thomas SJ, Cofield SS, Oparil S, Harding SM et al (2010) Spironolactone reduces severity of obstructive sleep apnoea in patients with resistant hypertension: a preliminary report. J Hum Hypertens 24(8):532–537. Epub 2009/12/18
49. Kato M, Roberts-Thomson P, Phillips BG, Haynes WG, Winnicki M, Accurso V et al (2000) Impairment of endothelium-dependent vasodilation of resistance vessels in patients with obstructive sleep apnea. Circulation 102(21):2607–2610. Epub 2000/11/22
50. Ip MS, Tse HF, Lam B, Tsang KW, Lam WK (2004) Endothelial function in obstructive sleep apnea and response to treatment. Am J Respir Crit Care Med 169(3):348–353. Epub 2003/10/11
51. Jelic S, Lederer DJ, Adams T, Padeletti M, Colombo PC, Factor PH et al (2010) Vascular inflammation in obesity and sleep apnea. Circulation 121(8):1014–1021. Epub 2010/02/18
52. Butt M, Khair OA, Dwivedi G, Shantsila A, Shantsila E, Lip GY (2011) Myocardial perfusion by myocardial contrast echocardiography and endothelial dysfunction in obstructive sleep apnea. Hypertension 58(3):417–424. Epub 2011/07/13
53. Jelic S, Padeletti M, Kawut SM, Higgins C, Canfield SM, Onat D et al (2008) Inflammation, oxidative stress, and repair capacity of the vascular endothelium in obstructive sleep apnea. Circulation 117(17):2270–2278. Epub 2008/04/17
54. Dyugovskaya L, Lavie P, Lavie L (2002) Increased adhesion molecules expression and production of reactive oxygen species in leukocytes of sleep apnea patients. Am J Respir Crit Care Med 165(7):934–939. Epub 2002/04/06
55. Minoguchi K, Yokoe T, Tazaki T, Minoguchi H, Tanaka A, Oda N et al (2005) Increased carotid intima-media thickness and serum inflammatory markers in obstructive sleep apnea. Am J Respir Crit Care Med 172(5):625–630. Epub 2005/08/27

56. Kanagy NL, Walker BR, Nelin LD (2001) Role of endothelin in intermittent hypoxia-induced hypertension. Hypertension 37(2 Part 2):511–515. Epub 2001/03/07
57. Ryan S, Taylor CT, McNicholas WT (2005) Selective activation of inflammatory pathways by intermittent hypoxia in obstructive sleep apnea syndrome. Circulation 112(17):2660–2667. Epub 2005/10/26
58. Shamsuzzaman AS, Winnicki M, Lanfranchi P, Wolk R, Kara T, Accurso V et al (2002) Elevated C-reactive protein in patients with obstructive sleep apnea. Circulation 105(21):2462–2464. Epub 2002/05/30
59. Yokoe T, Minoguchi K, Matsuo H, Oda N, Minoguchi H, Yoshino G et al (2003) Elevated levels of C-reactive protein and interleukin-6 in patients with obstructive sleep apnea syndrome are decreased by nasal continuous positive airway pressure. Circulation 107(8):1129–1134. Epub 2003/03/05
60. Ohga E, Nagase T, Tomita T, Teramoto S, Matsuse T, Katayama H et al (1999) Increased levels of circulating ICAM-1, VCAM-1, and L-selectin in obstructive sleep apnea syndrome. J Appl Physiol 87(1):10–14. Epub 1999/07/20
61. O'Rourke MF, Nichols WW (2005) Aortic diameter, aortic stiffness, and wave reflection increase with age and isolated systolic hypertension. Hypertension 45(4):652–658. Epub 2005/02/09
62. Mitchell GF, Lacourciere Y, Ouellet JP, Izzo JL Jr, Neutel J, Kerwin LJ et al (2003) Determinants of elevated pulse pressure in middle-aged and older subjects with uncomplicated systolic hypertension: the role of proximal aortic diameter and the aortic pressure-flow relationship. Circulation 108(13):1592–1598. Epub 2003/09/17
63. Schillaci G, Bilo G, Pucci G, Laurent S, Macquin-Mavier I, Boutouyrie P et al (2012) Relationship between short-term blood pressure variability and large-artery stiffness in human hypertension: findings from 2 large databases. Hypertension 60(2):369–377. Epub 2012/07/04
64. Doonan RJ, Scheffler P, Lalli M, Kimoff RJ, Petridou ET, Daskalopoulos ME et al (2011) Increased arterial stiffness in obstructive sleep apnea: a systematic review. Hypertens Res: Off J Jap Soc Hypertens 34(1):23–32. Epub 2010/10/22
65. Tsioufis C, Thomopoulos K, Dimitriadis K, Amfilochiou A, Tousoulis D, Alchanatis M et al (2007) The incremental effect of obstructive sleep apnoea syndrome on arterial stiffness in newly diagnosed essential hypertensive subjects. J Hypertens 25(1):141–146. Epub 2006/12/05
66. Drager LF, Bortolotto LA, Figueiredo AC, Silva BC, Krieger EM, Lorenzi-Filho G (2007) Obstructive sleep apnea, hypertension, and their interaction on arterial stiffness and heart remodeling. Chest 131(5):1379–1386. Epub 2007/05/15
67. Shiina K, Tomiyama H, Takata Y, Usui Y, Asano K, Hirayama Y et al (2006) Concurrent presence of metabolic syndrome in obstructive sleep apnea syndrome exacerbates the cardiovascular risk: a sleep clinic cohort study. Hypertens Res: Off J Jap Soc Hypertens 29(6):433–441. Epub 2006/08/31
68. Nagahama H, Soejima M, Uenomachi H, Higashi Y, Yotsumoto K, Samukawa T et al (2004) Pulse wave velocity as an indicator of atherosclerosis in obstructive sleep apnea syndrome patients. Intern Med 43(3):184–188. Epub 2004/04/22
69. Kohler M, Pepperell JC, Casadei B, Craig S, Crosthwaite N, Stradling JR et al (2008) CPAP and measures of cardiovascular risk in males with OSAS. Eur Res J Off J Eur Soc Clini Res Physiol 32(6):1488–1496. Epub 2008/07/26
70. Drager LF, Bortolotto LA, Figueiredo AC, Krieger EM, Lorenzi GF (2007) Effects of continuous positive airway pressure on early signs of atherosclerosis in obstructive sleep apnea. Am J Respir Crit Care Med 176(7):706–712. Epub 2007/06/09
71. Rasche K, Keller T, Tautz B, Hader C, Hergenc G, Antosiewicz J et al (2010) Obstructive sleep apnea and type 2 diabetes. Eur J Med Res 15(Suppl 2):152–156. Epub 2010/12/22
72. Basoglu OK, Sarac F, Sarac S, Uluer H, Yilmaz C (2011) Metabolic syndrome, insulin resistance, fibrinogen, homocysteine, leptin, and C-reactive protein in obese patients with obstructive sleep apnea syndrome. Ann Thor Med 6(3):120–125. Epub 2011/07/16

73. Zirlik S, Hauck T, Fuchs FS, Neurath MF, Konturek PC, Harsch IA (2011) Leptin, obestatin and apelin levels in patients with obstructive sleep apnoea syndrome. Med Sci Monit Inter Med J Exper Clini Res 17(3):CR159–CR164. Epub 2011/03/02
74. Bonsignore MR, Esquinas C, Barcelo A, Sanchez-de-la-Torre M, Paterno A, Duran-Cantolla J et al (2012) Metabolic syndrome, insulin resistance and sleepiness in real-life obstructive sleep apnoea. Eur Res J Off J Eur Soc Clini Res Physiol 39(5):1136–1143. Epub 2011/11/15
75. Phillips BG, Kato M, Narkiewicz K, Choe I, Somers VK (2000) Increases in leptin levels, sympathetic drive, and weight gain in obstructive sleep apnea. Am J Physiol Heart Circ Physiol 279(1):H234–H237. Epub 2000/07/19
76. McNicholas WT, Bonsigore MR (2007) Sleep apnoea as an independent risk factor for cardiovascular disease: current evidence, basic mechanisms and research priorities. Eur Res J Off J Eur Soc Clini Res Physiol 29(1):156–178. Epub 2007/01/02
77. Yaggi HK, Concato J, Kernan WN, Lichtman JH, Brass LM, Mohsenin V (2005) Obstructive sleep apnea as a risk factor for stroke and death. N Engl J Med 353(19):2034–2041. Epub 2005/11/12
78. Selim B, Won C, Yaggi HK (2010) Cardiovascular consequences of sleep apnea. Clin Chest Med 31(2):203–220. Epub 2010/05/22
79. Gottlieb DJ, Yenokyan G, Newman AB, O'Connor GT, Punjabi NM, Quan SF et al (2010) Prospective study of obstructive sleep apnea and incident coronary heart disease and heart failure: the sleep heart health study. Circulation 122(4):352–360. Epub 2010/07/14
80. Redline S, Yenokyan G, Gottlieb DJ, Shahar E, O'Connor GT, Resnick HE et al (2010) Obstructive sleep apnea-hypopnea and incident stroke: the sleep heart health study. Am J Respir Crit Care Med 182(2):269–277. Epub 2010/03/27
81. Capampangan DJ, Wellik KE, Parish JM, Aguilar MI, Snyder CR, Wingerchuk D et al (2010) Is obstructive sleep apnea an independent risk factor for stroke? A critically appraised topic. Neurologist 16(4):269–273. Epub 2010/07/02
82. Marshall NS, Wong KK, Liu PY, Cullen SR, Knuiman MW, Grunstein RR (2008) Sleep apnea as an independent risk factor for all-cause mortality: the Busselton Health Study. Sleep 31(8):1079–1085. Epub 2008/08/22
83. Young T, Finn L, Peppard PE, Szklo-Coxe M, Austin D, Nieto FJ et al (2008) Sleep disordered breathing and mortality: eighteen-year follow-up of the Wisconsin sleep cohort. Sleep 31(8):1071–1078. Epub 2008/08/22
84. Otto ME, Belohlavek M, Romero-Corral A, Gami AS, Gilman G, Svatikova A et al (2007) Comparison of cardiac structural and functional changes in obese otherwise healthy adults with versus without obstructive sleep apnea. Am J Cardiol 99(9):1298–1302. Epub 2007/05/05
85. Tavil Y, Kanbay A, Sen N, Ciftci TU, Abaci A, Yalcin MR et al (2007) Comparison of right ventricular functions by tissue Doppler imaging in patients with obstructive sleep apnea syndrome with or without hypertension. Int J Cardiovasc Imaging 23(4):469–477. Epub 2006/10/21
86. Agrawal V, Vanhecke TE, Rai B, Franklin BA, Sangal RB, McCullough PA (2009) Albuminuria and renal function in obese adults evaluated for obstructive sleep apnea. Nephron Clin Pract 113(3):c140–c147. Epub 2009/08/13
87. Sim JJ, Rasgon SA, Derose SF (2010) Review article: managing sleep apnoea in kidney diseases. Nephrology (Carlton) 15(2):146–152. Epub 2010/05/18
88. Persell SD (2011) Prevalence of resistant hypertension in the United States, 2003–2008. Hypertension 57(6):1076–1080. Epub 2011/04/20
89. Egan BM, Zhao Y, Axon RN, Brzezinski WA, Ferdinand KC (2011) Uncontrolled and apparent treatment resistant hypertension in the United States, 1988 to 2008. Circulation 124(9):1046–1058. Epub 2011/08/10
90. de la Sierra A, Segura J, Banegas JR, Gorostidi M, de la Cruz JJ, Armario P et al (2011) Clinical features of 8295 patients with resistant hypertension classified on the basis of ambulatory blood pressure monitoring. Hypertension 57(5):898–902. Epub 2011/03/30

91. James PA, Oparil S, Carter BL, Cushman WC, Dennison-Himmelfarb C, Handler J et al (2014) 2014 evidence-based guideline for the management of high blood pressure in adults: report from the panel members appointed to the Eighth Joint National Committee (JNC 8). JAMA 311(5):507–520. Epub 2013/12/20
92. Mancia G, Fagard R, Narkiewicz K, Redon J, Zanchetti A, Bohm M et al (2013) 2013 ESH/ESC Guidelines for the management of arterial hypertension: the Task Force for the management of arterial hypertension of the European Society of Hypertension (ESH) and of the European Society of Cardiology (ESC). J Hypertens 31(7):1281–1357. Epub 2013/07/03
93. Wolf J, Hering D, Narkiewicz K (2010) Non-dipping pattern of hypertension and obstructive sleep apnea syndrome. Hypertens Res: Off J Jap Soc Hypertens 33(9):867–871. Epub 2010/09/08
94. Lavie-Nevo K, Pillar G (2006) Evening-morning differences in blood pressure in sleep apnea syndrome: effect of gender. Am J Hypertens 19(10):1064–1069. Epub 2006/10/10
95. Muxfeldt ES, Cardoso CR, Salles GF (2009) Prognostic value of nocturnal blood pressure reduction in resistant hypertension. Arch Intern Med 169(9):874–880. Epub 2009/05/13
96. Muxfeldt ES, Bloch KV, Nogueira AR, Salles GF (2003) Twenty-four hour ambulatory blood pressure monitoring pattern of resistant hypertension. Blood Press Monit 8(5):181–185. Epub 2003/11/19
97. Staessen JA, Thijs L, Fagard R, O'Brien ET, Clement D, de Leeuw PW et al (1999) Predicting cardiovascular risk using conventional vs ambulatory blood pressure in older patients with systolic hypertension. Systolic Hypertension in Europe Trial Investigators. JAMA 282(6):539–546. Epub 1999/08/18
98. Sega R, Facchetti R, Bombelli M, Cesana G, Corrao G, Grassi G et al (2005) Prognostic value of ambulatory and home blood pressures compared with office blood pressure in the general population: follow-up results from the Pressioni Arteriose Monitorate e Loro Associazioni (PAMELA) study. Circulation 111(14):1777–1783. Epub 2005/04/06
99. Kikuya M, Ohkubo T, Asayama K, Metoki H, Obara T, Saito S et al (2005) Ambulatory blood pressure and 10-year risk of cardiovascular and noncardiovascular mortality: the Ohasama study. Hypertension 45(2):240–245. Epub 2004/12/15
100. Fagard RH, Celis H, Thijs L, Staessen JA, Clement DL, De Buyzere ML et al (2008) Daytime and nighttime blood pressure as predictors of death and cause-specific cardiovascular events in hypertension. Hypertension 51(1):55–61. Epub 2007/11/28
101. Boggia J, Li Y, Thijs L, Hansen TW, Kikuya M, Bjorklund-Bodegard K et al (2007) Prognostic accuracy of day versus night ambulatory blood pressure: a cohort study. Lancet 370(9594):1219–1229. Epub 2007/10/09
102. Hansen TW, Li Y, Boggia J, Thijs L, Richart T, Staessen JA (2011) Predictive role of the nighttime blood pressure. Hypertension 57(1):3–10. Epub 2010/11/17
103. Clement DL, De Buyzere ML, De Bacquer DA, de Leeuw PW, Duprez DA, Fagard RH et al (2003) Prognostic value of ambulatory blood-pressure recordings in patients with treated hypertension. N Engl J Med 348(24):2407–2415. Epub 2003/06/13
104. Fagard RH, Van Den Broeke C, De Cort P (2005) Prognostic significance of blood pressure measured in the office, at home and during ambulatory monitoring in older patients in general practice. J Hum Hypertens 19(10):801–807. Epub 2005/06/17
105. Redon J, Campos C, Narciso ML, Rodicio JL, Pascual JM, Ruilope LM (1998) Prognostic value of ambulatory blood pressure monitoring in refractory hypertension: a prospective study. Hypertension 31(2):712–718. Epub 1998/02/14
106. Dolan E, Stanton A, Thijs L, Hinedi K, Atkins N, McClory S et al (2005) Superiority of ambulatory over clinic blood pressure measurement in predicting mortality: the Dublin outcome study. Hypertension 46(1):156–161. Epub 2005/06/09
107. Hansen TW, Jeppesen J, Rasmussen S, Ibsen H, Torp-Pedersen C (2005) Ambulatory blood pressure and mortality: a population-based study. Hypertension 45(4):499–504. Epub 2005/03/09

108. Sander D, Kukla C, Klingelhofer J, Winbeck K, Conrad B (2000) Relationship between circadian blood pressure patterns and progression of early carotid atherosclerosis: a 3-year follow-up study. Circulation 102(13):1536–1541. Epub 2000/09/27
109. Lurbe E, Redon J, Kesani A, Pascual JM, Tacons J, Alvarez V et al (2002) Increase in nocturnal blood pressure and progression to microalbuminuria in type 1 diabetes. N Engl J Med 347(11):797–805. Epub 2002/09/13
110. Metoki H, Ohkubo T, Kikuya M, Asayama K, Obara T, Hashimoto J et al (2006) Prognostic significance for stroke of a morning pressor surge and a nocturnal blood pressure decline: the Ohasama study. Hypertension 47(2):149–154. Epub 2005/12/29
111. Parati G, Lombardi C, Hedner J, Bonsignore MR, Grote L, Tkacova R et al (2012) Position paper on the management of patients with obstructive sleep apnea and hypertension: joint recommendations by the European Society of Hypertension, by the European Respiratory Society and by the members of European COST (COoperation in Scientific and Technological research) ACTION B26 on obstructive sleep apnea. J Hypertens 30(4):633–646. Epub 2012/03/13
112. Parati G, Lombardi C, Hedner J, Bonsignore M, Grote L, Tkacova R et al (2013) Recommendations for the management of patients with obstructive sleep apnoea and hypertension. Eur Res J Off J Eur Soc Clini Res Physiol 41(3):523–538
113. O'Brien E, Asmar R, Beilin L, Imai Y, Mallion JM, Mancia G et al (2003) European Society of Hypertension recommendations for conventional, ambulatory and home blood pressure measurement. J Hypertens 21(5):821–848. Epub 2003/04/26
114. Oikawa T, Obara T, Ohkubo T, Kikuya M, Asayama K, Metoki H et al (2006) Characteristics of resistant hypertension determined by self-measured blood pressure at home and office blood pressure measurements: the J-HOME study. J Hypertens 24(9):1737–1743. Epub 2006/08/18
115. de la Sierra A, Banegas JR, Oliveras A, Gorostidi M, Segura J, de la Cruz JJ et al (2012) Clinical differences between resistant hypertensives and patients treated and controlled with three or less drugs. J Hypertens 30(6):1211–1216. Epub 2012/04/25
116. Pickering TG, Davidson K, Gerin W, Schwartz JE (2002) Masked hypertension. Hypertension 40(6):795–796. Epub 2002/12/07
117. Parati G, Ulian L, Santucciu C, Omboni S, Mancia G (1998) Difference between clinic and daytime blood pressure is not a measure of the white coat effect. Hypertension 31(5):1185–1189. Epub 1998/05/12
118. Muxfeldt ES, Bloch KV, Nogueira Ada R, Salles GF (2005) True resistant hypertension: is it possible to be recognized in the office? Am J Hypertens 18(12 Pt 1):1534–1540. Epub 2005/12/21
119. Oliveras A, Armario P, Hernandez-Del Rey R, Arroyo JA, Poch E, Larrousse M et al (2010) Urinary albumin excretion is associated with true resistant hypertension. J Hum Hypertens 24(1):27–33. Epub 2009/05/08
120. Pierdomenico SD, Lapenna D, Bucci A, Di Tommaso R, Di Mascio R, Manente BM et al (2005) Cardiovascular outcome in treated hypertensive patients with responder, masked, false resistant, and true resistant hypertension. Am J Hypertens 18(11):1422–1428. Epub 2005/11/11
121. Salles GF, Cardoso CR, Muxfeldt ES (2008) Prognostic influence of office and ambulatory blood pressures in resistant hypertension. Arch Intern Med 168(21):2340–2346. Epub 2008/11/26
122. Cuspidi C, Macca G, Sampieri L, Michev I, Salerno M, Fusi V et al (2001) High prevalence of cardiac and extracardiac target organ damage in refractory hypertension. J Hypertens 19(11):2063–2070. Epub 2001/10/26
123. Moser M, Setaro JF (2006) Clinical practice. Resistant or difficult-to-control hypertension. N Engl J Med 355(4):385–392. Epub 2006/07/28
124. Johansson K, Hemmingsson E, Harlid R, Trolle Lagerros Y, Granath F, Rossner S et al (2011) Longer term effects of very low energy diet on obstructive sleep apnoea in cohort derived

from randomised controlled trial: prospective observational follow-up study. BMJ 342:d3017. Epub 2011/06/03
125. Yee BJ, Phillips CL, Banerjee D, Caterson I, Hedner JA, Grunstein RR (2007) The effect of sibutramine-assisted weight loss in men with obstructive sleep apnoea. Int J Obes (Lond) 31(1):161–168. Epub 2006/05/03
126. Pannain S, Mokhlesi B (2010) Bariatric surgery and its impact on sleep architecture, sleep-disordered breathing, and metabolism. Best Pract Res Clin Endocrinol Metab 24(5):745–761. Epub 2010/11/30
127. Buchwald H, Avidor Y, Braunwald E, Jensen MD, Pories W, Fahrbach K et al (2004) Bariatric surgery: a systematic review and meta-analysis. JAMA 292(14):1724–1737. Epub 2004/10/14
128. Leech JA, Onal E, Lopata M (1992) Nasal CPAP continues to improve sleep-disordered breathing and daytime oxygenation over long-term follow-up of occlusive sleep apnea syndrome. Chest 102(6):1651–1655. Epub 1992/12/01
129. Kribbs NB, Pack AI, Kline LR, Getsy JE, Schuett JS, Henry JN et al (1993) Effects of one night without nasal CPAP treatment on sleep and sleepiness in patients with obstructive sleep apnea. Am Rev Respir Dis 147(5):1162–1168. Epub1993/05/01
130. Bradley TD, Floras JS (2009) Obstructive sleep apnoea and its cardiovascular consequences. Lancet 373(9657):82–93. Epub2008/12/23
131. Alajmi M, Mulgrew AT, Fox J, Davidson W, Schulzer M, Mak E et al (2007) Impact of continuous positive airway pressure therapy on blood pressure in patients with obstructive sleep apnea hypopnea: a meta-analysis of randomized controlled trials. Lung 185(2):67–72. Epub2007/03/30
132. Haentjens P, Van Meerhaeghe A, Moscariello A, De Weerdt S, Poppe K, Dupont A et al (2007) The impact of continuous positive airway pressure on blood pressure in patients with obstructive sleep apnea syndrome: evidence from a meta-analysis of placebo-controlled randomized trials. Arch Intern Med 167(8):757–764. Epub2007/04/25
133. Bazzano LA, Khan Z, Reynolds K, He J (2007) Effect of nocturnal nasal continuous positive airway pressure on blood pressure in obstructive sleep apnea. Hypertension 50(2):417–423. Epub2007/06/06
134. Becker HF, Jerrentrup A, Ploch T, Grote L, Penzel T, Sullivan CE et al (2003) Effect of nasal continuous positive airway pressure treatment on blood pressure in patients with obstructive sleep apnea. Circulation 107(1):68–73. Epub2003/01/08
135. Logan AG, Tkacova R, Perlikowski SM, Leung RS, Tisler A, Floras JS et al (2003) Refractory hypertension and sleep apnoea: effect of CPAP on blood pressure and baroreflex. Eur Res J Off J Eur Soc Clini Res Physiol 21(2):241–247. Epub2003/03/01
136. Dernaika TA, Kinasewitz GT, Tawk MM (2009) Effects of nocturnal continuous positive airway pressure therapy in patients with resistant hypertension and obstructive sleep apnea. J Clini Sleep Med JCSM Official Pub Am Ac Sleep Med 5(2):103–107. Epub2009/12/09
137. Barbe F, Duran-Cantolla J, Capote F, de la Pena M, Chiner E, Masa JF et al (2010) Long-term effect of continuous positive airway pressure in hypertensive patients with sleep apnea. Am J Respir Crit Care Med 181(7):718–726. Epub2009/12/17
138. Lozano L, Tovar JL, Sampol G, Romero O, Jurado MJ, Segarra A et al (2010) Continuous positive airway pressure treatment in sleep apnea patients with resistant hypertension: a randomized, controlled trial. J Hypertens 28(10):2161–2168. Epub2010/06/26
139. Hu X, Fan J, Chen S, Yin Y, Zrenner B (2015) The role of continuous positive airway pressure in blood pressure control for patients with obstructive sleep apnea and hypertension: a meta-analysis of randomized controlled trials. J Clin Hypertens (Greenwich) 17(3):215–222. Epub2015/01/15
140. Martinez-Garcia MA, Capote F, Campos-Rodriguez F, Lloberes P, Diaz de Atauri MJ, Somoza M et al (2013) Effect of CPAP on blood pressure in patients with obstructive sleep apnea and resistant hypertension: the HIPARCO randomized clinical trial. JAMA 310(22):2407–2415. Epub2013/12/12

141. Muxfeldt ES, Margallo V, Costa LM, Guimaraes G, Cavalcante AH, Azevedo JC et al (2015) Effects of continuous positive airway pressure treatment on clinic and ambulatory blood pressures in patients with obstructive sleep apnea and resistant hypertension: a randomized controlled trial. Hypertension 65(4):736–742. Epub2015/01/21
142. DiBona GF, Kopp UC (1997) Neural control of renal function. Physiol Rev 77(1):75–197. Epub1997/01/01
143. Doumas M, Faselis C, Papademetriou V (2011) Renal sympathetic denervation in hypertension. Curr Opin Nephrol Hypertens 20(6):647–653. Epub2011/09/03
144. Schlaich MP, Sobotka PA, Krum H, Lambert E, Esler MD (2009) Renal sympathetic-nerve ablation for uncontrolled hypertension. N Engl J Med 361(9):932–934. Epub2009/08/28
145. Witkowski A, Prejbisz A, Florczak E, Kadziela J, Sliwinski P, Bielen P et al (2011) Effects of renal sympathetic denervation on blood pressure, sleep apnea course, and glycemic control in patients with resistant hypertension and sleep apnea. Hypertension 58(4):559–565. Epub 2011/08/17
146. Ziegler MG, Milic M, Sun P (2011) Antihypertensive therapy for patients with obstructive sleep apnea. Curr Opin Nephrol Hypertens 20(1):50–55. Epub 2011/02/18
147. Pimenta E, Calhoun DA (2010) Treatment of resistant hypertension. J Hypertens 28(11): 2194–2195. Epub 2010/10/16

Part III

Interventions for Essential Hypertension

The Impact of Uncontrolled Hypertension on the Cerebrovascular System

6

Mónica Domenech and Antonio Coca

Abbreviations

BMI	Body mass index
BP	Blood pressure
CCB	Calcium channel blocker
CI	Confidence interval
DBP	Diastolic blood pressure
INVEST	INternational VErapamil SR-Trandolapril
MI	Myocardial infarction
NEMESIS	North East Melbourne Stroke Incidence Study
ONTARGET	Ongoing Telmisartan Alone and in combination with Ramipril Global Endpoint Trial
SBP	Systolic blood pressure
SHOT	Stroke in hypertension optimal treatment
SMMSE	Standardized Mini-Mental State Exam
Syst-Eur	Systolic Hypertension in Europe trial

6.1 Introduction

Stroke is one of the major causes not only of mortality but also of the disease burden worldwide, due to residual disability and cognitive decline. In the European Union, stroke is the second cause of mortality (10.9 %), immediately after coronary heart

M. Domenech, MD, PhD • A. Coca, MD, PhD, FRCP, FESC (✉)
Hypertension and Vascular Risk Unit, Department of Internal Medicine, Hospital Clínic, IDIBAPS, University of Barcelona, Barcelona, Spain
e-mail: acoca@clinic.ub.es

C. Tsioufis et al. (eds.), *Interventional Therapies for Secondary and Essential Hypertension*, Updates in Hypertension and Cardiovascular Protection,
DOI 10.1007/978-3-319-34141-5_6

disease (18.1 %), and accounts for approximately 200,000 deaths yearly. In Europe, stroke accounts for 5.3 % of the total burden of illness, but, due to aging of the population, it has been calculated that, by the year 2020, stroke will account for 6.2 % of the total illness burden [1]. These data emphasize the importance of stroke prevention, when the frequent post-stroke disability is taken into account: among stroke survivors aged ≥65 years, 50 % have some residual hemiparesis, 30 % are unable to walk without assistance, 26 % are dependent on others for help with daily living, 19 % have aphasia, 35 % have depressive symptoms, and 26 % are being cared for in a nursing home [2]. Although stroke mortality is high, the majority of stroke patients survive although survivors have a high risk of stroke recurrence, which account for 15–20 % of all strokes, as well as a high risk for other cardiovascular events, such as myocardial infarction [3]. Therefore, the population of patients with a history or risk of stroke is large, and primary and secondary prevention of stroke is of the greatest importance.

6.2 Blood Pressure Targets in Stroke Prevention

The relationship between stroke mortality and both systolic blood pressure (SBP) and diastolic BP (DBP) has been demonstrated in observational studies including more than one million individuals. The results of the INTERSTROKE study, an epidemiological survey in 22 countries (four of which were European), confirmed that hypertension (HTN) is the most important risk factor for stroke (with a population attributable risk of over 50 %) and is more important than other objectively measured risk factors such as lipids or glucose [4]. Therefore, one of the most important unresolved questions is how far BP should be lowered to prevent the first stroke and recurrences.

As mentioned in the European Hypertension Guidelines [5], the major body of evidence confirming the beneficial effect of BP reduction in stroke prevention comes from observational studies and, to a lesser extent, from clinical trials. On the other hand, stroke is particularly frequent in the elderly, and in all trials in elderly hypertensive patients that have shown a significant benefit of BP lowering, the mean SBP achieved remained well over 140 mmHg, whereas the two trials in which SBP values lower than 140 mmHg were achieved in the more intensely treated group failed to show significant evidence of benefits [6] (Fig. 6.1).

A *post hoc* analysis of individuals with HTN and coronary artery disease enrolled in the INternational VErapamil SR-Trandolapril (INVEST) trial showed that both the proportion of visits with BP control (SBP <140 mmHg) and mean follow-up SBP were independently related to the risk of death, nonfatal MI, and nonfatal stroke [7]. Likewise, a recent *post hoc* analysis of the Vitamin Intervention for Stroke Prevention trial [8], which included 3,680 individuals with recent (<120 days) stroke, followed for 2 years, showed that among subjects with elevated baseline SBP >75th percentile (>153 mmHg), the risks of primary and secondary outcomes were lower in those with BP-controlled ≥75 % versus <25 % of visits (adjusted hazard ratio, 0.46; 95 % confidence interval [CI], 0.26–0.84 and adjusted hazard

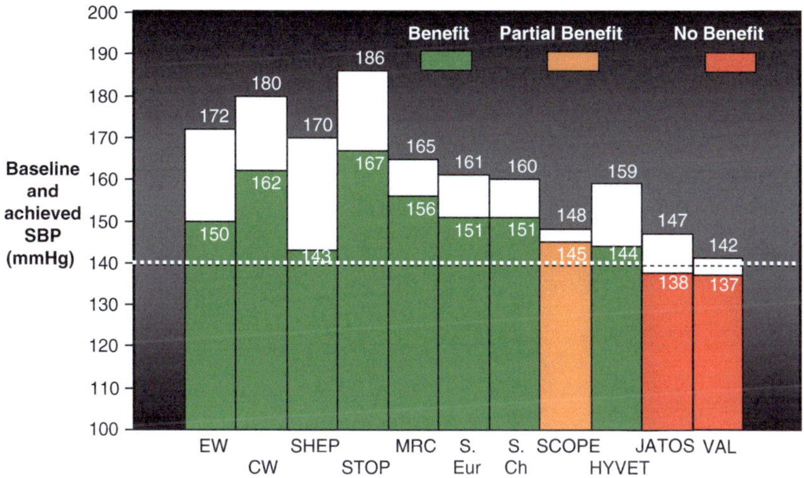

Fig. 6.1 Systolic BP achieved in elderly hypertension trials. Abbreviations: *EW* European Working Party on Hypertension in the Elderly trial, *CW* Coope and Warrander study, *SHEP* Systolic Hypertension in the Elderly Program, *STOP* Swedish Trial in Old Patients with Hypertension, *MRC* Medical Research Council trial on treatment of hypertension, *Syst-Eur* Systolic Hypertension in Europe trial, *Syst-China* Systolic Hypertension in China Trial, *SCOPE* Study on Cognition and Prognosis in the Elderly, *HYVET* Hypertension in the Very Elderly Trial, *JATOS* the Japanese Trial to Assess Optimal Systolic BP in Elderly Hypertensive Patients, *VALISH* Valsartan in Elderly Isolated Systolic Hypertension Study (Adapted from Ref. [11])

ratio, 0.51; 95 % CI, 0.32–0.82). Individuals with mean follow-up BP <140/90 mmHg had a lower risk of primary and secondary outcomes than those with BP ≥140/90 mmHg (adjusted hazard ratio, 0.76; 95 % CI, 0.59–0.98 and adjusted hazard ratio, 0.76; 95 % CI, 0.62–0.92). These data confirm that the consistency of BP control among subjects with elevated baseline SBP was linked to a reduction in the risk of recurrent stroke, myocardial infarction (MI), and vascular death (Fig. 6.2).

Similar data were published recently by Verdecchia et al. [9] where, of the 25,620 patients randomized in the Ongoing Telmisartan Alone and in combination with Ramipril Global Endpoint Trial (ONTARGET) study, 19,102 patients with coronary artery disease at baseline were selected for the analysis. The study found that, after adjustment for several potential determinants of reverse causality, a change in BP from baseline of −34/−21 mmHg (tenth percentile) was associated with a lesser risk of stroke, without any significant increase in the risk of myocardial infarction. In contrast, a rise in systolic or diastolic BP from baseline of 20/10 mmHg (90th percentile) was associated with an increased risk of stroke, while the risk of myocardial infarction increased with systolic BP but not with diastolic BP, confirming that the relationships between BP and risk are much steeper for stroke than for myocardial infarction.

However, the results of the North East Melbourne Stroke Incidence Study (NEMESIS) [10], which assessed the relationship between BP and long-term outcomes, suggest that after 5 years of follow-up of stroke survivors, those with SBP

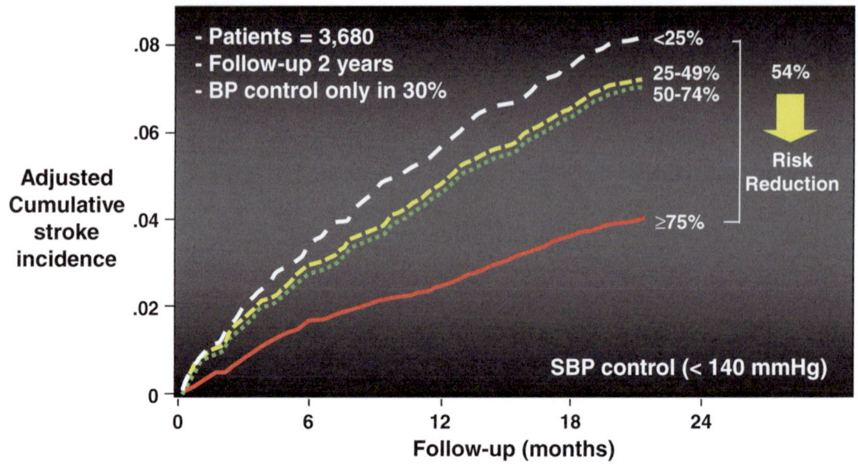

Fig. 6.2 Cumulative probability of recurrent stroke by BP control category (<25 %, 25–49 %, 50–74 %, and ≥75 %) in patients with baseline SBP >153 mmHg and recent ischemic stroke (Adapted from Ref. [8])

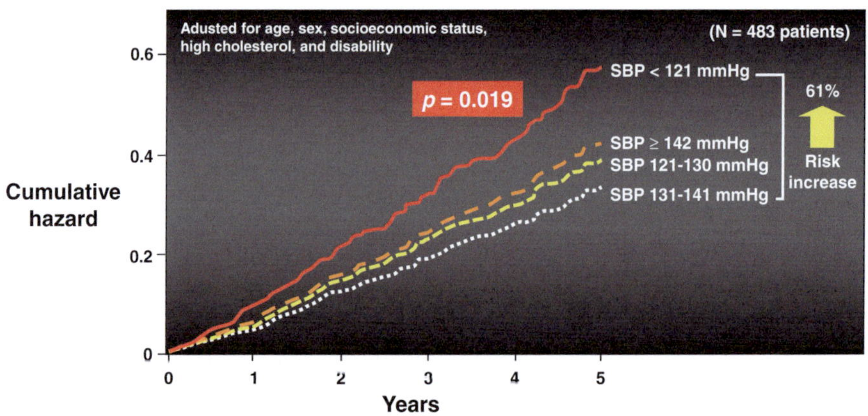

Fig. 6.3 Cumulative hazard of composite endpoint of death or nonfatal vascular event 5 years after NEMESIS entry. Adjusted for age, sex, socioeconomic status, history of high cholesterol, disability, and domicile. Years refer to the number of years between 5 and 10 years after stroke (Adapted from Ref. [10])

≤120 mmHg had a 61 % greater risk of recurrent stroke, acute myocardial infarction, and death (hazard ratio, 1.61; 95% CI, 1.08–2.41; *p=0.019*) compared with those with SBP 131–141 mmHg (Fig. 6.3). Compared with the reference category of SBP 131–141 mmHg, there were no differences in outcomes in patients with SBP 121–130 mmHg (*p = 0.491*) or 142–210 mmHg (*p = 0.313*). These findings were not modified after adjustment for the prescription of antihypertensive medications.

Therefore, there are two contrasting hypotheses with respect to BP targets: first, the lower the BP after treatment, the better the outcome and, second, the hypothesis that too low BP values are accompanied by a lower benefit and even higher risk. No specific randomized clinical trial that could answer this question has been carried out so far. For this reason, the European Society of Hypertension and the Chinese Hypertension League have designed the SHOT [11], a prospective, multinational, randomized trial with a 3×2 factorial design comparing three different SBP targets: (1) <145–135, (2) <135–125, and (3) <125 mmHg in 7,500 patients aged ≥65 years (2,500 in Europe, 5,000 in China) with hypertension and stroke or transient ischemic attack 1–6 months before randomization. It is hoped that the results of this trial will shed light on these opposing hypotheses.

6.3 Uncontrolled BP and Cognitive Decline and Dementia

There is growing awareness that vascular risk factors increase the risk of dementia, with plentiful evidence linking HTN to a later risk of cognitive decline and dementia [12]. Placebo-controlled clinical trials of antihypertensive drugs have, however, found little evidence to suggest that BP lowering reduces the risk of cognitive decline and dementia [13, 14]. In addition, the benefit observed in several trials seems to be similar for different antihypertensive strategies, regardless of the drug class, with the beneficial effects being on overall cognition (effect size, 0.05; 95 % CI, 0.02–0.07) and all cognitive functions except language [15]. In the meta-analysis by Levi et al. [15] of all clinical trials with antihypertensive drugs in which the incidence of dementia during treatment was assessed, antihypertensive treatment reduced the risk of all-cause dementia by 9 % compared to the control group (hazard ratio, 0.91; 95 % CI, 0.89–0.94), when randomized trials and observational studies were combined ($n = 15$).

The best results were observed in the Systolic Hypertension in Europe (Syst-Eur) trial [16, 17], which found a 50 % reduction in the incidence of dementia (vascular and Alzheimer's disease), over a median 2-year follow-up in participants aged ≥60 years. The treatment strategy was based on a CCB, although a combination with an angiotensin-converting enzyme inhibitor was needed in more than 80 % of patients to achieve BP control, suggesting that CCBs may have neuroprotective effects in addition to the BP lowering effect, protecting against calcium dysregulation, reducing neuronal calcium influx and consequent neuronal damage [18, 19]. However, this supposed beneficial effect has not been confirmed in all studies, and some have even suggested that CCBs are associated with a lesser decline in cognitive function [20, 21], whereas others found the opposite [22]. A recent review [23] that included nine studies (only one clinical trial that compared CCBs with placebo) concluded that there is no clear evidence to suggest that CCB use increases or decreases the risk of cognitive decline or dementia in the very elderly.

Finally, in a very recent population-based cohort study, the Newcastle 85+ Study [24], which included 238 hypertensive patients on antihypertensive treatment, an association between CCB use and less cognitive decline over the 3-year follow-up was found: the rate of decline was lower by 1.29 Standardized Mini-Mental State Exam (SMMSE) points (95 % CI, 0.16–2.42; $p=0.03$) in patients receiving CCBs compared with those taking other antihypertensive classes after adjustment for age, sex, years of education, baseline SMMSE score, smoking, body mass index (BMI), baseline BP, and incident cerebrovascular events. This finding was even stronger in the cognitively intact (SMMSE >24), in whom the rate of cognitive decline was 1.33 SMMSE points lower (95 % CI, 0.30–2.37; $p=0.01$). These results provide partial support for an association between CCB use and a lower rate of cognitive decline in very old adults with hypertension, emphasizing the need for robust clinical trials to determine which BP thresholds and targets are appropriate for a number of patient groups with increased cardiovascular risk, including those with stroke. Meanwhile, it would seem prudent to achieve strict BP control with values lower than 140/90 mmHg in the majority of patients in order to reduce the risk of the first stroke and cognitive decline and, perhaps, to lower values in secondary stroke prevention in patients with lacunar stroke [25].

References

1. Murray CJ, Lopez A (2006) The global burden of disease. Harvard University Press, Boston
2. Di Carlo A, Baldereschi M, Gandolfo C, Candelise L, Ghetti A, Maggi S et al (2003) Stroke in an elderly population: Incidence and impact on survival and daily function. The Italian Longitudinal Study on Aging. Cerebrovasc Dis 16:141–150
3. Touze' E, Varenne O, Chatellier G, Peyrard S, Rothwell PM, Mas JL (2005) Risk of myocardial infarction and vascular death after transient ischaemic attack and ischaemic stroke: a systematic review and meta-analysis. Stroke 36:2748–2755
4. O'Donnell MJ, Xavier D, Liu L, Zhang H, Chin SL, Rao-Melacini P et al (2010) Risk factors for ischaemic and intracerebral haemorrhagic stroke in 22 countries (the INTERSTROKE study): a case-control study. Lancet 376:112–123
5. Mancia G, Fagard R, Narkiewicz K, Redon J, Zanchitti A, Bohm M et al (2013) The task force for the management of arterial hypertension of the European Society of Hypertension (ESH) and of the European Society of Cardiology (ESC). 2013 ESH/ESC guidelines for the management of arterial hypertension. J Hypertens 31:1281–1357
6. Zanchetti A, Grassi G, Mancia G (2009) When should antihypertensive drug treatment be initiated and to what level should systolic blood pressure be lowered? A critical reappraisal. J Hypertens 27:923–934
7. Mancia G, Messerli F, Bakris G, Zhou Q, Champion A, Pepine CJ (2007) Blood pressure control and improved cardiovascular outcomes in the International Verapamil SR-Trandolapril Study. Hypertension 50:299–305
8. Towfighi A, Markovic D, Ovbiagele B (2014) Consistency of blood pressure control after ischemic stroke: prevalence and prognosis. Stroke 45(5):1313–1317
9. Verdecchia P, Reboldi G, Angeli F, Trimarco B, Mancia G, Pogue J, Gao P, Sleight P, Teo K, Yusuf S (2015) Systolic and diastolic blood pressure changes in relation with myocardial infarction and stroke in patients with coronary artery disease. Hypertension 65(1):108–114
10. Kim J, Gall SL, Nelson MR, Sharman JE, Thrift AG (2014) Lower systolic blood pressure is associated with poorer survival in long-term survivors of stroke. J Hypertens 32(4):904–911
11. Zanchetti A, Liu L, Mancia G, Parati G, Grassi G, Stramba-Badiale M et al (2014) Blood pressure and LDL-cholesterol targets for prevention of recurrent strokes and cognitive decline in the hypertensive patient: design of the European Society of Hypertension-Chinese Hypertension

League Stroke in Hypertension Optimal Treatment randomized trial. J Hypertens 32(9):1888–1897
12. Tzourio C, Dufouil C, Ducimetie're P, Alpe'rovitch A, The EVA study group (1999) Cognitive decline in individuals with high blood pressure: a longitudinal study in the elderly. Neurology 53:1948–1952
13. Peters R, Beckett N, Forette F, Tuomilehto J, Clarke R, Ritchie C et al (2008) Incident dementia and blood pressure lowering in the hypertension in the very elderly trial cognitive function assessment (HYVET-COG): a double-blind, placebo-controlled trial. Lancet Neurol 7:683–689
14. Shah K, Qureshi S, Johnson M, Parikh N, Schulz P, Kunik M (2009) Does use of antihypertensive drugs affect the incidence or progression of dementia? A systematic review. Am J Geriatr Pharmacother 7:v250–v261
15. Levi Marpillat N, Macquin-Mavier I, Tropeano AI, Bachoud-Levi AC, Maison P (2013) Antihypertensive classes, cognitive decline and incidence of dementia: a network meta-analysis. J Hypertens 31(6):1073–1082
16. Forette F, Seux M, Staessen J, Thijs L, Birkenha¨ger W, Babarskiene MR et al (1998) Prevention of dementia in a randomised double-blind placebo-controlled systolic hypertension in Europe (SYST-EUR) trial. Lancet 352:1347–1351
17. Forette F, Seux M, Staessen J, Thijs L, Babarskiene M, Babeanu S et al (2002) Systolic hypertension in Europe investigators. The prevention of dementia with antihypertensive treatment. Arch Int Med 162:2046–2052
18. Mason R, Leeds P, Jacob R, Hough C, Zhang K, Mason P et al (1999) Inhibition of excessive neuronal apoptosis by the calcium antagonist amlodipine and antioxidants in cerebellar granule cells. J Neurochem 72:1448–1456
19. Tomassioni D, Lanari A, Silvestrelli G, Traini E, Amenta F (2008) Nimodipine and its use in cerebrovascular disease: evidence from recent preclinical and controlled clinical studies. Clin Exp Hypertens 30:744–766
20. Trompet S, Westendorp R, Kamper A, Craen A (2008) Use of calcium antagonists and cognitive decline in old age. The Leiden 85-plus study. Neurobiol Aging 29:306–308
21. Paran E, Anson O, Lowenthal D (2010) Cognitive function and antihypertensive treatment in the elderly: a 6-year follow-up study. Am J Ther 17:358–364
22. Maxwell C, Hogan D, Ebly E (1999) Calcium-channel blockers and cognitive function in elderly people: results from the Canadian study of health and aging. Can Med Assoc J 161:501–506
23. Peters R, Booth A, Peters J (2014) A systematic review of calcium channel blocker use and cognitive decline/dementia in the elderly. J Hypertens 32:1945–1958
24. Peters R, Collerton J, Granic A, Davies K, Kirkwood T, Jagger C (2015) Antihypertensive drug use and risk of cognitive decline in the very old: an observational study: the New castle 85+ Study. J Hypertens 33:2156–2164
25. Odden MC, McClure LA, Sawaya BP, White CL, Peralta CA, Field TS et al (2016) Achieved blood pressure and outcomes in the secondary prevention of small subcortical strokes trial. Hypertension 67:63–69

The Impact of Uncontrolled Hypertension on the Heart

7

Enrico Agabiti Rosei and Massimo Salvetti

Abbreviations

LVH	Left ventricular hypertrophy
BP	Blood pressure
CHD	Coronary heart disease
DBP	Diastolic blood pressure
HTN	Hypertension
LV	Left ventricular
SBP	Systolic blood pressure
CV	Cardiovascular

Available data indicate that raised blood pressure (BP) represents the greatest single contributor to the global burden of disease and to global mortality [1]. According to the results of a large meta-analysis that included about one million adults, each increase in systolic BP (SBP) of 20 mm Hg and/or each 10 mm Hg increase in diastolic BP (DBP) doubles the risk of fatal coronary events [2]. The relationship between BP and coronary heart disease (CHD) mortality may be recognized even below the traditional thresholds for hypertension (HTN), being evident over the BP

E. Agabiti Rosei (✉)
Department of Clinical and Experimental Sciences, University of Brescia, Owensboro, KY, USA

Department of Medicine, Azienda Spedali Civili di Brescia, European Society of Hypertension, Gardone Val Trompia, Italy
e-mail: enrico.agabitirosei@unibs.it

M. Salvetti
Department of Clinical and Experimental Sciences, University of Brescia, Owensboro, KY, USA

C. Tsioufis et al. (eds.), *Interventional Therapies for Secondary and Essential Hypertension*, Updates in Hypertension and Cardiovascular Protection,
DOI 10.1007/978-3-319-34141-5_7

range of 115/75–185/115 mm Hg; the increased risk is evident for all ages, although the absolute risk increases with increasing age. Several risk factors for CHD, such as dyslipidemia, diabetes mellitus, obesity, and sedentary habits, are frequently associated with HTN and contribute to the increased risk of CHD.

7.1 Mechanisms

Several mechanisms contribute to the pathogenesis of cardiac damage in HTN.

Hypertension favors the development of *atherosclerosis* in several vascular beds and in particular in the coronary vasculature, thereby favoring acute and chronic myocardial ischemia. In hypertensive patients, *endothelial dysfunction* may reduce the vasodilator capacity and contribute to thrombosis. In addition, in hypertensive patients, *alterations of the microcirculation* are frequently observed. Perivascular fibrosis, media hypertrophy with increase of vascular media to lumen ratio, and capillary rarefaction may all favor the occurrence of myocardial ischemia, also in the absence of epicardial coronary artery disease. Myocardial ischemia may also be favored by the development of *left ventricular hypertrophy (LVH)*. LVH is not uncommon in hypertensive patients: using the echocardiographic technique, it has been demonstrated that the prevalence of LVH in the Framingham population increases from 5 % in subjects younger than 30 years to 50 % in those older than 70 years [3]. LVH is initially a useful compensatory process that represents an adaptation to increased ventricular wall stress but is also the first step toward the development of an overt clinical disease in hypertensive patients. In fact, the increase in left ventricular (LV) mass leads to an imbalance of myocardial oxygen demand and supply and to a reduction in coronary flow reserve. Furthermore, LVH in hypertensive patients represents an important step toward the development of overt congestive heart failure. Hypertension is the most important modifiable risk factor for *heart failure* [4, 5] and increases the risk for heart failure in all age groups. It has been calculated that in subjects aged 40 years or older with increased BP, the lifetime risk of developing heart failure is double than that of subjects with BP lower than 140/90 mm Hg. For congestive heart failure occurring in the absence of myocardial infarction, it has been calculated that lifetime risk is one in nine for men and one in six for women, which indicates that the risk of heart failure is largely attributable to HTN. Hypertension can lead directly to the development of heart failure by several mechanisms, alone or in combination, such as hemodynamic load, decreased intrinsic myocardial contractility, adverse chamber remodeling and LVH, coronary microvascular disease with impaired coronary hemodynamics, and ventricular fibrosis.

7.2 Detection of Cardiac Damage in Hypertension

Early detection of preclinical cardiac damage is crucial for the maximal reduction of cardiovascular (CV) risk. In fact, organ damage represents an intermediate step in the chain of events that, from high BP values, often associated to other CV risk factors leads to clinical complications.

Electrocardiography represents a simple and inexpensive tool for the detection of LVH; several diagnostic criteria can be used, and, despite the low sensitivity, LVH diagnosed by the Sokolow-Lyon index or the Cornell voltage-duration product has been shown to be an independent predictor of cardiovascular events [4, 6]. Electrocardiography can also be used to detect patterns of repolarization abnormalities and arrhythmias, including atrial fibrillation [4]. Echocardiography is a specific, repeatable, and far more sensitive measure of LVH in comparison with *Electrocardiography*. The accuracy of echocardiography has been validated with measurements obtained by necroscopic examination. Left ventricular hypertrophy is usually diagnosed when LV mass exceeds 115 g/m^2 in men and 95 g/m^2 in women [7], but the relationship between LV mass and incidence of cardiovascular events is continuous. Concentric LV hypertrophy is associated with the highest risk of cardiovascular events. Indices of systolic and diastolic function (as assessed by 2-D, Doppler, and tissue Doppler echocardiography) and left atrial volume may also add further prognostic information. Also segmental wall motion abnormalities have been shown to be predictive of cardiovascular events, being a possible manifestation of coronary heart disease. If present, they require testing for CHD. It is well known that the noninvasive *detection of cardiac ischemia* may be challenging in hypertensive patients. Exercise treadmill test remains the first step also in hypertensive patients, but the specificity and sensitivity is lower as compared to the majority of patients, although substantial variation exists in different studies (sensitivity and specificity of 68 % and 77 % in a large meta-analysis, but with very large variability, i.e., from 17 to 100 %) [8, 9]. Therefore, when the exercise treadmill test is positive or non-diagnostic, a stress echocardiogram (exercise or, as an alternative, pharmacological) may be useful in order to further refine the diagnosis. Stress echocardiography should be considered as first line test when baseline electrocardiographic abnormalities and/or LVH is present. As an alternative, myocardial perfusion scintigraphy may be used: in hypertensive patients a sensitivity of 85–90 % and a specificity of about 70 % have been reported, but the presence of LVH may reduce its overall accuracy. Multi-detector computer tomography allows the direct evaluation of the coronary vascular bed, but the issue of radiation risk should be taken into account. Indication for coronary angiography should be always carefully evaluated, in consideration of its invasive nature, of the possible complications, and of the peculiar pathophysiological characteristics of these patients.

7.3 Treatment

Five decades of randomized clinical trials and a number of meta-analyses performed after 1990 [10–13] have clearly demonstrated that BP lowering reduces cardiovascular events and mortality, with relative risk reductions that are proportional to the magnitude of the BP lowering achieved. As also shown in the first, pioneering clinical trials, antihypertensive treatment is capable of reducing all types of complications associated with raised BP. A recent large meta-analysis [12] has further confirmed that stroke and heart failure are the events most effectively prevented by BP lowering (heart failure to an even larger extent than stroke) and has also shown that CHD and cardiovascular and all-cause mortality are also significantly reduced. A reduction of 10 mm Hg SBP and 5 mm Hg DBP was found to be associated with a reduction in the risk of heart failure of 43 % and of CHD of 16 %. Similarly, in another very recent meta-analysis [13] for a 10 mm Hg reduction in systolic BP, a 28 % reduction in the risk of heart failure and a 17 % reduction in the risk of CHD were observed.

Importantly, antihypertensive treatment has also been found very effective in regressing LVH [4, 9], an intermediate phenotype in the progression of hypertensive heart disease that is associated to an increased risk of adverse outcomes. Treatment-induced regression of LVH has been found associated to a reduced risk of future cardiovascular complications, independently of possible confounders [4, 9] and may be considered among the goals of antihypertensive treatment.

7.4 What Is Uncontrolled Hypertension for Cardiac Complications?

Despite increased awareness of the importance of BP lowering and the availability of effective and well-tolerated antihypertensive drugs, BP values remain above target in a significant proportion of hypertensive patients in Europe and worldwide [14–16]; in particular, European data indicate that BP is controlled in less than one third of treated hypertensives. Inadequate BP control is likely to be responsible for a remarkable excess of morbid events; despite this, only few studies have specifically analyzed the additional CV risk related to poor BP control. In a group of 4714 French men treated for hypertension (mean age 50 years, mainly uncomplicated hypertensives) [17], those with uncontrolled BP (i.e., BP ≥140/90 mm Hg) had a statistically significant increase in relative risk for CV mortality (1.66; 95 % CI, 1.04–2.64) and for CHD mortality (2.35; 95 % CI, 1.03–5.35) as compared with subjects with controlled BP values, even after adjustment for possible confounders. In this study, the relationship between on-treatment SBP and CV disease risk was linear (Fig. 7.1); the relative risk (RR) for adjusted CV disease and CHD mortality was approximately 2.5 times higher in treated hypertensive men with SBP values over 160 mm Hg than those with SBP values <140 mm Hg.

Another study from the same authors evaluated a large group of 8,893 treated hypertensives and 25,880 age and gender matched untreated normotensive and hypertensive subjects. Treated hypertensives had higher BP values (SBP + 15 mm Hg, DBP + 9 mm Hg), a higher prevalence of associated comorbidities and concomitant CV risk factors, including an increased prevalence of LVH. After a follow-up of 8–12 years, 2,317 fatal events were observed. Treated hypertensive subjects had an almost twofold increase in CV disease and CHD mortality compared with untreated subjects. In a multivariable model that adjusted for associated risk factors, the increased mortality in treated subjects persisted: relative risk (RR) 1.52; 95 % CI, 1.33–1.74 for cardiovascular mortality and RR 1.49, 95 % CI, 1.19–1.86 for coronary mortality. Interestingly, when authors introduced SBP in the statistical model (Fig. 7.2), the difference between treated and untreated subjects was

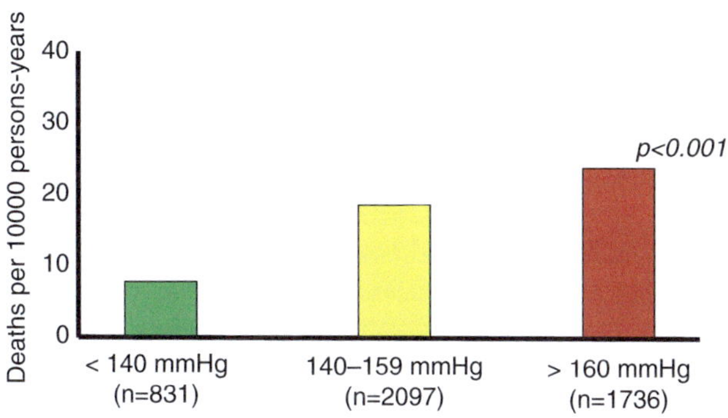

Fig. 7.1 Age-adjusted CHD mortality rates according to SBP in men treated for hypertension (Data from Ref. [17])

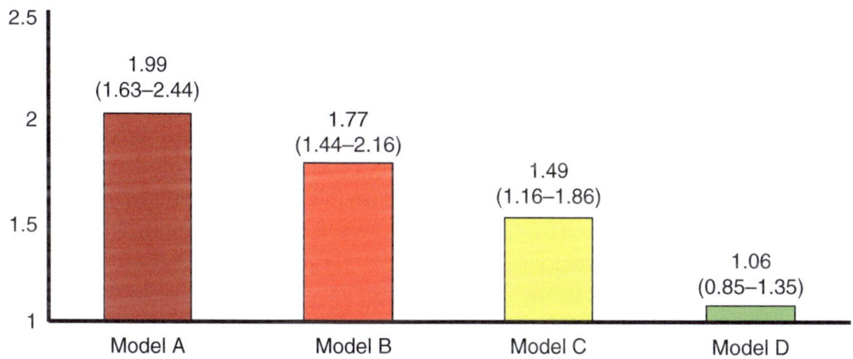

Fig. 7.2 Risk ratios for CHD mortality in treated versus untreated subjects. *Model A* unadjusted RR, *Model B* adjusted for unmodifiable CVD risk factors. *Model C* includes Model B plus modifiable CVD risk factors, *Model D* includes Model C, plus adjustment for systolic blood pressure (Adapted from Ref. [18])

nonsignificant (CV disease (RR, 1.10; 95 % CI, 0.88–1.33) and CHD (RR, 1.08; 95 % CI, 0.85–1.32)) [18]. These results indicate that uncontrolled BP plays a major role in the excess risk of cardiac events observed in treated hypertensive individuals.

More recently, Benner and coworkers applied the Framingham risk equations in order to calculate a 4-year risk of CHD in the population included in the 1999–2002 National Health and Nutrition Examination Survey (NHANES) datasets [19]. Hypertension and cholesterol levels were then statistically "controlled" to ideal levels, and risks were recalculated. When BP and cholesterol were statistically "controlled," the 4-year risk of CHD events declined from 7.3 to 3.5 %. The analysis suggested that 64 % of 4-year risk of CHD was attributable to uncontrolled BP and lipids.

As far as the risk of congestive heart failure is concerned, an analysis performed in the Cardiovascular Health Study population showed that uncontrolled HTN was highly prevalent (54 %) and was associated with older age and LVH [20]. After propensity score matching, when uncontrolled HTN was compared with controlled HTN, the matched hazard ratio of congestive heart failure during 13 years of follow-up was 1.39 (95 % CI 1.12–1.73; $p = .003$) (Fig. 7.3). The persistence of an increased risk for heart failure after propensity score matching suggests that the increased incidence of heart failure observed in patients with uncontrolled HTN in this study may not be explained by imbalances in baseline characteristics.

Uncontrolled HTN has been found associated with subsequent increased risk of cardiac complications also in patients with resistant HTN. In the population-based Reasons for Geographic And Racial Differences in Stroke (REGARDS) Study [21], in uncontrolled patients with apparent treatment-resistant HTN) (≥3 medication classes and BP ≥140/90 mm Hg), as compared to patients with controlled resistant HTN (≥4 medication classes and BP <140/90 mm Hg), a significantly increased risk of CHD (hazzard ratio (HR), 2.33; 95 % CI, 1.21–4.48) was observed (Fig. 7.4) during a follow-up period of 4.4 years, after full multivariable adjustment. Similarly, in patients included in the Antihypertensive and Lipid-Lowering Treatment to Prevent Heart Attack Trial (ALLHAT) study [22], participants with true resistant HTN and BP not at goal had a higher incidence rate of various outcomes, and in particular of CHD (HR 1.43, 95 % CI 1.16–1.76) and congestive heart failure (CHF) (HR 1.91 95 % CI 1.53–2.39). Interestingly, achievement of target BP in patients previously diagnosed as having resistant HTN is associated to a better prognosis. Fatemi et al. [23] identified a group of veterans with resistant HTN at a first visit. At a second follow-up visit, after 3 years, patients were divided into two groups: those in whom BP was still uncontrolled and those with controlled BP. After further 6 years, patients with controlled BP at the second visit had a 46 % lower risk of all-cause mortality; authors, however, did not report specific cause mortality and CV event rates.

7.5 The Issue of BP Target

Another relevant aspect is related to the optimal BP target to be reached in hypertensive patients in order to obtain the maximal prevention of cardiac complications.

Very recently the results of the systolic blood pressure intervention trial (SPRINT) study [24], which enrolled high risk patients with an age of >55 years, with BP values >130 mm Hg, have suggested that targeting an SBP of less than 120 mm Hg may result in lower rates of fatal and nonfatal major CV events and death from any cause. Considering cardiac events, the analysis of the pre-specified secondary outcomes of acute myocardial infarction and acute coronary syndromes did not show any significant difference between groups (HR 0.83, 95 % CI 0.64–1.09 and HR 1.00, 95 % CI 0.64–1.55 for the two outcomes, respectively, p = n.s.).On the contrary, authors reported a statistically significant difference in the risk of heart failure, being less 38 % in favor of the intensive treatment strategy, which also strongly contributed to the difference in the primary outcome. Recent interesting findings might support a more intensive strategy for the reduction of heart failure in hypertensive patients: a post hoc analysis of the Action to Control Cardiovascular Risk in

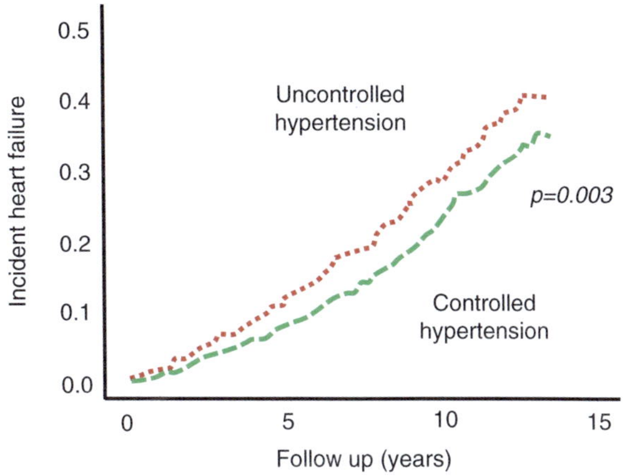

Fig. 7.3 Kaplan-Meier plots for incident heart failure by uncontrolled hypertension (BP ≥ 140 and or 90 mm Hg) in a propensity-matched cohort of Cardiovascular Health Study participants (Adapted form Ref. [20])

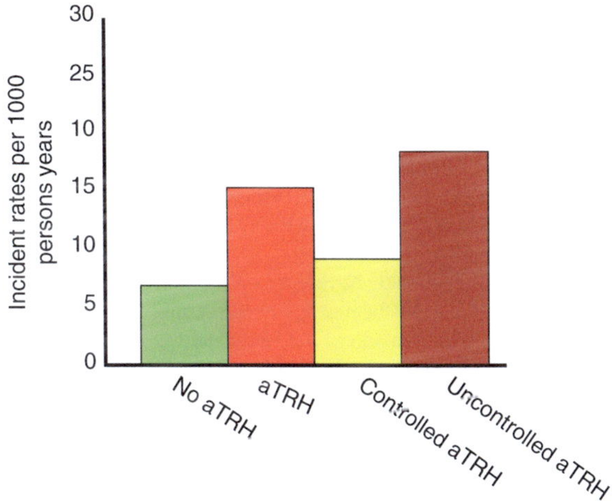

Fig. 7.4 Incidence rates of stroke, coronary heart disease, and all-cause mortality among REGARDS participants with and without apparent treatment-resistant hypertension (Adapted from Ref. [21])

Diabetes (ACCORD) trial has shown that targeting a systolic BP of <120 mm Hg as compared with <140 mm Hg produces a greater reduction in electrocardiographic indices of LVH [25]. In fact, after a median follow-up of 4.4 years, intensive, compared with standard, BP lowering was associated with a 39 % lower risk of LVH (OR 0.61, 95 % CI 0.43–0.88; $p=0.008$) [26]. Similarly, in the Cardio-Sis trial, in hypertensive nondiabetic patients, lowering of SBP to <130 mm Hg decreased the likelihood of electrocardiographic LVH by 39 %, compared with usual lowering to SBP <140 mm Hg [26]. These results could give some pathophysiological background to the consistent reduction in the incidence of heart failure observed in SPRINT.

Conclusions

Epidemiological data indicate that HTN remains one of the most important precursors to the development of cardiac complications. Blood pressure control is largely insufficient and is responsible for an excess risk of cardiac complications and death. Improvement of BP control is likely to represent the most effective strategy for the prevention of cardiac complication in the population.

References

1. Global Burden of Metabolic Risk Factors for Chronic Diseases Collaboration (2014) Cardiovascular disease, chronic kidney disease, and diabetes mortality burden of cardiometabolic risk factors from 1980 to 2010: a comparative risk assessment. Lancet Diabetes Endocrinol 2(8):634–647
2. Lewington S, Clarke R, Qizilbash N, Peto R, Collins R, Prospective Studies Collaboration (2002) Age-specific relevance of usual blood pressure to vascular mortality: a meta-analysis of individual data for one million adults in 61 prospective studies [published correction appears in Lancet. 2002;361:1060]. Lancet 360:1903–1913
3. Kaplan NM (1995) Multiple risk factors for coronary heart disease in patients with hypertension. J Hypertens 13(Suppl 2):S1–S5
4. Agabiti Rosei E, Muiesan ML (2011) Hypertension and left ventricular hypertrophy. Eur Soc Hypertens Sci Newslet 2:No. 10R. www.eshonline.org
5. Kazzam E, Ghurbana BA, Obineche EN, Nicholls MG (2005) Hypertension: still an important cause of heart failure ? J Hum Hypert 19:267–275
6. Vakili B, Okin P, Devereux RB (2001) Prognostic implications of left ventricular hypertrophy. Am Heart J 141:334–341
7. Mancia G, Fagard R, Narkiewicz K, Redon J, Zanchetti A, Bohm M et al (2013) 2013 ESH/ESC guidelines for the management of arterial hypertension: the task force for the management of arterial hypertension of the European Society of Hypertension (ESH) and of the European Society of Cardiology (ESC). J Hypertens 31(7):1281–1357
8. Tsioufis C, Dimitriadis K, Thomopoulos C, Manolis A, Agabiti Rosei E (2012) How to identify coronary artery disease in an asymptomatic hypertensive patient? Eur Soc Hypertens Sci Newslet 13:No. 54. www.eshonline.org
9. Agabiti Rosei E, de Simone G, Mureddu G et al (2008) Arterial hypertension and cardiac damage. Diagnostic and therapeutic guidelines. High Blood Press Cardiovasc Prev 15:141–170
10. Zanchetti A (2005) Evidence-based medicine in hypertension: what type of evidence? J Hypertens 23:1113–1120
11. Collins R, Peto R, MacMahon S, Godwin J, Qizilbash N, Hebert P et al (1990) Blood pressure, stroke, and coronary heart disease. Part 2. Short-term reductions in blood pressure: overview of randomised drug trials in their epidemiological context. Lancet 335:827–839
12. Thomopoulos C, Parati G, Zanchetti A (2014) Effects of blood pressure lowering on outcome incidence in hypertension. 1. Overview, meta-analyses, and meta-regression analyses of randomized trials. J Hypertens 32:2285–2295
13. Ettehad D, Emdin CA, Kiran A, Anderson SG, Callender T, Emberson J, Chalmers J, Rodgers A, Rahimi K (2015) Blood pressure lowering for prevention of cardiovascular disease and death: a systematic review and meta-analysis. Lancet 387:957–967 [Epub ahead of print]
14. Grassi G, Cifkova R, Laurent S, Narkiewicz K, Redon J, Farsang C, Viigimaa M, Erdine S, Brambilla G, Bombelli M, Dell'Oro R, Notari M, Mancia G (2011) Blood pressure control and cardiovascular risk profile in hypertensive patients from central and eastern European countries: results of the BP-CARE study. Eur Heart J 32(2):218–225

15. Tocci G, Ferrucci A, Pontremoli R, Ferri C, Rosei EA, Morganti A, Trimarco B, Mancia G, Borghi C, Volpe M (2015) Blood pressure levels and control in Italy: comprehensive analysis of clinical data from 2000–2005 and 2005–2011 hypertension surveys. J Hum Hypertens 29(11):696–701
16. American Heart Association Statistics Committee and Stroke Statistics Subcommittee (2015) Heart disease and stroke statistics – 2015 update: a report from the American Heart Association. Circulation 131(4):e29–e322
17. Benetos A, Thomas F, Bean K, Gautier S, Smulyan H, Guize L (2002) Prognostic value of systolic and diastolic blood pressure in treated hypertensive men. Arch Intern Med 162(5):577–581
18. Benetos A, Thomas F, Bean KE, Guize L (2003) Why cardiovascular mortality is higher in treated hypertensives versus subjects of the same age, in the general population. J Hypertens 21(9):1635–1640
19. Benner J, Smith T, Petrilla A, Klingman D, Goel S, Tang S, Wong N (2008) Estimated prevalence of uncontrolled hypertension and multiple cardiovascular risk factors and their associated risk of coronary heart disease in the United States. J Am Soc Hypertens 2(1):44–53
20. Iyer A, Ahmed M, Filippatos G, Ekundayo J, Aban I, Love T, Nanda N, Bakris G, Fonarow G, Aronow W, Ahmed A (2010) Uncontrolled hypertension and increased risk for incident heart failure in older adults with hypertension: findings from a propensity-matched prospective population study. J Am Soc Hypertens 4(1):22–31
21. Irvin M, Booth J, Shimbo D, Lackland D, Oparil S, Howard G, Safford M, Muntner P, Calhoun D (2014) Apparent treatment-resistant hypertension and risk for stroke, coronary heart disease, and all-cause mortality. J Am Soc Hypertens 8(6):405–413
22. Muntner P, Davis B, Cushman W, Bangalore S, Calhoun D, Pressel S, Black H, Kostis J, Probstfield J, Whelton P, Rahman M, ALLHAT Collaborative Research Group (2014) Treatment-resistant hypertension and the incidence of cardiovascular disease and end-stage renal disease: results from the Antihypertensive and Lipid-Lowering Treatment to Prevent Heart Attack Trial (ALLHAT). Hypertension 64(5):1012–1021
23. Fatemi O, Faselis C, Kokkinos P, Papademetriou V (2016) Improvement in all-cause mortality with blood pressure control in a group of US Veterans with drug-resistant hypertension. J Clin Hypertens (Greenwich) 18(1):33–39
24. SPRINT Research Group (2015) A randomized trial of intensive versus standard blood-pressure control. N Engl J Med 373:2103–2116 [Epub ahead of print]
25. Soliman E, Byington R, Bigger T, Evans G, Okin P, David C, Goff DC Jr, Chen H (2015) Effect of intensive blood pressure lowering on left ventricular hypertrophy in patients with diabetes mellitus. Action to control cardiovascular risk in diabetes blood pressure trial. Hypertension 66:1123–1129
26. Verdecchia P, Staessen JA, Angeli F, de Simone G, Achilli A, Ganau A, Mureddu G, Pede S, Maggioni AP, Lucci D, Reboldi G, Cardio-Sis Investigators (2009) Usual versus tight control of systolic blood pressure in nondiabetic patients with hypertension (Cardio-Sis): an open-label randomised trial. Lancet 374:525–533

Optimization of Antihypertensive Drug Treatment in Resistant Hypertension

8

Giuseppe Mancia

Abbreviations

ACE	Angiotensin-converting enzyme
BP	Blood pressure
DBP	Diastolic blood pressure
dRHTN	Drug-resistant hypertension
RAS	Renin-angiotensin system
SBP	Systolic blood pressure

8.1 Introduction

When a truly drug-resistant hypertension (dRHTN) has been identified [1], physicians have to decide which therapeutic option might offer the best chance to effectively lower the elevated blood pressure (BP) values, hopefully leading the patient's status to BP control (<140/90 mmHg) [1, 2]. Although invasive procedures such as renal denervation and carotid baroreflex stimulation can achieve this goal in a number of patients [3, 4], there is no question that the first treatment approach to consider is the (1) removal of lifestyle factors that may oppose the BP lowering effect of the administered drugs, such as a high intake of salt, abuse of alcohol, obesity [5, 6] or co-treatments that have direct or indirect pressor effects [7] and (2) modification of the existing treatment regimen by an increase of the dose or the extension of the

G. Mancia
IRCCS Istituto Auxologico Italiano and Policlinico di Monza,
University of Milano-Bicocca, Milan, Italy
e-mail: giuseppe.mancia@unimib.it

C. Tsioufis et al. (eds.), *Interventional Therapies for Secondary and Essential Hypertension*, Updates in Hypertension and Cardiovascular Protection,
DOI 10.1007/978-3-319-34141-5_8

medicaments already prescribed. This chapter will discuss how to make the best use of the medicament option.

8.2 Rationalization of the Three Drug Treatment Regimen

Hypertension guidelines emphasize the need for combination treatment to be based on drugs with different and complementary mechanisms of the BP lowering effect. They recommend a three drug combination to make use of a diuretic, a blocker of the renin-angiotensin system (RAS), be it an angiotensin-converting enzyme (ACE) inhibitor or an angiotensin receptor antagonist and a calcium channel blocker because this fulfils the above requirement and has been shown to markedly reduce BP (up to 30–40 mmHg reduction of systolic values) in hypertensive patients with a variety of clinical characteristics [8–10]. In resistant hypertensive patients under treatment with three drugs, a therapeutic option is thus to ensure that a diuretic/RAS blocker/calcium channel blocker combination is used, provided that (1) no contra-indication to one or another of these drugs exists or (2) the clinical condition of the patient requires other drugs to be part of the combination, such as a beta-blocker in patients with a history of coronary disease or heart failure. Of special importance is the inclusion of a diuretic in the three drug treatment regimen because diuretics enhance the antihypertensive effect of most antihypertensive agents, and difficult-to-treat hypertension may not rarely be associated with sodium and fluid retention as well as hypervolemia [11].

8.3 Increasing the Dose of the Prescribed Three Drugs

Drug underdosing is frequent in treated hypertensive patients; its high prevalence is one of the factors responsible for the low rate of BP control exhibited by the hypertensive population worldwide [12]. Careful checking of the drug doses prescribed (or assumed) is thus mandatory when dealing with a BP that remains uncontrolled under a three drug therapeutic regimen, an adequate dose of each of them being indeed a prerequisite for patient inclusion in the dRHTN category. Once this is established, however, a further increase in the dose of the prescribed drugs does not appear to be particularly helpful because (1) the shape of the dose/effect relationship can make the additional BP lowering effect far from substantial and (2) there may be with a number of drug classes (e.g., calcium channel blockers) a more prominent increase in the drug-related side effects [13]. It should nevertheless be emphasized that this may not be entirely true for diuretics because, as shown in Fig. 8.1, increasing the dose of hydrochlorothiazide beyond the usual 25 mg daily has been associated with a clear-cut further BP reduction; that is also the case for an increase of the thiazide-like diuretic chlorthalidone beyond the usual 12.5 mg, daily [14]. Along this line, several studies have shown an increase in the usual dose of diuretics to be accompanied by an increase in the number of resistant hypertensive patients reaching BP control. For

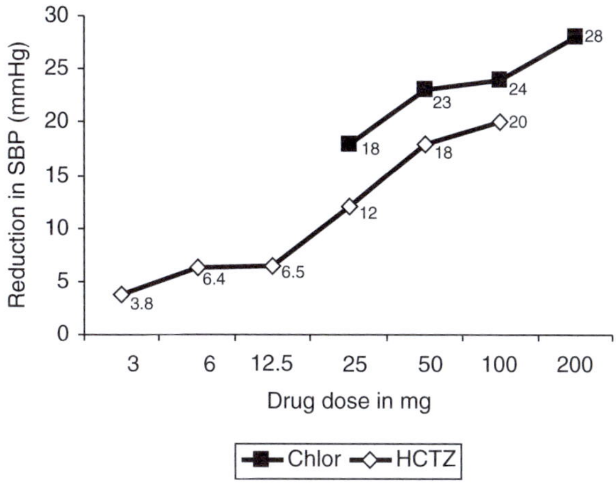

Fig. 8.1 Effect of hydrochlorothiazide (*HCTZ*) and chlorthalidone (*chlor*) on systolic blood pressure (*SBP*) as a function of the daily dose (mg) (From Carter et al. [14], by permission)

example, in an American study on a cohort of about 150 resistant hypertensive patients, optimization of the existing treatment regimen that included an increase of the dose of diuretic was followed by BP control (<140/90 mmHg) in more than 50 % of the cases [15].

8.4 Addition of a Fourth Drug

The drugs that are available as fourth step treatment of dRHTN have mechanisms of action that are only partly different from those of the drugs included in the background of three drug treatment regimen. Beta-blockers, alpha-I blockers and central agents, for example, share their sympatho-moderating influence with RAS blockers [16]. Beta-blockers and mineralocorticoid receptor antagonists share their opposition to the pressor and sodium retaining the effect of angiotensin II with RAS blockers. Direct vasodilators share their ability to reduce vasomotor tone with calcium channel blockers. Despite this potential mechanistic overlapping, however, addition of any fourth drug to the existing drug regimen stands a chance to lower BP and achieve control in a number of resistant hypertensive patients, which makes this approach the preferable one in this clinical condition.

Which drug to select among the available options is difficult to decide on an evidence basis because very few studies have addressed this issue by a randomized double-blind design, making the present fourth drug choice largely empiric. In this context, however, mineralocorticoid receptor antagonists and alpha-I blockers should probably be regarded as the preferred choice for pathophysiological considerations as well as for the extent of therapeutic data. Pathophysiological evidence leaves no doubt that hypertension is accompanied by (1) a sympathetic activation that is increased with the degree of BP elevation [17] and is particularly pronounced in patients whose BP is resistant to treatment (Fig. 8.2) [18] and (2) a

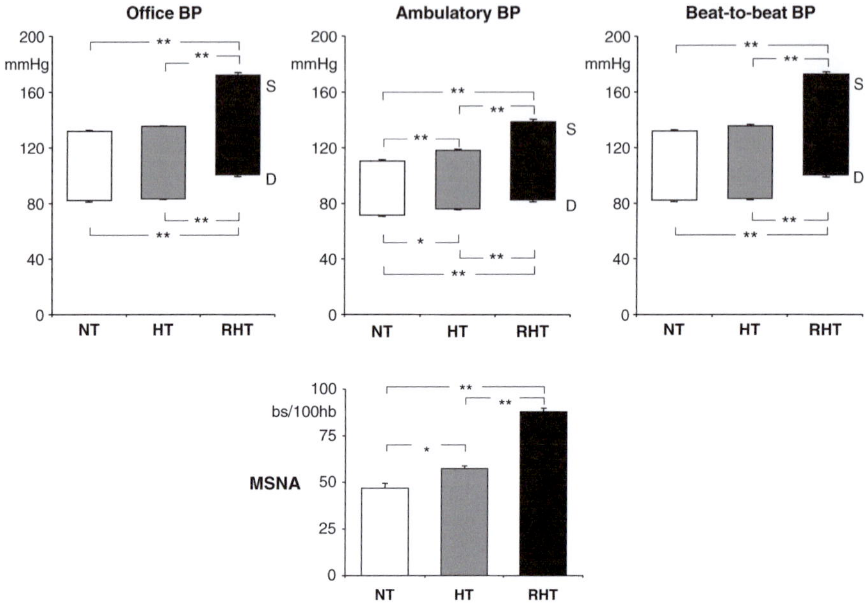

Fig. 8.2 Office, ambulatory and beat-to-beat (finger) blood pressure (*BP*) in normotensives (*NT*), non-resistant hypertensives (*HT*) and resistant hypertensives (*RHT*). Muscle sympathetic nerve traffic (MSNA) measured by microneurography in the three groups is also shown. $*P<0.05$; $**P<0.01$ (From Grassi et al. [18], by permission)

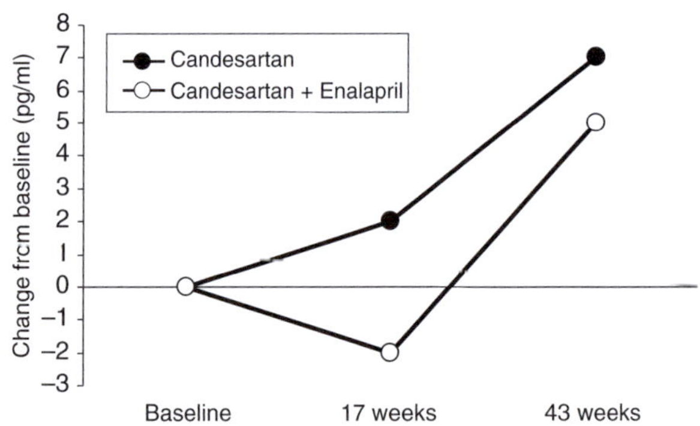

Fig. 8.3 Escape of aldosterone (serum concentration) in patients under treatment with an angiotensin receptor antagonist or an angiotensin receptor antagonist/ACE inhibitor combination (From McKelvie et al. [19], by permission)

plasma and tissue elevation of aldosterone whose secretion by the adrenal glands escapes, for a variety of reasons, the inhibitory effect of RAS blockers even when combined to oppose the production or influence of angiotensin II more effectively [19] (Fig. 8.3). Therapeutic evidence shows that these two drug classes lower BP in patients in whom multidrug treatment did not achieve control. This is exemplified by the Anglo-Scandinavian Cardiac Outcomes Trial (ASCOT) in which the addition of the alpha-I blocker doxazosin in a large

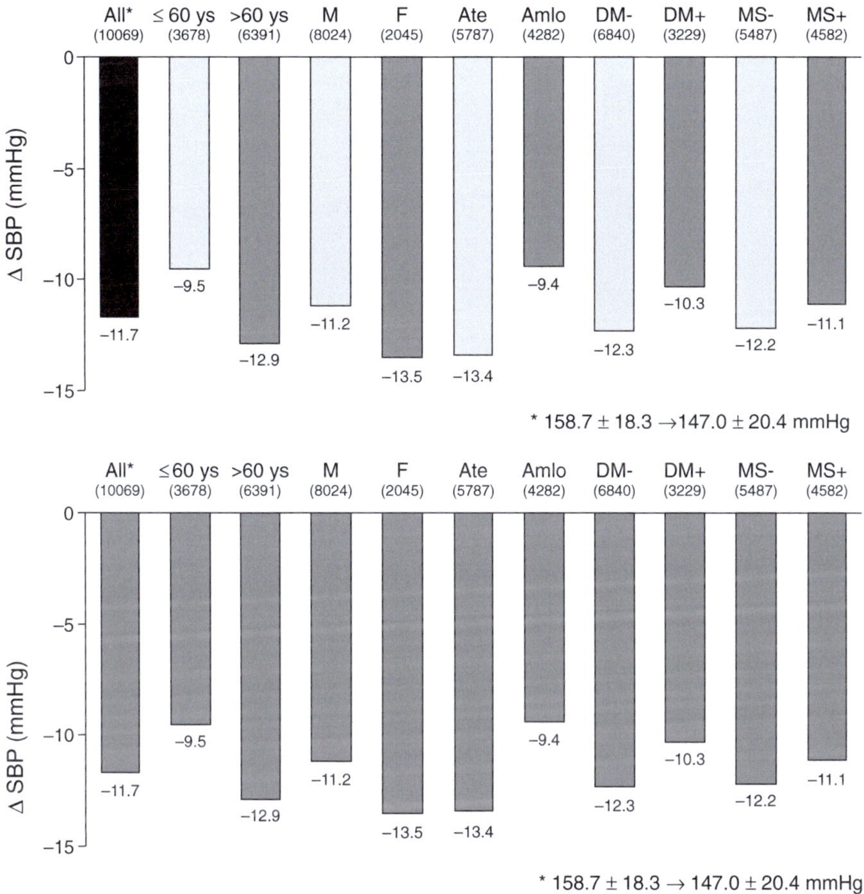

Fig. 8.4 Systolic blood pressure (*SBP*) reduction induced by doxazosin administration in patients in whom SBP was not controlled by multiple drug treatment. Data from different patient subgroups. *Ys* years, *M* males, *F* females, *Ate* group initially treated with atenolol, *Amlo* group initially treated with amlodipine, *DM* diabetes mellitus, *MS* metabolic syndrome (From Chapman et al. [20], by permission)

number of hypertensives uncontrolled by combination of various drugs lowered systolic BP by about 13–14 mm Hg, this being the case in a variety of clinical or demographic conditions (Fig. 8.4) [20]. Interestingly, the BP lowering effect was associated with no major side effect and no increased risk of heart failure, at variance from what has been reported in the doxazosin-treated hypertensive patients of the Antihypertensive and Lipid-Lowering Treatment to Prevent Heart Attack Trial (ALLHAT) [21]. It is further exemplified by the BP reduction observed in the same trial when a similarly large number of patients in whom multidrug treatment had failed to achieve BP control were given spironolactone (Fig. 8.5) [22].

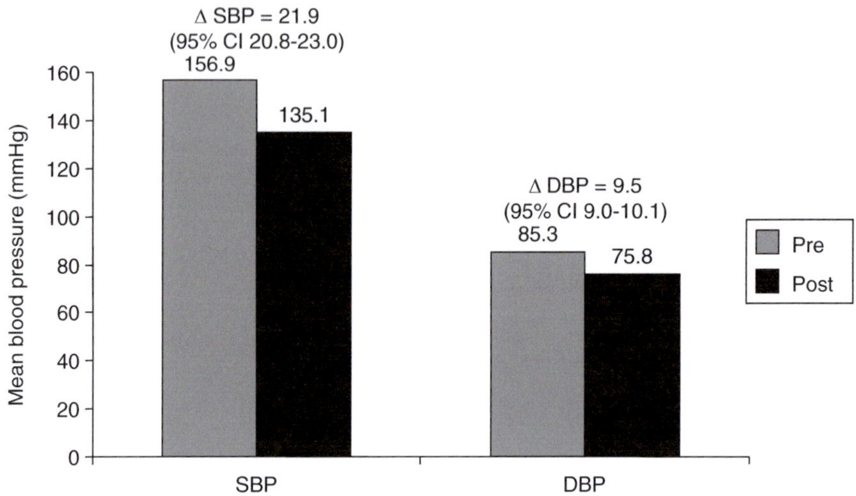

Fig. 8.5 Systolic blood pressure (*SBP*) and diastolic blood pressure (*DBP*) before (pre) and after (post) administration of spironolactone in patients in whom BP was not controlled by multiple drug treatment. Treatment-induced changes are shown at the top of the histograms. *CI* confidence intervals (From Davis et al. [21], by permission)

8.5 Mineralocorticoid Receptor Antagonists: Further Evidence

Support to use of mineralocorticoid receptor antagonists as the fourth drug to be administered in dRHTN can be found in several other studies that have shown, in some instances via a randomized, placebo-controlled design, the BP lowering ability of this class to include not only spironolactone but also eplerenone at adequate doses [23–30]. The most important documentation of the effectiveness of these drugs, however, comes from the recently published The Prevention and Treatment of Hypertension with Algorithm-based therapy (PATHWAY-2) study in which several hundred patients with a BP uncontrolled by the recommended three drug treatment regimen were randomized to the addition of spironolactone, bisoprolol, doxazosin or placebo. Following a few months of treatment, patients taking spironolactone showed a significantly greater BP reduction than patients taking doxazosin or bisoprolol, whose effect was modestly, albeit significantly, more evident than placebo. This was the case not only for office but also for home BP whose treatment-induced modification was the primary end point of the study (Fig. 8.6) [31]. This will probably lead future guidelines to privilege mineralocorticoid receptor antagonists over other drug options as the preferred fourth choice in dRHTN and perhaps also to define hypertension as resistant to treatment only after administration of a drug of this class has proven ineffective.

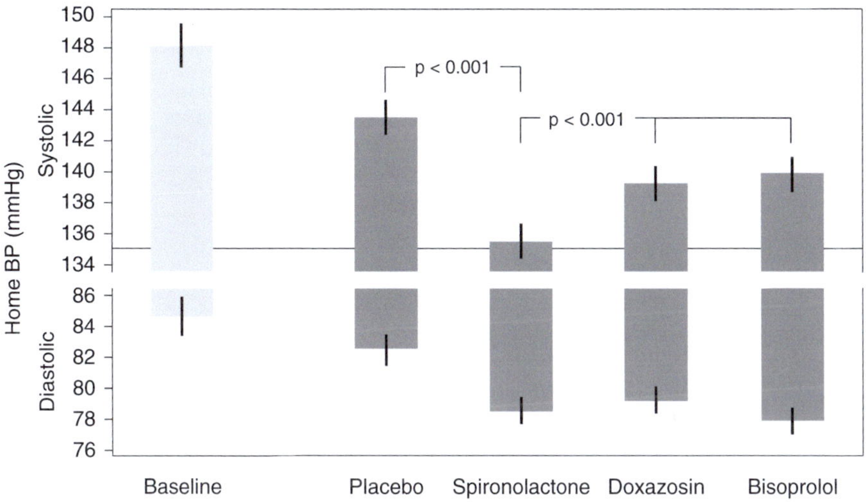

Fig. 8.6 Home blood pressure (*BP*) values at baseline and during treatment with placebo, spironolactone, doxazosin and bisoprolol (From Williams et al. [31], by permission)

8.6 Unmet Needs

Although more effective than any other added drug currently available, mineralocorticoid receptor antagonists by no means take care of all the problems posed by treatment of dRHTN. First, these drugs are associated with a number of serious side effects such as hyperkalemia and reduction of renal function [22, 32]. Second, both hyperkalemia and reduction of renal function are more frequent and severe in patients with a seriously impaired glomerular filtration, a condition that was excluded in the patients enrolled for the PATHWAY-2 study but that is not at all uncommon in dRHTN [33]. Third, despite the greater BP lowering effect in the PATHWAY-2 study, spironolactone failed to effectively lower BP in about 40 % of the study population, i.e. those with a high renin level, and perhaps a concomitant sympathetic hyperactivity (Fig. 8.7) [31]. Thus, more than a single drug class appears to be needed as fourth choice in order to extend effective treatment to the vast majority of resistant hypertensive individuals.

Future studies will have to address this issue by comparing the addition of a fourth drug with the combination of two or more additional agents, hopefully clarifying which combinations have the greatest potential to extend BP control. They may also, however, elect to address alternative possibilities, namely, whether (1) BP can be reduced in a larger number of resistant hypertensive patients by the use of drugs belonging to the same class but having a different site of action [34], an approach that sequential administration of a thiazide diuretic, a loop diuretic and amiloride has proven effective [35], or (2) a more precise assessment of the resistant hypertension phenotype. The latter approach will mean to (1) identify as precisely as possible the nature and extent

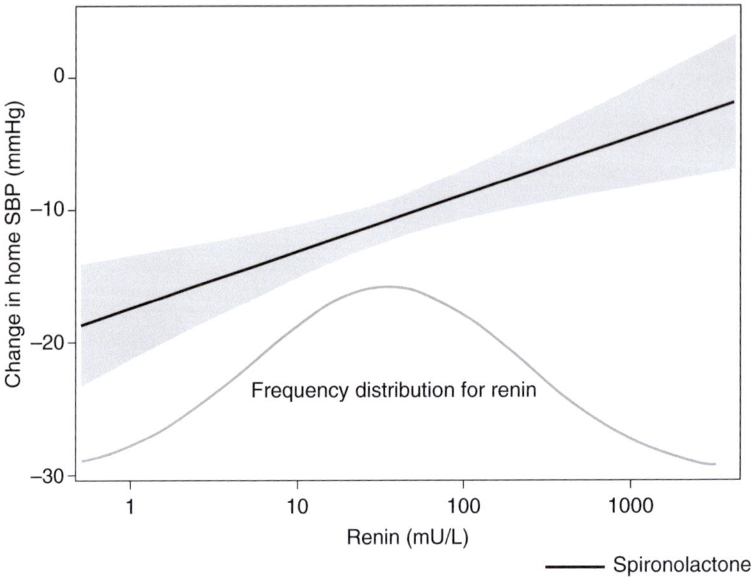

Fig. 8.7 Relationship between the home systolic blood pressure (*SBP*) change induced by spironolactone and plasma renin activity in the PATHWAY-2 study (From Williams et al. [31], by permission)

of the alterations of the structure and function of the organs (the heart, brain, kidney and vessels) targeted by the uncontrolled BP status and (2) determine which among the multiple neural and humoral mechanisms controlling circulation is more severely deranged, in order to try to individualize treatment and increase its success rate.

Finally, drug treatment of dRHTN may in the future count on new effective BP lowering agents. In the past, the use of endothelin antagonists has been disappointing because their BP lowering effect turned out to be questionable and accompanied by an unfavourable side effect profile [36]. Drugs targeting arterial stiffening (a structural alteration majorly responsible for the difficulty of lowering systolic values) have also met with difficulties that have prevented their extensive testing in humans. However, new dual-acting molecules as well as new powerful and better tolerated vasodilators are promising medicaments that may allow to more successfully face therapeutic control of a condition that may have a prevalence greater than 5 % of the overall hypertensive population [1], thereby involving in Europe several hundred thousand individuals.

References

1. Mancia G, Fagard R, Narkiewicz K, Redon J, Zanchetti A, Böhm M, Christiaens T, Cifkova R, De Backer G, Dominiczak A, Galderisi M, Grobbee DE, Jaarsma T, Kirchhof P, Kjeldsen SE, Laurent S, Manolis AJ, Nilsson PM, Ruilope LM, Schmieder RE, Sirnes PA, Sleight P,

Viigimaa M, Waeber B, Zannad F (2013) The Task Force for the management of arterial hypertension of the European Society of Hypertension (ESH) and of the European Society of Cardiology (ESC). 2013 ESH/ESC Guidelines for the management of arterial hypertension. J Hypertens 31:1281–1357
2. Burnier M, Pechere Bertschi A, Wuezner G (2013) Treatment of resistant hypertension. Which additional antihypertensive drugs. In: Mancia G (Ed). Resistant Hypertension. Springer, Milan. pp 115–126
3. Schmieder RE, Redon J, Grassi G, Kjeldsen SE, Mancia G, Narkiewicz K, Parati G, Ruilope L, van de Borne P, Tsioufis C (2012) ESH position paper: renal denervation – an interventional therapy of resistant hypertension. J Hypertens 30:837–841
4. Bakris GL, Nadim MK, Haller H, Lovett EG, Schafer JE, Bisognano JD (2012) Baroreflex activation therapy provides durable benefit in patients with resistant hypertension: results of long-term follow-up in the Rheos Pivotal Trial. J Am Soc Hypertens 6:152–158
5. Florczak E, Prejbisz A, Szwench-Pietrasz E, Sliwiński P, Bieleń P, Klisiewicz A, Michałowska I, Warchoł E, Januszewicz M, Kała M, Witkowski A, Więcek A, Narkiewicz K, Somers VK, Januszewicz A (2013) Clinical characteristics of patients with resistant hypertension: the RESIST-POL study. J Hum Hypertens 27:678–685
6. Pimenta E, Gaddam KK, Oparil S, Aban I, Husain S, Dell'Italia LJ, Calhoun DA (2009) Effects of dietary sodium reduction on blood pressure in subjects with resistant hypertension: results from a randomized trial. Hypertension 54:475–481
7. Forman JP, Rimm EB, Curhan GC (2007) Frequency of analgesic use and risk of hypertension among men. Arch Intern Med 167:394–399
8. Tóth K, PIANIST Investigators (2014) Antihypertensive efficacy of triple combination perindopril/indapamide plus amlodipine in high-risk hypertensives: results of the PIANIST study (Perindopril-Indapamide plus AmlodipiNe in high rISk hyperTensive patients). Am J Cardiovasc Drugs 14:137–145
9. Calhoun DA, Lacourcière Y, Chiang YT, Glazer RD (2009) Triple antihypertensive therapy with amlodipine, valsartan, and hydrochlorothiazide: a randomized clinical trial. Hypertension 54:32–39
10. Kjeldsen SE, Messerli FH, Chiang CE, Meredith PA, Liu L (2012) Are fixed-dose combination antihypertensives suitable as first-line therapy? Curr Med Res Opin 28:1685–1697
11. Rossi GP (2013) Resistant hypertension. Neurohumoral aspects. In: Mancia G (ed) Resistant hypertension. Springer, Milan, pp 11–21
12. Pereira M, Lunet N, Azevedo A, Barros H (2009) Differences in prevalence, awareness, treatment and control of hypertension between developing and developed countries. J Hypertens 27:963–975
13. Law MR, Wald NJ, Morris JK, Jordan RE (2003) Value of low dose combination treatment with blood pressure lowering drugs: analysis of 354 randomised trials. BMJ 326:1427
14. Carter BL, Ernst ME, Cohen JD (2004) Hydrochlorothiazide versus chlorthalidone: evidence supporting their interchangeability. Hypertension 43:4–9
15. Garg JP, Elliott WJ, Folker A, Izhar M, Black HR, RUSH University Hypertension Service (2005) Resistant hypertension revisited: a comparison of two university-based cohorts. Am J Hypertens 18:619–626
16. Saino A, Pomidossi G, Perondi R, Valentini R, Rimini A, Di Francesco L, Mancia G (1997) Intracoronary angiotensin II potentiates coronary sympathetic vasoconstriction in humans. Circulation 96:148–153
17. Mancia G, Grassi G (2014) The autonomic nervous system and hypertension. Circ Res 114: 1804–1814
18. Grassi G, Seravalle G, Brambilla G, Pini C, Alimento M, Facchetti R, Spaziani D, Cuspidi C, Mancia G (2014) Marked sympathetic activation and baroreflex dysfunction in true resistant hypertension. Int J Cardiol 177:1020–1025
19. McKelvie RS, Yusuf S, Pericak D, Avezum A, Burns RJ, Probstfield J, Tsuyuki RT, White M, Rouleau J, Latini R, Maggioni A, Young J, Pogue J (1999) Comparison of candesartan, enalapril, and their combination in congestive heart failure: randomized evaluation of strategies for

left ventricular dysfunction (RESOLVD) pilot study. The RESOLVD Pilot Study Investigators. Circulation 100:1056–1064
20. Chapman N, Chang CL, Dahlöf B, Sever PS, Wedel H, Poulter NR, ASCOT Investigators (2008) Effect of doxazosin gastrointestinal therapeutic system as third-line antihypertensive therapy on blood pressure and lipids in the Anglo-Scandinavian Cardiac Outcomes Trial. Circulation 118:42–48
21. Davis BR, Kostis JB, Simpson LM, Black HR, Cushman WC, Einhorn PT, Farber MA, Ford CE, Levy D, Massie BM, Nawaz S, ALLHAT Collaborative Research Group (2008) Heart failure with preserved and reduced left ventricular ejection fraction in the antihypertensive and lipid-lowering treatment to prevent heart attack trial. Circulation 118:2259–2267
22. Chapman N, Dobson J, Wilson S, Dahlöf B, Sever PS, Wedel H, Poulter NR, Anglo-Scandinavian Cardiac Outcomes Trial Investigators (2007) Effect of spironolactone on blood pressure in subjects with resistant hypertension. Hypertension 49:839–845
23. Azizi M, Sapoval M, Gosse P, Monge M, Bobrie G, Delsart P, Midulla M, Mounier-Véhier C, Courand PY, Lantelme P, Denolle T, Dourmap-Collas C, Trillaud H, Pereira H, Plouin PF, Chatellier G, Renal Denervation for Hypertension (DENERHTN) investigators (2015) Optimum and stepped care standardised antihypertensive treatment with or without renal denervation for resistant hypertension (DENERHTN): a multicentre, open-label, randomised controlled trial. Lancet 385:1957–1965
24. Rosa J, Widimský P, Toušek P, Petrák O, Čurila K, Waldauf P, Bednář F, Zelinka T, Holaj R, Štrauch B, Šomlóová Z, Táborský M, Václavík J, Kociánová E, Branny M, Nykl I, Jiravský O, Widimský J Jr (2015) Randomized comparison of renal denervation versus intensified pharmacotherapy including spironolactone in true-resistant hypertension: six-month results from the Prague-15 study. Hypertension 65:407–413
25. Václavík J, Sedlák R, Plachy M, Navrátil K, Plásek J, Jarkovsky J, Václavík T, Husár R, Kociánová E, Táborsky M (2011) Addition of spironolactone in patients with resistant arterial hypertension (ASPIRANT): a randomized, double-blind, placebo-controlled trial. Hypertension 57:1069–1075
26. Nishizaka MK, Zaman MA, Calhoun DA (2003) Efficacy of low-dose spironolactone in subjects with resistant hypertension. Am J Hypertens 16:925–930
27. Pitt B, Reichek N, Willenbrock R, Zannad F, Phillips RA, Roniker B, Kleiman J, Krause S, Burns D, Williams GH (2003) Effects of eplerenone, enalapril, and eplerenone/enalapril in patients with essential hypertension and left ventricular hypertrophy: the 4E-left ventricular hypertrophy study. Circulation 108:1831–1838
28. de Souza F, Muxfeldt E, Fiszman R, Salles G (2010) Efficacy of spironolactone therapy in patients with true resistant hypertension. Hypertension 55:147–152
29. Rodilla E, Costa JA, Pérez-Lahiguera F, Baldó E, González C, Pascual JM (2009) Spironolactone and doxazosin treatment in patients with resistant hypertension. Rev Esp Cardiol 62:158–166
30. Ramsay LE, Silas JH, Freestone S (1980) Diuretic treatment of resistant hypertension. Br Med J 281:1101–1103
31. Williams B, MacDonald TM, Morant S, Webb DJ, Sever P, McInnes G, Ford I, Cruickshank JK, Caulfield MJ, Salsbury J, Mackenzie I, Padmanabhan S, Brown MJ, British Hypertension Society's PATHWAY Studies Group (2015) Spironolactone versus placebo, bisoprolol, and doxazosin to determine the optimal treatment for drug-resistant hypertension (PATHWAY-2): a randomised, double-blind, crossover trial. Lancet 386:2059–2068
32. Bianchi S, Bigazzi R, Campese VM (2006) Long-term effects of spironolactone on proteinuria and kidney function in patients with chronic kidney disease. Kidney Int 70:2116–2123
33. Daugherty SL, Powers JD, Magid DJ, Tavel HM, Masoudi FA, Margolis KL, O'Connor PJ, Selby JV, Ho PM (2012) Incidence and prognosis of resistant hypertension in hypertensive patients. Circulation 125:1635–1642
34. Mancia G (2012) Additional drug treatment in resistant hypertension: need for randomized studies. J Hypertens 30:1514–1515

35. Bobrie G, Frank M, Azizi M, Peyrard S, Boutouyrie P, Chatellier G, Laurent S, Menard J, Plouin PF (2012) Sequential nephron blockade versus sequential renin-angiotensin system blockade in resistant hypertension: a prospective, randomized, open blinded endpoint study. J Hypertens 30:1656–1664
36. Weber MA, Black H, Bakris G, Krum H, Linas S, Weiss R, Linseman JV, Wiens BL, Warren MS, Lindholm LH (2009) A selective endothelin-receptor antagonist to reduce blood pressure in patients with treatment-resistant hypertension: a randomised, double-blind, placebo-controlled trial. Lancet 374:1423–1431

9 Blood Pressure Measurement Before and After Intervention

J. Redon

Abbreviations

ABPM	Ambulatory blood pressure monitoring
BP	Blood pressure
DBP	Diastolic blood pressure
HTN	Hypertension
PWV	Pulse wave velocity
RDN	Renal denervation
SBP	Systolic blood pressure

9.1 Resistant Hypertension

The complexity and the uncertainties about long-term effect of the invasive interventions to treat essential hypertension (HTN) require a precise diagnosis about the real "resistance" to the antihypertensive treatment given, and it is defined when a therapeutic strategy that includes appropriate lifestyle measures plus a diuretic and two other antihypertensive drugs belonging to different classes at adequate doses fails to lower systolic blood pressure (SBP) and diastolic blood pressure (DBP) values to <140 and 90 mmHg, respectively. Consequently, in the process of diagnosis and follow-up, blood pressure (BP) measurement is the first step that is not exempt of difficulties due to the variability of BP as a parameter. It has long been known that BP is characterized by an array of spontaneous variations. BP

J. Redon
INCLIVA, Research Institute, University of Valencia and CIBERObn Health Institute Carlos III, Madrid, Spain
e-mail: Josep.Redon@uv.es

C. Tsioufis et al. (eds.), *Interventional Therapies for Secondary and Essential Hypertension*, Updates in Hypertension and Cardiovascular Protection,
DOI 10.1007/978-3-319-34141-5_9

values vary markedly within the 24 h because of day-night changes but also because of differences among hours, minutes, and even adjacent beats. They also show variations over more prolonged periods because of differences among days, months, and season [1]. Even though it has been discussed, the prognostic relevance of the different kinds of variability in the case of resistant hypertension is a challenge at the time of evaluation. Several factors have been associated to the high day-to-day variability of patients with resistant hypertension and among them the number of drugs prescribed [2]. Therefore, more precise BP is mandatory in order to take the right decisions.

Limitations of office BP are well known due to the reduced number of BP readings and the white-coat effect. Then, out-of-office BP measurements, by using 24-h ambulatory blood pressure monitoring (24-h ABPM) or by home self-BP measurements, can provide more precise values avoiding "false" resistance due to persistence of alerting reaction to the BP measurement action, the so-called "white-coat" reaction.

The fundamentals of out-of-office BP are based on a more reliable estimation of BP values by increasing the number of BP readings and measuring them under regular living conditions, coupled with the observation of dynamic behaviour during the entire day. As a consequence of the better estimation of BP, the relationship with HTN-induced organ damage and the prognostic value for cardiovascular/renal disease is significantly better when compared to office BP values. Moreover, clinically relevant discrepancies between office and ambulatory BP are identified in treated subjects with apparent resistant HTN.

In 1998 our group found that in the absence or in the presence of a previous cardiovascular event, ambulatory BP was an independent marker of risk for new cardiovascular events, demonstrating for the first time that ABPM was useful in stratifying the risk in patients with resistant HTN [3]. Afterward, two studies [4, 5] have confirmed our initial results and reinforced the superiority of ambulatory BP over office BP for stratifying risk. More recently, our group conducted a study repeating monitoring during the follow-up. Awake BP >135 mmHg was significantly associated with cardiovascular risk in a time-derived analysis [6].

Once pseudoresistance due to white-coat effect is identified, patients require fur ther follow-up with ambulatory monitoring since qualification of patients can change with the subsequent monitoring. In fact, one study demonstrated that among those with a diagnosis of pseudoresistance, one third of the subjects were true resistant after a second monitoring three months apart. When repeated every six months, 1 out of 7 subjects were resistant in each monitoring [7]. No studies systematically analysed the opposite phenomenon, how many true resistant can be considered white coat when repeating monitoring.

Over the last years, noninvasive indirect assessment of aortic BP has become widely performed in hypertension clinics [3] and seems to be superior to peripheral BP in correlating with severity of existing cardiovascular disease and prediction of subsequent events [4]. Indirect aortic BP measurements have been introduced in the field of HTN based on (a) differences between brachial and aortic BP existing due to the pressure amplification and (b) higher damaging effect of local BP than brachial

BP, closer to the target organs in hypertensive patients. Measurement of BP parameters can provide additional information to those obtained with peripheral BP values. The potential utility at the time of evaluating resistant HTN has not been tested although it has been measured as a part of the evaluation of organ damage in the large vessels simultaneously to the pulse wave velocity (PWV).

9.2 Recommendations at the Evaluation

9.2.1 Office BP Measurements

Despite the high variability and the potential problems, office BP is still the cornerstone for the diagnosis of HTN. Consequently, office BP should be measured in the best conditions possible, measuring several times in the visit and in several visits before considering a patient as apparently resistant hypertension.

A protocol including at least three BP measuring in the conditions recommended by the ESH-ESC Guidelines and repeated in at least three visits should be recommended.

- *Average of higher or equal to 140 mmHg systolic and/or 90 mmHg are the thresholds accepted to define lack of control.*

9.2.2 Aortic BP

Aortic BP is not recommended to be assessed as a part of the study of resistant HTN.

9.2.3 Out-of-Office BP

The 2013 ESH-ESC Guidelines in the evaluation and treatment of HTN, as well as many other position statements from Scientific Societies, recommend the use of out-of-office BP, mainly 24-h ABPM, to assess patients with apparent resistant HTN, and they put it as a mandatory in the process of selecting patients for invasive procedures. As the advantage in reproducibility, defined as the degree of variation between two recording sessions, depends on the number of readings, current guidelines have recommended collecting at least one reading every 20 minutes in order to create a BP profile. Due to the potential variability of BP values, more than one 24-h monitoring should be recommended before defining a patient as really resistant to treatment if no urgency exists at the time to take decisions.

Home self-BP measurements can be used as an auxiliary method at the time of diagnosis by using the protocol recommended by the Working Group on ABPM of the ESH, in which one week of monitoring, excluding the first day, with at least two daily BP measurements is recommended [5].

- More than one 24-h monitoring one month apart.
- HSBP should be used as an auxiliary method but should not be considered the reference.
- Average of higher or equal to 135 mmHg systolic and/or 85 mmHg for awake ABMP or self-BP measurements are the thresholds accepted to define lack of control.

9.3 BP After Renal Denervation

Measurement of BP values after the renal denervation (RDN) procedure should be performed taking advantage not only of the conventional office values but also of out-of-office and aortic BP measurements. Discrepant reductions, however, can be observed between office and ambulatory BP. In our hands, a large reduction of both systolic and diastolic BP values was observed after the initial BP assessment, which was even more evident in ambulatory BP values than in the office counterparts. While office BP tended to have closer values, a large reduction was observed in ambulatory BP. The discrepancies in the trend between office and ambulatory BP during the study can be explained by the persistence of the white-coat effect on office BP measurements, by the real impact of the treatment changes on ambulatory BP or by regression to the mean [8, 9].

Besides the important significance of BP parameters other than office BP, previous observations about the impact of RDN on these parameters raise the necessity of having adequate evaluation [10]. In the first published studies, doubts have been raised about the lesser out-of-office BP reduction compared to the reduction of office BP after RDN. In fact, in a multicentre observational study, ambulatory BP was obtained after 3, 6 and 12 months in 303 subjects after RDN. Office and ambulatory BP reduction after 6 months (−24/−10 mmHg and−10/−5 mmHg, respectively) showed discrepancies in BP response. There was no effect on ambulatory BP monitoring in pseudoresistant patients, whereas office BP was reduced to a similar extent [11]. Discrepancies, however, have been observed in the reported results. While some studies have demonstrated that ambulatory BP reduction is around one third of the office BP reduction [5, 12], others observed more relevant reductions [13].

The ABPM report of the SYMPLICITY HTN-3 did not demonstrate a benefit of RDN on reduction in ambulatory BP in either the 24-h or day or night periods compared with the sham procedure [14]. Two major underlying mechanisms that may contribute to explain the different responses in office and ambulatory BP, when present, were white-coat effect of office measurements and the larger number of BP readings available with ambulatory BP monitoring, with the consequence of a narrower distribution of the values, although a placebo effect and a regression to the mean phenomenon, both affecting only office and not ambulatory BP, may also play a role [15].

The impact in arterial stiffness and central hemodynamic has been reported in 110 patients who underwent RDN. Besides the known effect of RDN on brachial BP, the study showed that RDN significantly improves arterial stiffness and central hemodynamic [16]. Other studies have also reported the reduction of aortic BP in parallel to the brachial BP [17, 18]. Likewise, PWV, the gold standard to assess aortic compliance, was significantly reduced. Although the initial effect is BP-related in the long term, 6 months, seems to be independent of lowering BP [17]. The potential benefits of this reduction should be established in the future, but aortic BP and PWV may be monitored in subjects after RDN.

9.4 Recommendations in the Evaluation

9.4.1 Office BP Measurements

Despite the high variability and the potential problems, office BP is still the cornerstone for the evaluation of antihypertensive treatment. Consequently, office BP should be measured in the best conditions possible, being measured several times during the visit.

- Daily measurement during the first week after hospital release.
- Weekly office BP during the first month and thereafter monthly until six months.
- The goal should be BP <140/90 mmHg.

9.4.2 Aortic BP

Aortic BP is not recommended to be calculated as a part of the study of resistant hypertension. In those centres where aortic BP and PWV are available, they can be measured at the end of the first and the sixth month.

9.4.3 Out-of-Office BP

Out-of office is basic for the follow-up in order to assess the impact of the procedure, and both 24-h ABPM and home BP may be complementary.

- Once a month home BP.
- 24-h ABPM monitoring should be performed at the end of the first and the sixth month.
- Goal is average of home BP or awake BP <135/85 mmHg.

References

1. Mancia G (2012) Short- and Long-term blood pressure variability. Hypertension 60:512–517
2. Howard JP, Patel H, Shun-Shin MJ, Mourad JJ, Blacher J, Mahfoud F et al (2015) Impact of number of prescribed medications on visit-to-visit variability of blood pressure: implications for design of future trials of renal denervation. J Hypertens 33:2359–2367
3. Herbert A, Cruickshank JK, Laurent S, Boutouyrie P, Reference Values for Arterial Measurements Collaboration (2014) Establishing reference values for central blood pressure and its amplification in a general healthy population and according to cardiovascular risk factors. Eur Heart J 35:3122–3133
4. Mancia G, Fagard R, Narkiewicz K, Redón J, Zanchetti A, Böhm M, Task Force Members et al (2013) 2013 ESH/ESC Guidelines for the management of arterial hypertension: the Task Force for the management of arterial hypertension of the European Society of Hypertension (ESH) and of the European Society of Cardiology (ESC). J Hypertens 31:1281–1357
5. Parati G, Stergiou GS, Asmar R, Bilo G, de Leeuw P, Imai Y, ESH Working Group on Blood Pressure Monitoring et al (2010) European Society of Hypertension practice guidelines for home blood pressure monitoring. J Hum Hypertens 24:779–785
6. Pascual JM, Rodilla E, Costa JA, Garcia-Escrich M, Gonzalez C, Redon J (2014) Prognostic value of microalbuminuria during antihypertensive treatment in essential hypertension. Hypertension 64:1228–1234
7. Muxfeldt ES, Fiszman R, de Souza F, Viegas B, Oliveira FC, Salles GF (2012) Appropriate time interval to repeat ambulatory blood pressure monitoring in patients with white-coat resistant hypertension. Hypertension 59:384–389
8. Persu A, Jin Y, Azizi M, Baelen M, Völz S, Elvan A, European Network COordinating research on Renal Denervation (ENCOReD) et al (2014) Blood pressure changes after renal denervation at 10 European expert centers. J Hum Hypertens 28:150–156
9. Rohla M, Nahler A, Lambert T, Reiter C, Gammer V, Grund M et al (2016) Predictors of response to renal denervation for resistant arterial hypertension: a single center experience. J Hypertens 34:123–129
10. Doumas M, Anyfanti P, Bakris G (2012) Should ambulatory blood pressure monitoring be mandatory for future studies in resistant hypertension: a perspective. J Hypertens 30:874–876
11. Mahfoud F, Ukena C, Schmieder RE, Cremers B, Rump LC, Vonend O et al (2013) Ambulatory blood pressure changes after renal sympathetic denervation in patients with resistant hypertension. Circulation 128:132–140
12. Lambert T, Blessberger H, Gammer V, Nahler A, Grund M, Kerschner K et al (2014) Effects of renal denervation on ambulatory blood pressure measurements in patients with resistant arterial hypertension. Clin Cardiol 37:307–311
13. Ott C, Mahfoud F, Schmid A, Ditting T, Sobotka PA, Veelken R, Spies A, Ukena C, Laufs U, Uder M, Böhm M, Schmieder RE (2013) Renal denervation in moderate treatment-resistant hypertension. J Am Coll Cardiol 62:1880–1886
14. Bakris GL, Townsend RR, Liu M, Cohen SA, D'Agostino R, Flack JM, SYMPLICITY HTN-3 Investigators et al (2014) Impact of renal denervation on 24-hour ambulatory blood pressure: results from SYMPLICITY HTN-3. J Am Coll Cardiol 64:1071–1078
15. Mancia G, Parati G (2004) Office compared with ambulatory blood pressure in assessing response to antihypertensive treatment: a meta-analysis. J Hypertens 22:435–445
16. Brandt MC, Reda S, Mahfoud F, Lenski M, Böhm M, Hoppe UC (2012) Effects of renal sympathetic denervation on arterial stiffness and central hemodynamics in patients with resistant hypertension. J Am Coll Cardiol 60:1956–1965
17. Mortensen K, Franzen K, Himmel F, Bode F, Schunkert H, Weil J, Reppel M (2012) Catheter-based renal sympathetic denervation improves central hemodynamics and arterial stiffness: a pilot study. J Clin Hypertens 14:861–870
18. Ott C, Janka R, Schmid A, Titze S, Ditting T, Sobotka PA et al (2013) Vascular and renal hemodynamic changes after renal denervation. Clin J Am Soc Nephrol 8:1195–1201

Novel Drugs in the Treatment of Hypertension

10

Reinhold Kreutz and Engi Abdel-Hady Algharably

Abbreviations

ACE	Angiotensin-converting enzyme
ACE2	Angiotensin-converting enzyme 2
Ala	Alamandine
Ang 1–7	Angiotensin 1–7
Ang 1–9	Angiotensin 1–9
Ang II	Angiotensin II
Ang III	Angiotensin III
Ang IV	Angiotensin IV
ANP	Atrial natriuretic peptide
APA	Aminopeptidase A
APN	Aminopeptidase N
ARB	Angiotensin receptor blockers
ARNI	Angiotensin receptor–neprilysin inhibitor
AT1	Angiotensin II type 1
AT2	Angiotensin II type 2
ATryn	Recombinant human antithrombin
BNP	B-type natriuretic peptide
BP	Blood pressure
C21	Compound 21
cGMP	Cyclic guanosine monophosphate
CINOD	Cyclooxygenase-inhibiting nitric oxide donator

R. Kreutz (✉) • E. Abdel-Hady Algharably
Department of Clinical Pharmacology and Toxicology, Institut für Klinische Pharmakologie und Toxikologie, Charité – Universitätsmedizin Berlin,
Charitéplatz 1, Berlin 10117, Germany
e-mail: reinhold.keutz@charite.de

C. Tsioufis et al. (eds.), *Interventional Therapies for Secondary and Essential Hypertension*, Updates in Hypertension and Cardiovascular Protection,
DOI 10.1007/978-3-319-34141-5_10

CYP	Cytochrome P450
DIF	Digoxin antibody fab
DN	Diabetic nephropathy
DβH	Dopamine β-hydroxylase
ECE	Endothelin-converting enzyme
EDLF	Endogenous digitalis-like factors
ENaC	Epithelial sodium channel
EO	Endogenous ouabain
ET-1	Endothelin-1
ETA	Endothelin A
ETB	Endothelin B
GWAS	Genome-wide association studies
HF	Heart failure
HFrEF	Heart failure with reduced ejection fraction
HP-β-CD	Hydroxypropyl-β-cyclodextrin
HTN	Hypertension
IRAP	Insulin-regulated membrane aminopeptidase/insulin-responsive aminopeptidase
MHS	Milan hypertensive
MR	Mineralocorticoid receptor
NAT2	N-acetyltransferase 2
NEP	Neutral endopeptidase 24.11
NHE	Na+/H+ exchangers
NHE3	NHE isoform 3
NO	Nitric oxide
NPR	Natriuretic peptide receptor
RAAS	Renin–angiotensin–aldosterone system
rhACE2	Recombinant human angiotensin-converting enzyme
sEH	Soluble epoxide hydrolase
SGC	Soluble guanylate cyclase
SHR	Spontaneously hypertensive rats
VIP	Vasoactive intestinal polypeptide

Pharmacological therapy in combination with lifestyle changes represents the backbone of the therapeutic management of arterial hypertension (HTN) [1]. The recent European guidelines of the European Society of Hypertension and the European Society of Cardiology for the management of HTN recommend with class I and evidence level A the use of diuretics (including thiazides, chlorthalidone, and indapamide), beta-blockers, calcium antagonists, angiotensin-converting enzyme (ACE) inhibitors, and angiotensin receptor blockers (ARB) for the initiation and maintenance of antihypertensive treatment, either as monotherapy or in some combinations with each other [1]. The impressive prognostic value of blood pressure (BP) lowering in hypertensive patients by using treatment algorithms that are based on the use of these drugs has been demonstrated in multiple trials [1] including the recent Randomized Trial of Intensive versus Standard Blood-Pressure Control (SPRINT) [2]. In addition, further drugs including mineralocorticoid receptor (MR) antagonists, amiloride, and the alpha-1-blocker doxazosin are available for treatment of patients with resistant hypertension [1]. Nevertheless, there is still a need for additional novel BP-lowering drugs, e.g., in the latter patients, in individuals with special conditions (comorbidities), or in patients not responding or tolerating the available drugs. Accordingly, several novel drugs for the treatment of HTN are being currently developed either at the preclinical or clinical stage. They will be summarized in this short overview, and a summary of the compounds and their status of development is given in the Table 10.1.

10.1 Drugs Acting on the Renin–Angiotensin–Aldosterone System

The renin–angiotensin–aldosterone system (RAAS) is a major regulator of cardiovascular function including BP control and is important for cardiovascular and renal organ damage as well as repair [3, 4]. In the classical concept, one principal effector of the RAAS is the angiotensin II (Ang II) acting on Ang II type 1 receptors (AT1) to mediate its main vascular effects as well as secretion of the other principal effector aldosterone from the adrenals [3]. The RAAS is, however, a much more complex system with additional sites recently identified that influence either BP homeostasis or cardiovascular function and structure, thereby representing potential targets for therapy [4] (Fig. 10.1). A crucial question during the development of novel drugs interfering with the RAAS is whether novel compounds could provide improved cardiovascular and renal protection beyond that provided by ACE inhibitors or angiotensin receptor blockers (ARB) [4].

10.1.1 Activators of the ACE2/Angiotensin 1–7/Mas Receptor Axis (RAAS Counter-Regulatory System)

An important counter-regulatory pathway within the RAAS involves angiotensin-converting enzyme 2 (ACE2), angiotensin-1–7 (Ang 1–7), and the Mas receptor that interacts with the classical angiotensinogen–Ang II–AT1–aldosterone axis of the RAAS (Fig. 10.1) [4, 5]. ACE2 is a carboxypeptidase that converts Ang I to angiotensin 1–9 (Ang 1–9) and Ang II to Ang 1–7; Ang 1–9 is also converted to Ang 1-7 by ACE. Therefore, ACE2 induces vasodilation by reducing Ang II effects and by increasing Ang 1–7 synthesis. The latter binds to the Mas receptor and thereby exhibits antifibrotic, anti-inflammatory, and antiproliferative effects in addition to nitric oxide (NO) release and activation of baroreflex sensitivity [4]. Thus

Table 10.1 Selected novel drugs in the treatment of hypertension and their status of development

Therapeutic group/category	Drug	Status	Selected clinical trial number	Pharmaceutical industry/ developer
ACE2 activator	XNT	Preclinical	n.a.	–
ACE2 activator	DIZE	Preclinical	n.a.	–
ACE2 activator	APN01 (rhACE2) GSK 2586881 (rhACE2)	Phase I Phase II	NCT00886353 NCT01597635	Apeiron Biologics GlaxoSmithKline
Ang 1–7 analog	HP-β-CD/Ang 1–7	Preclinical	n.a.	–
Mas-related G-protein-coupled receptor, member D agonist	Alamandine/HPβCD	Preclinical	n.a.	–
AT2 receptor agonist	C21	Preclinical	n.a.	Vicore Pharma
Mas agonist Non-peptide Peptide	AVE0991 CGEN-856S	Preclinical Preclinical	n.a. n.a.	– –
Aldosterone synthase inhibitor	LCI699 (Osilodrostat)	Stopped at phase II	NCT00817635 NCT00817414 NCT00732771 NCT00758524	Novartis Pharmaceuticals
Mineralocorticoid receptor antagonist	BAY 94–8862 (Finerenone)	Phase IIb Phase III[b]	NCT01807221 NCT01874431 NCT02540993 NCT02545049	Bayer HealthCare
Aminopeptidase N inhibitor	PC18	Preclinical	n.a.	–
Aminopeptidase A inhibitor	RB150 (QGC001)	Phase IIa	NCT02322450	Quantum Genomics SA
IRAP inhibitors	HFI-419	Preclinical	n.a.	–
Dual-acting angiotensin receptor–neprilysin inhibitor	LCZ696 (Sacubitril/Valsartan)	Approved Phase III	NCT00549770 NCT01785472 NCT01920711	Novartis Pharmaceuticals
Dual-acting endothelin-converting enzyme–neprilysin inhibitor	SLV-306 (Daglutril)	Phase II	NCT00160212 NCT00160225	Solvay pharmaceuticals
Natriuretic peptide A agonist	PL-3994	Phase II	NCT00686803	Palatin Technologies

ANP analog, selective for NPR-C	C-ANP4-23	Preclinical	n.a.	–
Vasoactive intestinal peptide receptor 2 (VPAC2) agonist	PB1046 (Vasomera)	Phase I	NCT01523067 NCT01873885	PhaseBio Pharmaceuticals Inc.
Nitric oxide-donor CINOD Soluble guanylate cyclase stimulator	AZD 3582 (Naproxcinod) YC-1 BAY-63-2521 (Riociguat)	Phase III[c] Preclinical Phase III	NCT00662896 NCT00662610 n.a. NCT00810693 NCT00863681	NicOx – Bayer HealthCare
Endothelin antagonist	Bosentan Darusentan	Phase II Stopped at phase III	Krum et al. 1998 NCT00389675 NCT00353574	Actelion Pharmaceuticals Gilead Sciences
Soluble epoxide hydrolase inhibitors	AR9281	Stopped at phase II	NCT00847899	Arete Therapeutics
Intestinal Na+/H+ exchanger 3 inhibitor	AZD1722 (Tenapanor) SAR218034	Phase II Preclinical	NCT01847092 NCT02675998 n.a.	Ardelyx –
Dopamine β-hydroxylase inhibitor	BIA 5–453 (Etamicastat)	Phase I	2008-002789-09[a]	BIAL-Portela & Ca., SA
Vaccine against angiotensin II	CYT006-AngQβ AngII-KLH pHAV-4AngIIs	Phase II Preclinical Preclinical	NCT00500786 n.a. n.a.	Cytos Biotechnology AG –
Vaccine against angiotensin II type 1 receptor	ATRQβ-001 ATR12181	Preclinical Preclinical	n.a. n.a.	– –
Vaccine against angiotensin I/II	Anti-angiotensin peptide (AngI-R)	Preclinical	n.a.	–
Preeclampsia drugs Anti-digoxin antibody fragment Recombinant antithrombin	DIF ATryn	Phase II expedited Phase III	NCT00158743 NCT02059135	BTG; Glenveigh Pharmaceuticals rEVO Biologics

NCT indicates the clinical trial number registered at ClinicalTrials.gov, *CINOD* cyclooxygenase-inhibiting nitric oxide donator. Read labeling of compounds indicates ongoing clinical investigation in 2015 and 2016

[a]Indicates the clinical trial number registered at EudraCT trial registration

[b]In diabetic kidney disease

[c]In arthritis; n.a., not applicable

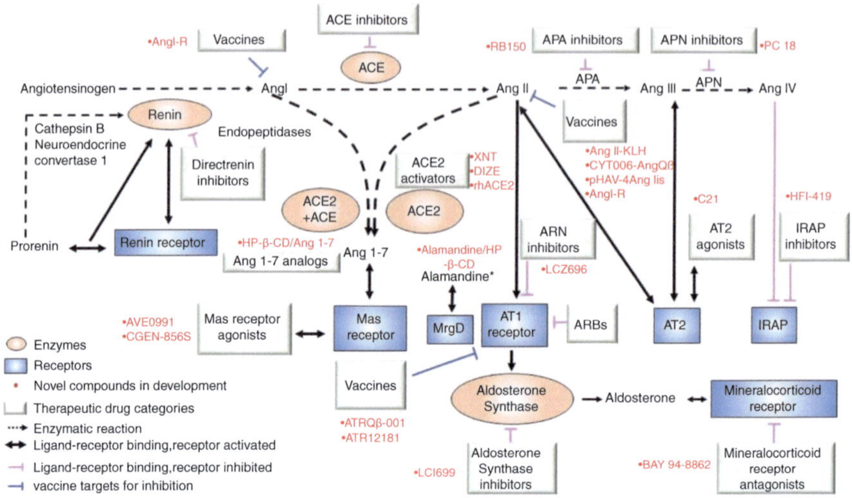

Fig. 10.1 The renin–angiotensin–aldosterone (RAAS) system and its possibilities for pharmacological intervention for antihypertensive treatment (modified according to Romero et al. 2015). The core of the classical RAAS is the conversion of angiotensinogen to angiotensin I by renin. Ang I is cleaved to angiotensin II (Ang II) by the angiotensin-converting enzyme. Ang II activates angiotensin II receptor type 1 to stimulate aldosterone release, increasing water and sodium retention and increasing BP. Novel antihypertensive agents aim to activate the counter-regulatory RAAS including ACE2–Ang 1-7–Mas, Ang II-AT2, and Ang IV–IRAP pathways. An alternative inhibitory strategy within the RAAS includes aldosterone blockade at the receptor level such as by the mineralocorticoid receptor antagonists (finerenone) or through inhibiting its synthesis by aldosterone synthase inhibitors such as by LCI699. Abbreviations: *ACE* angiotensin-converting enzyme, *ACE2* angiotensin-converting enzyme 2, *Ang* angiotensin, *ARB* angiotensin receptor blocker, *ARN* angiotensin receptor–neprilysin, *AT1* type 1 Ang II receptor, *AT2* type 2 Ang II receptor, *APA* aminopeptidase A inhibitor, *APN* aminopeptidase N inhibitor, *IRAP* leucyl-cystinyl aminopeptidase (also known as insulin-regulated membrane aminopeptidase or insulin-responsive aminopeptidase), *Mas* proto-oncogene Mas, *MrgD* Mas-related G-protein-coupled receptor, member D, *rh* recombinant human

augmentation of ACE2/Ang 1–7/Mas signaling counteracts several of the detrimental effects of the classical RAAS axis as shown in animal models of HTN [4, 5].

(i) *XNT and DIZE* are small-molecule ACE2 activator compounds that were synthesized based on the crystal structure of the ACE2 enzyme [5, 6]. Studied in spontaneously hypertensive rats (SHR), XNT was found to lower BP, improve cardiac function, and reverse myocardial, perivascular, and renal fibrosis [6, 7].

(ii) *Recombinant human ACE2 (rhACE2)* was studied as an alternative to pharmacological activation of ACE2 in SHR and was capable of lowering BP, inducing anti-inflammatory effects in a model of lipopolysaccharide-induced lung injury and slowing the progression of diabetic nephropathy (DN) in animal models [8, 9]. In a phase I clinical study in healthy and normotensive subjects, rhACE2 exhibited a sustained (>24 h) lowering of circulating Ang II levels without effects on BP and with a good safety profile [10]. A modified rhACE2 compound (GSK2586881) has been evaluated in acute lung injury or acute respiratory distress syndrome (Table 10.1).

(iii) *HP-β-CD/Ang 1–7* representing a hydroxypropyl-β-cyclodextrin incorporated Ang [1–7] formulation and a cyclic Ang 1–7 analog containing a thioester bridge were both designed to protect Ang 1–7 against degradation and thus to prolong its half-life in vivo [11, 12]. Hence, Ang 1–7 with its short half-life has been studied even in clinical phase I/II studies but not further developed due to its limitation. Treatment of SHR with the orally active HP-β-CD/Ang 1–7 formulation demonstrated antihypertensive effects [13] and beneficial effects in animal models of myocardial infarction [12], atherosclerosis [14], and diabetes [15].

(iv) *Alamandine (*Ala[1]-Ang 1–7) is a novel identified component of the RAAS with similar structure and biological activity as Ang 1–7 except for replacement of the N-terminal Asp residue by Ala [16]. In addition, it exerts its action through a different receptor by binding to the Mas-related G-protein-coupled receptor, member D. An orally active inclusion complex of almandine/HP-β-CD reduced BP in SHR and inhibited cardiac fibrosis in isoproterenol-treated rats [16].

(v) *Compound 21 (C21)* is a selective non-peptide agonist on the Ang II type 2 receptor (AT2) [17]. In animal models, C21 alone does not decrease BP but exerts anti-inflammatory, antifibrotic, and antiapoptotic properties, supporting a role for C21 in preventing hypertension-induced target organ damage [17]. In addition, more recent data in rodents indicate that AT2 stimulation by C21 could modulate fluid retention and hypertension [18].

(vi) *AVE0991* and *CGEN-856S* are other non-peptide and peptide agonists of the Mas receptor, respectively. Experimental studies with AVE0991 indicated its BP-lowering and cardiovascular protective effects in rats with renovascular hypertension [19]. CGEN-856S exhibited also vasorelaxing, antihypertensive, and cardioprotective effects in animal studies [20, 21].

10.1.2 Anti-Aldosterone Agents

Aldosterone acts primarily in renal collecting ducts where it binds to the MR. The activation of MR increases the expression of epithelial sodium channel (ENaC) which stimulates Na^+ reabsorption and consecutively secretion of K^+ and thereby affects water retention and extracellular volume expansion [22]. Aldosterone also exerts a number of non-epithelial effects such as induction of inflammation, vascular stiffening, and myocardial fibrosis delineating its role in the development and progression of HTN and related target organ damage [4, 22].

10.1.2.1 Aldosterone Synthase Inhibitors

Blocking MR can cause reactive increase in RAAS components and particularly in aldosterone levels that limit their efficacy, e.g., by activation of non-genomic aldosterone signaling pathways [23]. In addition, tissues not protected by MR receptor blockade such as the brain could be adversely affected [24]. In contrast, inhibiting aldosterone synthesis can prevent these effects by reducing aldosterone concentrations [23].

Osilodrostat (LCI699) was the first orally active aldosterone synthase [cytochrome P450 (CYP) 11B2] inhibitor developed for human use and structurally related to FAD286. The latter is the enantiomer of fadrozole that harbors minimal aromatase activity while retaining potent aldosterone synthase inhibitory activity and was found to attenuate myocardial and renal injury in preclinical studies [25]. LCI699 decreased plasma and urine aldosterone concentrations and increased plasma renin activity in a dose-dependent manner in animal models of HTN and heart failure (HF) [26, 27]. The challenge in the development of CYP11B2 inhibitors results from the fact that CYP11B2 shares an enzymatic 11ß-hydroxylase activity and thus a high sequence homology with the corresponding 11ß-hydroxylase, i.e., CYP11B1, enzyme [24]. The early clinical development of LCI699 included four phase II studies in patients with primary aldosteronism, resistant and uncontrolled HTN, and essential HTN as recently summarized [24]. An extensive endocrine biomarker analysis of the hypothalamic–pituitary–adrenal axis in these studies indicated that interference of LCI699 in the RAAS occurred with limited target selectivity. Thus, the inhibition of 11ß-hydroxylase reaction in the adrenal gland, leading to supraphysiological levels of 11-deoxycortiscosterone, represented a disadvantage of this compound that may explain the blunted BP response observed for LCI699 [24]. Consequently, because of these observations further development of LCI699 in aldosterone-related hypertensive and cardiovascular diseases was terminated [5]. Nevertheless, the studies with LCI699 emphasized the importance of selectivity for the development of other novel aldosterone synthase inhibitors over other steroidogenic CYP enzymes, in particular CYP11B1. Recently, novel second-generation aldosterone synthase inhibitors with greater selectivity, e.g., N-(pyridin-3-yl) benzamides, have been reported, which could be promising drug candidates for the treatment of aldosterone-related hypertensive and cardiovascular diseases [28].

10.1.2.2 Mineralocorticoid Receptor Antagonists

Finerenone (BAY 94–8862) is a novel nonsteroidal MR antagonist with greater selectivity than spironolactone for the MR over other steroid hormone receptors and greater affinity than eplerenone for the MR [29]. Finerenone reduced cardiac hypertrophy, plasma prohormone of brain natriuretic peptide, and proteinuria more efficiently than the steroidal MR antagonist eplerenone when comparing equinatriuretic doses in a rat model of HTN-related heart failure and renal dysfunction [30]. Subsequently, the mineralocorticoid receptor antagonist tolerability study (ARTS) trial program with several phase II studies were designed to assess the safety and tolerability of finerenone and to select doses for the pivotal phase III clinical trials [4, 5]. The first completed ARTS trial assessed in two sub-studies the efficacy and safety of finerenone in patients with systolic HF and mild chronic kidney disease. Taken together, finerenone was at least as effective as spironolactone in decreasing B-type natriuretic peptide (BNP), N-terminal proBNP, and albuminuria; it was also associated with lower incidences of hyperkalemia and worsening of renal function

[31]. Overall, adverse effects were infrequent and mostly mild [31]. Finerenone has completed phase IIb clinical trials in patients with worsening chronic HF and type 2 diabetes mellitus and/or chronic kidney disease (ARTS-HF) and in patients with type 2 diabetes mellitus and DN (ARTS-DN), respectively (Table 10.1). The published data of the ARTS-DN study indicated that the addition of finerenone compared with placebo resulted in improvement in the urinary albumin–creatinine ratio in patients with DN [32]. Two phase III studies involving overall an estimated number of more than 11,000 patients with type 2 diabetes mellitus and diabetic kidney disease are currently ongoing (Table 10.1).

10.1.3 Centrally Acting Aminopeptidase Inhibitors

Activation of the RAAS in the brain has been implicated in the pathogenesis of hypertension in experimental studies [3, 33]. In the brain, Ang II and Ang III are converted by two membrane-bound zinc metalloproteases, i.e., aminopeptidase A (APA) and aminopeptidase N (APN) [5, 33]. Ang II is metabolized to angiotensin III (Ang III) by APA which is then converted into angiotensin IV (Ang IV) by APN. The development of the selective APA and APN inhibitors EC33 and PC18, respectively, has allowed the demonstration that brain Ang III generated by APA is one of the main effector peptides in the brain RAS by exerting a tonic stimulatory control of BP in conscious hypertensive rats [33].

RB150 (QGC001) is an orally active dimer of EC33 that crosses the blood–brain barrier. In animal studies, RB150 generates two active molecules of EC33 in the brain, where it inhibits brain APA and reduces Ang III formation thereby normalizing BP in hypertensive rats [33]. The decrease in BP involves two different mechanisms: (i) a decrease in vasopressin release into the bloodstream, which in turn increases diuresis resulting in blood volume reduction and (ii) a decrease in sympathetic tone decreasing vascular resistance [33]. Early clinical studies in healthy normotensive subjects showed that RB150 (renamed QGC001) did not significantly change BP or heart rate at any dose, while the drug was well tolerated as single dose or in multiple doses over a 7 day treatment period [34]. A phase IIa proof of concept exploratory study in 36 patients with essential hypertension was initiated with this prototype of a new class of centrally acting antihypertensive agents [34].

10.1.4 IRAP Inhibitors (Insulin-Regulated Membrane Aminopeptidase or Insulin-Responsive Aminopeptidase)

IRAP is a high-affinity receptor for Ang IV (Fig. 10.1). Ang IV inhibits the enzymatic activation of IRAP, and IRAP inhibition has been linked to NO release and anti-inflammatory and antifibrotic effects [4]. Non-peptide compounds inhibiting IRAP were developed including HFI-419 which was found to enhance memory in rats [35]. Early data from animal studies have shown that HFI-419 provides also cardiovascular protective effects opposing the detrimental influence of Ang II, independent of BP changes [36]. The potential role of IRAP inhibition in BP control has yet to be clarified.

10.2 Vasopeptidase Inhibitors

Neutral endopeptidase 24.11 (NEP) or neprilysin is the major enzymatic pathway for the degradation of natriuretic peptides including atrial natriuretic peptide (ANP) and BNP [37]. However, neprilysin inhibitors per se are ineffective in lowering BP probably attributable to the fact that neprilysin itself degrades also vasoconstrictor peptides such as Ang II and endothelin-1 [38]. Nevertheless, experimental studies have shown that adding a neprilysin inhibitor to a RAAS blocker or an endothelin-converting enzyme (ECE) inhibitor enhances vasodilatory, natriuretic, and beneficial effects on tissue remodeling [39]. Previously, single molecules that inhibit both ACE and NEP have been shown to be advantageous compared to ACE inhibitors as BP-lowering drugs owing to their greater potentiation of vasodilator/natriuretic effects including activation of bradykinin effects [37]. However, the latter also proved to be the Achilles heel of this combination therapy [40]. The first-generation compound omapatrilat with this dual mode of action exhibited greater antihypertensive efficacy and encouraging cardiovascular effects compared to conventional ACE inhibitors [41]. However, the drug was not approved for clinical use due to a high rate of angioedema observed in clinical studies that was attributed to bradykinin activation.

10.2.1 Dual-Acting Angiotensin Receptor–Neprilysin Inhibitors

LCZ696 is a first-in-class angiotensin receptor–neprilysin inhibitor (ARNI), composed of two molecular moieties in a single crystalline complex—the ARB valsartan and a NEP inhibitor prodrug AHU377 (sacubitril) in a 1:1 ratio. Sacubitril is a prodrug activated to sacubitril at (LBQ657) by demethylation via esterases [42]. In a proof of concept phase II trial LCZ696 produced significantly greater reductions than valsartan in office systolic and diastolic BP, 24-h ambulatory systolic BP and pulse pressure over the entire dose range tested [22]. Importantly, no cases of angioedema were reported, although only a few Black and Asian patients prone to develop this condition were included in this study. An even greater BP-lowering efficacy of the compound along with a favorable tolerability profile was subsequently also shown in mixed Asian [43] and Japanese [43] patient groups. Two interesting studies comparing the effects of treatment with the LCZ696 and the ARB olmesartan on arterial stiffness and vascular remodeling parameters in patients with HTN have been completed (NCT01692301 and NCT0187073). The prospective comparison of angiotensin receptor–neprilysin inhibitor with angiotensin receptor blocker measuring arterial stiffness in the elderly (PARAMETER) study [44] met its primary endpoint by showing that the ARNI group had a significantly greater reduction in central aortic systolic pressure after 12 weeks of treatment versus the comparator group treated with olmesartan [45]. The observed greater changes in 24-h brachial and central aortic systolic BP for the LCZ696 group, especially at night, seem also important since elevation of nighttime BP is more difficult to control and associated with increased cardiovascular risk. Although several trials with LCZ696 in HTN or HTN associated diseases have been initiated as recently summarized [46], there are currently no specific phase III trials initiated in patients with HTN. Moreover, a planned phase III study on the efficacy and safety of LCZ696 alone and in combination with amlodipine in patients with HTN was subsequently withdrawn (NCT01865188). The further clinical development program of LCZ696 from phase II to phase III has focused on patients with HF [46]. Meanwhile, LCZ696 was approved by the US Food and Drug Administration [47] and the European Medical Agency [48] for the treatment of adult patients with symptomatic chronic HF with reduced ejection fraction (HfrEF) in 2015. This resulted from the completion of a successful pivotal phase III trial (PARADIGM) in which the drug was tested in this condition [49]. In the PARADIGM trial, LCZ696 showed a striking reduction in cardiovascular mortality and morbidity in patients with HFrEF. The ongoing efficacy and safetyof LCZ696 compared to valsartan, on morbidity and mortality in HF patients with preserved ejection fraction (PARAGON-HF) phase III trial (NCT01920711) will address an important condition with an unmet medical need and frequent target organ damage observed in patients with HTN. Nevertheless, it would be important to conduct further studies comparing the antihypertensive efficacy and outcome of LCZ696 with other drug classes such as calcium channel blockers and diuretics in patients with HTN [46].

10.2.2 Dual-Acting Endothelin-Converting Enzyme–Neprilysin Inhibitors

Endothelin-converting enzyme (ECE) represents an important peptidase in the endothelin system. It cleaves inactive big endothelin-1 to active endothelin-1 (ET-1), which binds to endothelin type A receptors exerting vasopressor effects [50]. The combination of NEP and ECE inhibition has been also considered as an attractive therapeutic strategy in cardiovascular diseases [50].

Daglutril (SLV-306) is a first-in-class dual-acting neprilysin–ECE inhibitor [51]. The compound is hydrolyzed to the active metabolite KC-12615 after oral administration [52]. In rodent models of diabetes mellitus, daglutril reduced BP and proteinuria as effectively as captopril [53]. After the successful completion of phase I studies [5], clinical development included so far two phase II trials with relatively small number of patients, e.g., one in patients with hypertension [46] and one in hypertensive patients with type 2 diabetes and nephropathy [51]. The available data indicated that daglutril improved BP control with an acceptable safety profile supporting the combined neprilysin–ECE inhibition as a new treatment approach in this high-risk population [51].

10.3 Natriuretic Peptide Receptor Agonists

The biological actions of natriuretic peptides are mediated by activation of cell surface natriuretic peptide receptors (NPR) mainly NPR-A and NPR-B [54]. They activate membrane-associated guanylyl cyclases and production of the classical second messenger cyclic guanosine monophosphate (cGMP). In addition, NPR-C represents a clearance receptor that internalizes the natriuretic peptides and also inhibits adenylyl cyclase [54].

(i) *PL-3994* is an NPR-A agonist with reduced affinity for NPR-C and increased resistance to neprilysin [54]. A phase I and phase II trial have been successfully completed with PL-3994 with no safety concerns identified [5]. In the phase II study in subjects with hypertension who were receiving ≥1 antihypertensive medications, a significant reduction in BP compared with placebo was observed [5]. It appears that PL-3994 works synergistically with ACE inhibitors, which suggests its use as potential adjunct therapy in patients with resistant HTN or HF [5].

(ii) *C-ANP 4-23* is a ring-deleted analog of ANP that acts selectively on NPR-C, thereby decreasing the enhanced expression of Giα proteins which are involved in the pathogenesis of hypertension [55]. Early experimental studies with C-ANP 4–23 after parenteral application in SHR support a novel therapeutic role of NPR-C ligands as a potential target for the treatment of HTN and cardiovascular diseases that goes beyond the mechanisms attributable to the clearance receptor function as previously considered [55].

10.4 Vasoactive Intestinal Peptide Receptor Agonist

Vasoactive intestinal polypeptide (VIP) is a neuropeptide that functions as a neuromodulator and neurotransmitter [56]. It is a potent vasodilator and has positive inotropic/chronotropic properties mediated via the G-protein-coupled receptors VPAC1 and VPAC2. VIP has been suggested as a therapeutic target for both systemic and pulmonary hypertensions as well as HF although the peptide itself has a short half-life (<2 min) [5, 56].

Vasomera (PB1046) is a first-in-class long-acting biopolymer-based selective VPAC2 receptor agonist developed by fusing an analog of VIP with an elastin-like polypeptide [57]. Preclinical studies showed that Vasomera reduced BP and improved inotropic and lusitropic properties of the heart in animal models with hypertension and HF [5]. In early clinical phase I studies in patients with essential hypertension, parenteral application of Vasomera significantly decreased both systolic and diastolic BP in a dose-dependent manner with no clinically relevant dose-dependent increases in HR. In addition, the drug use was safe and well tolerated [58].

10.5 Drugs Acting on the NO and Soluble Guanylate Cyclase Pathway

Soluble guanylate cyclase (sGC) is a key enzyme of the NO signaling pathway and an attractive novel therapeutic target for hypertension and cardiopulmonary disease [59]. Impaired NO and cGMP signaling has been implicated in the pathogenesis of cardiovascular disease, including systemic arterial and pulmonary hypertension [59]. On binding of NO to a prosthetic heme group on sGC, the enzyme catalyzes synthesis of cGMP which produces vasorelaxation and inhibits smooth muscle proliferation, leukocyte recruitment, and platelet aggregation through a number of downstream mechanisms [59]. The time-honored pharmacological approach to use organic nitrates to treat cardiovascular diseases is limited by several vascular and extravascular changes that compromise their vasodilatory effects on long-term administration [60]. To overcome these shortcomings, new compounds have been developed as vasodilators for treating hypertension and other cardiovascular diseases including nitrosyl-cobinamide [61], nitric oxide-releasing pharmacodynamic hybrids of losartan [62] and telmisartan [63], respectively, and naproxcinod [64]. These agents directly release NO and potentially overcome the problems of long-acting nitrates such as the occurrence of tolerance [60].

(i) *Naproxcinod* is a cyclooxygenase-inhibiting nitric oxide-donating (CINOD) compound derived from naproxen. This compound has BP-lowering effects in patients with HTN as documented by 24-h ambulatory BP monitoring [65]. Naproxcinod may be therefore a beneficial alternative for patients with osteoarthritis requiring nonsteroidal anti-inflammatory drugs.

(ii) *YC-1* is a synthetic benzylindazole compound and a first sGC stimulator that stabilizes the enzyme in its active configuration [59]. Early studies demonstrated that intravenous YC-1 produced significant BP reductions in a rat model of HTN supporting sGC activators as BP-lowering compounds [66]. Subsequently, YC-1 has been shown to have additional cGMP-independent effects that limit its usefulness as a sGC stimulator [59].

(iii) *Riociguat (BAY 63–2521)* represents an orally bioavailable sGC stimulator that was subsequently developed after further research efforts and pharmacokinetic optimization with an investigation of>800 pyrimidine candidates [59]. Riociguat reduced BP and demonstrated renal and cardiac protective effects in a rat model of chronic renal failure [67]. The compound was the first sGC stimulator to make the transition into clinical research after showing promising results in the treatment of pulmonary hypertension [59]. Meanwhile it has been approved as a first-in-class compound for the treatment of pulmonary hypertension after the successful conduction of a pivotal phase III trial [68]. Although clinical research with sGC stimulators is currently focusing on pulmonary hypertension, sGC stimulators have clearly a potential for the treatment of systemic hypertension as evident from several experimental studies [59].

10.6 Endothelin Receptor Antagonists

Endothelin-1 is a potent endothelium-derived vasoconstrictor peptide that acts through endothelin-A (ETA) and endothelin-B receptors (ETB) mediating vasoconstriction and inflammation [69].

(i) *Bosentan* was the first-in-class non-peptidergic, orally active mixed ETA and ETB antagonist [64]. The systemic BP-lowering efficacy of bosentan was shown in early clinical trials [70]; however, the drug was further developed to gain market approval for the treatment of pulmonary hypertension but not for the treatment of systemic hypertension [64]. The latter was due to several side effects including hepatotoxicity, edema, and water retention that are associated with the use of the drug [70]. In addition, bosentan exhibits a potential for drug interactions mediated by CYP450 3A4 or p-glycoprotein.

(ii) *Darusentan* is a selective ETA antagonist that demonstrated beneficial effects in hypertensive animal models and particularly in salt-sensitive hypertension [66]. Despite promising preclinical data, further clinical development was not continued, because darusentan failed to meet the primary endpoint to lower sitting systolic BP more than the placebo in patients with resistant hypertension in a pivotal phase III trial [71]. Yet, in this study darusentan provided a greater reduction in systolic BP at ambulatory BP monitoring [71].

10.7 Soluble Epoxide Hydrolase Inhibitors

In mammals, soluble epoxide hydrolase (sEH) catalyzes the conversion of multiple lipid epoxides to the corresponding dihydroxy lipids and represents a novel drug target for the treatment of hypertension, inflammatory diseases, and cancer [72]. The available preclinical data indicated a beneficial effect of sEH inhibitors on BP, cardiac hypertrophy, and aneurysm formation [73].

AR9281 was developed as a potent and selective inhibitor of human sEH; however, a phase II trial showed that this compound was ineffective in lowering BP in patients with mild to moderate HTN and impaired glucose tolerance halting further clinical investigation in 2009 [5].

10.8 Intestinal Na+/H+ Exchanger 3 Inhibitor

High intestinal sodium absorption is linked to the pathogenesis of HTN and target organ damage. Inhibition of transmembrane Na+/H+ exchangers (NHE) that are located at the apical membrane of the enterocyte represents a novel strategy to lower BP by impairing intestinal sodium absorption [74]. Genetic studies implicate the NHE isoform 3 (NHE3) as the major absorptive sodium transporter [74].

(i) *Tenapanor* is a selective inhibitor of NHE3 (SLC9A3) that acts locally in the intestine because of its negligible bioavailability after oral application [74]. Tenapanor reduced urinary sodium and increased stool sodium in a dose-dependent manner in rodents and in humans. It reduced also BP in rat models of chronic kidney disease, and clinical trials in patients with chronic kidney disease and associated conditions are ongoing [74].

(ii) *SAR218034 (SAR)* is another orally non-absorbable specific NHE3 inhibitor that was found to reduce intestinal sodium absorption and to lower BP in hypertensive animal models [75].

10.9 Dopamine β-Hydroxylase (DβH) Inhibitor

DβH catalyzes the hydroxylation of dopamine into noradrenaline in the sympathetic nervous system. Unlike adrenergic receptor blockade, inhibition of DβH may cause a more gradual sympathetic slowdown and increases dopamine levels thereby stimulating renal vasodilation and diuresis [76].

Etamicastat (*BIA 5-453)* is an oral, potent, and reversible inhibitor of DβH that does not pass the blood–brain barrier and thus is selective for peripheral DβH when administered orally [5]. Animal studies in SHR and models of HF were promising supporting clinical development of etamicastat. Phase I studies in healthy subjects and in patients with mild to moderate hypertension showed good tolerability and dose-dependent decreases in 24-h ambulatory BP [77] supporting further development. However, the pharmacokinetics of the drug is significantly influenced by N-acetylation by the polymorphic N-acetyltransferase 2 (NAT2), which requires consideration during further clinical development [77].

10.10 Vaccines

Immunization strategies appear as an attractive treatment approach in HTN because they offer the advantage of long-term efficacy after short-term administration. Thus, they reduce the need for daily dosing as necessary with conventional drugs. This is particularly relevant, since low adherence represents a significant barrier in the successful management of hypertension in clinical practice [1]. Proof of concept studies using vaccines targeting renin in animal studies have been already reported in 1958 [78]. Recent immunization strategies are also targeting the RAAS [5]. Although an Ang I vaccine (*PMD3117*) lowered BP in animal models, this strategy was ineffective in hypertensive patients [79]. Currently investigated vaccines are targeted against Ang I/II (*AngI-R*) [80], Ang II (*AngII-KLH, pHAV-4AngIIs*), and AT1R (*ATRQβ-001, ATR12181*) [5].

CYT006-AngQb is a vaccine against an Ang II-derived peptide conjugated to a viruslike particle derived from the bacteriophage Qß [81]. It lowered BP in SHR animals and was subsequently evaluated in clinical phase I and IIa (study 01) studies in which the BP-lowering potential was demonstrated [81]. Of interest, a subsequent phase IIa trial (study 02), which used an accelerated immunization schedule in an attempt to induce higher antibody titers, was successful in boosting the antibody titer fivefold, but resulted contrary to the expectation in smaller BP reductions and lower antibody affinities to Ang II [5, 82]. These studies highlighted the need for a better understanding of the mechanism that affect antibody titers and affinities by applying different dosing and timing regimens for the development of effective vaccines for hypertension therapy. No further development in clinical studies has been documented after completion of a third phase IIa trial (study 03) in 2009 with CYT006-AngQb (Table 10.1). Nevertheless, as summarized in the Table, several vaccines are still in development; however, they are still at the preclinical stage.

10.11 Drugs for Treatment of Preeclampsia

Endogenous digitalis-like factors (EDLF) represent a family of circulating Na+/K+-ATPase inhibitors that have been implicated in the pathogenesis of HTN and are elevated in preeclampsia [83]:

(i) *DIF* representing anti-digoxin antibody Fab fragments that bind to EDLF, thereby causing a decrease in serum EDLF levels, has been suggested as a therapeutic approach in preeclampsia [83]. A clinical phase II trial that evaluated whether a commercially available DIF (Digibind) can delay delivery in patients with severe preeclampsia demonstrated beneficial effects on renal function and a trend toward reduction in antihypertensive drug usage [83]; however, no prolongation of pregnancy or improvement of maternal outcome in women with severe preeclampsia was observed [83]. In 2015, the currently only available DigiFab compound has been granted both orphan drug and fast-track review designations by FDA for the use in the treatment of severe preeclampsia. Thus, the company involved is planning a dose ranging and a phase IIb/IIIa clinical study using this DIF compound [5].

(ii) *ATryn* representing recombinant human antithrombin has been proposed as another therapeutic approach in preeclampsia, because proof of concept studies with antithrombin replacement reduced BP and proteinuria in women with early-onset severe preeclampsia [84]. Therefore, a randomized placebo-controlled phase III trial that will assess the efficacy, safety, and pharmacokinetics of ATryn in addition to expectant management for the treatment of preterm preeclampsia (PRESERVE-1) has been initiated and is expected to be completed in 2016 (Table 10.1).

10.12 Outlook: Novel Targets and Drugs Delivered from Genomics and Pharmacogenomics

Genomic studies in hypertensive animal models, characterization of human monogenetic hypertension disorders, and identification of rare and common variants related to BP control and hypertension have significantly enriched our understanding of BP regulation [85]. Furthermore, an important expectation of these studies and of additional pharmacogenomic research is their potential to identify novel targets for antihypertensive treatment [85–87].

Rostafuroxin is a digitoxigenin derivative which selectively antagonizes the effects of endogenous ouabain (EO) on Na+/K+-ATPase and mutated adducin [85]. The identification of mutations in the heterodimeric cytoskeleton protein adducin and the development of this compound resulted from a comprehensive analysis of the genetic mechanism in the Milan hypertensive (MHS) rat model [85]. This analysis suggested that an interaction between adducin and EO represents a triggering mechanism for hypertension in MHS and in some patients with a genetic profile affecting this interaction. Rostafuroxin selectively displaces ouabain from the Na+/K+-ATPase and was shown to lower BP in MHS and in humans [85]. In a randomized placebo-controlled phase II dose-finding study, rostafuroxin did not reduce BP at any dose in an overall cohort of newly recruited, never-treated patients, while the tolerability of the drug was good compared to placebo [88]. In additional phase II study analysis, a significant BP-lowering effect was, however, shown in carriers of a genetic profile affecting the EO-adducin pathway, whereas the presence of this profile did not affect the BP response to losartan or hydrochlorothiazide [85]. Currently, a confirmatory phase IIb trial is ongoing to further validate this potential pharmacogenetic and personalized treatment approach and to detect the dose of rostafuroxin that could be evaluated in phase III trials [85].

In contrast to this candidate gene-driven approach, genome-wide association studies (GWAS) have so far identified over 60 genetic loci influencing BP and HTN [87]. Taken together, this genetic information has not led to a personalized or precision medicine approach in hypertensive disease. Thus, this genetic knowledge has so far no impact on HTN management in clinical practice either at the diagnostic or therapeutic level. Nevertheless, among these associations detected in GWAS, evidence has been obtained that multiple genes are either current drug targets or are druggable based on the predicted potential of a protein to be modified by a small molecule drug [87, 89]. To move forward from this genetic basis into further translational research and hopefully development of novel antihypertensive drugs is the next important pending step, although to make this progress is a challenging task [90, 91].

References

1. Mancia G, Fagard R, Narkiewicz K, Redon J, Zanchetti A, Bohm M et al (2013) 2013 ESH/ESC guidelines for the management of arterial hypertension: the task force for the management of arterial hypertension of the European Society of Hypertension (ESH) and of the European Society of Cardiology (ESC). J Hypertens 31(7):1281–1357
2. Wright JT Jr, Williamson JD, Whelton PK, Snyder JK, Sink KM, Rocco MV et al (2015) A randomized trial of intensive versus standard blood-pressure control. N Engl J Med 373(22):2103–2116
3. Paul M, Poyan Mehr A, Kreutz R (2006) Physiology of local renin-angiotensin systems. Physiol Rev 86(3):747–803

4. Romero CA, Orias M, Weir MR (2015) Novel RAAS agonists and antagonists: clinical applications and controversies. Nat Rev Endocrinol 11(4):242–252
5. Oparil S, Schmieder RE (2015) New approaches in the treatment of hypertension. Circ Res 116(6):1074–1095
6. Hernandez Prada JA, Ferreira AJ, Katovich MJ, Shenoy V, Qi Y, Santos RA et al (2008) Structure-based identification of small-molecule angiotensin-converting enzyme 2 activators as novel antihypertensive agents. Hypertension 51(5):1312–1317
7. Ferreira AJ, Shenoy V, Qi Y, Fraga-Silva RA, Santos RA, Katovich MJ et al (2011) Angiotensin-converting enzyme 2 activation protects against hypertension-induced cardiac fibrosis involving extracellular signal-regulated kinases. Exp Physiol 96(3):287–294
8. Treml B, Neu N, Kleinsasser A, Gritsch C, Finsterwalder T, Geiger R et al (2010) Recombinant angiotensin-converting enzyme 2 improves pulmonary blood flow and oxygenation in lipopolysaccharide-induced lung injury in piglets. Crit Care Med 38(2):596–601
9. Oudit GY, Liu GC, Zhong J, Basu R, Chow FL, Zhou J et al (2010) Human recombinant ACE2 reduces the progression of diabetic nephropathy. Diabetes 59(2):529–538
10. Haschke M, Schuster M, Poglitsch M, Loibner H, Salzberg M, Bruggisser M et al (2013) Pharmacokinetics and pharmacodynamics of recombinant human angiotensin-converting enzyme 2 in healthy human subjects. Clin Pharmacokinet 52(9):783–792
11. Kluskens LD, Nelemans SA, Rink R, de Vries L, Meter-Arkema A, Wang Y et al (2009) Angiotensin-(1-7) with thioether bridge: an angiotensin-converting enzyme-resistant, potent angiotensin-(1-7) analog. J Pharmacol Exp Ther 328(3):849–854
12. Marques FD, Melo MB, Souza LE, Irigoyen MC, Sinisterra RD, de Sousa FB et al (2012) Beneficial effects of long-term administration of an oral formulation of Angiotensin-(1-7) in infarcted rats. Int J Hypertens 2012:795452
13. Bertagnolli M, Casali KR, De Sousa FB, Rigatto K, Becker L, Santos SH et al (2014) An orally active angiotensin-(1-7) inclusion compound and exercise training produce similar cardiovascular effects in spontaneously hypertensive rats. Peptides 51:65–73
14. Fraga-Silva RA, Savergnini SQ, Montecucco F, Nencioni A, Caffa I, Soncini D et al (2014) Treatment with angiotensin-(1-7) reduces inflammation in carotid atherosclerotic plaques. Thromb Haemost 111(4):736–747
15. Santos SH, Giani JF, Burghi V, Miquet JG, Qadri F, Braga JF et al (2014) Oral administration of angiotensin-(1-7) ameliorates type 2 diabetes in rats. J Mol Med (Berl) 92(3):255–265
16. Lautner RQ, Villela DC, Fraga-Silva RA, Silva N, Verano-Braga T, Costa-Fraga F et al (2013) Discovery and characterization of alamandine: a novel component of the renin-angiotensin system. Circ Res 112(8):1104–1111
17. Foulquier S, Steckelings UM, Unger T (2012) Impact of the AT(2) receptor agonist C21 on blood pressure and beyond. Curr Hypertens Rep 14(5):403–409
18. Kemp BA, Howell NL, Gildea JJ, Keller SR, Padia SH, Carey RM (2014) AT(2) receptor activation induces natriuresis and lowers blood pressure. Circ Res 115(3):388–399
19. Cunha TM, Lima WG, Silva ME, Souza Santos RA, Campagnole-Santos MJ, Alzamora AC (2013) The Nonpeptide ANG-(1-7) mimic AVE 0991 attenuates cardiac remodeling and improves baroreflex sensitivity in renovascular hypertensive rats. Life Sci 92(4-5):266–275
20. Savergnini SQ, Beiman M, Lautner RQ, de Paula-Carvalho V, Allahdadi K, Pessoa DC et al (2010) Vascular relaxation, antihypertensive effect, and cardioprotection of a novel peptide agonist of the MAS receptor. Hypertension 56(1):112–120
21. Savergnini SQ, Ianzer D, Carvalho MB, Ferreira AJ, Silva GA, Marques FD et al (2013) The novel Mas agonist, CGEN-856S, attenuates isoproterenol-induced cardiac remodeling and myocardial infarction injury in rats. PLoS One 8(3):e57757
22. Ruilope LM (2008) Aldosterone, hypertension, and cardiovascular disease: an endless story. Hypertension 52(2):207–208
23. Hargovan M, Ferro A (2014) Aldosterone synthase inhibitors in hypertension: current status and future possibilities. JRSM Cardiovasc Dis. 2014 Feb 5;3:2048004014522440. doi:10.1177/2048004014522440. eCollection 2014.

24. Schumacher CD, Steele RE, Brunner HR (2013) Aldosterone synthase inhibition for the treatment of hypertension and the derived mechanistic requirements for a new therapeutic strategy. J Hypertens 31(10):2085–2093
25. Menard J, Pascoe L (2006) Can the dextroenantiomer of the aromatase inhibitor fadrozole be useful for clinical investigation of aldosterone-synthase inhibition? J Hypertens 24(6):993–997
26. Menard J, Gonzalez MF, Guyene TT, Bissery A (2006) Investigation of aldosterone-synthase inhibition in rats. J Hypertens 24(6):1147–1155
27. Lea WB, Kwak ES, Luther JM, Fowler SM, Wang Z, Ma J et al (2009) Aldosterone antagonism or synthase inhibition reduces end-organ damage induced by treatment with angiotensin and high salt. Kidney Int 75(9):936–944
28. Hu Q, Yin L, Hartmann RW (2014) Aldosterone synthase inhibitors as promising treatments for mineralocorticoid dependent cardiovascular and renal diseases. J Med Chem 57(12):5011–5022
29. Barfacker L, Kuhl A, Hillisch A, Grosser R, Figueroa-Perez S, Heckroth H et al (2012) Discovery of BAY 94-8862: a Nonsteroidal antagonist of the mineralocorticoid receptor for the treatment of cardiorenal diseases. ChemMedChem 7(8):1385–1403
30. Kolkhof P, Delbeck M, Kretschmer A, Steinke W, Hartmann E, Barfacker L et al (2014) Finerenone, a novel selective Nonsteroidal mineralocorticoid receptor antagonist protects from rat cardiorenal injury. J Cardiovasc Pharmacol 64(1):69–78
31. Pitt B, Kober L, Ponikowski P, Gheorghiade M, Filippatos G, Krum H et al (2013) Safety and tolerability of the novel non-steroidal mineralocorticoid receptor antagonist BAY 94-8862 in patients with chronic heart failure and mild or moderate chronic kidney disease: a randomized, double-blind trial. Eur Heart J 34(31):2453–2463
32. Bakris GL, Agarwal R, Chan JC, Cooper ME, Gansevoort RT, Haller H et al (2015) Effect of finerenone on albuminuria in patients with diabetic nephropathy: a randomized clinical trial. JAMA 314(9):884–894
33. Gao J, Marc Y, Iturrioz X, Leroux V, Balavoine F, Llorens-Cortes C (2014) A new strategy for treating hypertension by blocking the activity of the brain renin-angiotensin system with aminopeptidase a inhibitors. Clin Sci (Lond) 127(3):135–148
34. Balavoine F, Azizi M, Bergerot D, De Mota N, Patouret R, Roques BP et al (2014) Randomised, double-blind, placebo-controlled, dose-escalating phase I study of QGC001, a centrally acting aminopeptidase a inhibitor prodrug. Clin Pharmacokinet 53(4):385–395
35. Albiston AL, Morton CJ, Ng HL, Pham V, Yeatman HR, Ye S et al (2008) Identification and characterization of a new cognitive enhancer based on inhibition of insulin-regulated aminopeptidase. FASEB J 22(12):4209–4217
36. Lee HWR, Chai S, Pong W, Welungoda I, Gaspari T (2014) AT4 receptor/insulin regulated aminopeptidase inhibition protects against angiotensin II induced cardic fibrosis and vascular dysfunction. J Hypertens 32(Suppl 1): e551 [abstract 33.39]
37. Corti R, Burnett JC Jr, Rouleau JL, Ruschitzka F, Luscher TF (2001) Vasopeptidase inhibitors: a new therapeutic concept in cardiovascular disease? Circulation 104(15):1856–1862
38. von Lueder TG, Sangaralingham SJ, Wang BH, Kompa AR, Atar D, Burnett JC Jr et al (2013) Renin-angiotensin blockade combined with natriuretic peptide system augmentation: novel therapeutic concepts to combat heart failure. Circ Heart Fail 6(3):594–605
39. Rademaker MT, Charles CJ, Espiner EA, Nicholls MG, Richards AM, Kosoglou T (1998) Combined neutral endopeptidase and angiotensin-converting enzyme inhibition in heart failure: role of natriuretic peptides and angiotensin II. J Cardiovasc Pharmacol 31(1):116–125
40. Boix F (2002) Vasopeptidase inhibitors: a bradykinin link. Lancet 359(9312):1157–1158
41. Campese VM, Lasseter KC, Ferrario CM, Smith WB, Ruddy MC, Grim CE et al (2001) Omapatrilat versus Lisinopril: efficacy and neurohormonal profile in salt-sensitive hypertensive patients. Hypertension 38(6):1342–1348
42. Vardeny O, Miller R, Solomon SD (2014) Combined neprilysin and renin-angiotensin system inhibition for the treatment of heart failure. JACC Heart Fail 2(6):663–670

43. Kario K, Tamaki Y, Okino N, Gotou H, Zhu M, Zhang J (2015) LCZ696, a First-in-Class Angiotensin Receptor-Neprilysin Inhibitor: The first clinical experience in patients with severe hypertension. J Clin Hypertens (Greenwich) 18(4):308–14
44. Williams B, Cockcroft JR, Kario K, Zappe DH, Cardenas P, Hester A et al (2014) Rationale and study design of the prospective comparison of angiotensin receptor neprilysin inhibitor with angiotensin receptor blocker MEasuring arterial sTiffness in the eldERly (PARAMETER) study. BMJ Open 4(2):e004254
45. Williams B, Cockcroft JR, Kario K, Zappe D, Wang Q, Guo W (2015) Principal results of the prospective comparison of angiotensin receptor neprilysin inhibitor with angiotensin receptor blocker measuring arterial stiffness in the elderly (PARAMETER) study. In: European society of cardiology 2015 congress, London; A4143
46. Bavishi C, Messerli FH, Kadosh B, Ruilope LM, Kario K (2015) Role of neprilysin inhibitor combinations in hypertension: insights from hypertension and heart failure trials. Eur Heart J 36(30):1967–1973
47. FDA (2016) http://www.fda.gov/NewsEvents/Newsroom/PressAnnouncements/ucm453845.htm. Accessed Feb 2016
48. EMA (2016) http://www.ema.europa.eu/ema/index.jsp?curl=pages/medicines/human/medicines/004062/smops/Positive/human_smop_000874.jsp&mid=WC0b01ac058001d127. Accessed Feb 2016
49. McMurray JJ, Packer M, Desai AS, Gong J, Lefkowitz MP, Rizkala AR et al (2014) Angiotensin-neprilysin inhibition versus enalapril in heart failure. N Engl J Med 371(11):993–1004
50. Seed A, Kuc RE, Maguire JJ, Hillier C, Johnston F, Essers H et al (2012) The Dual endothelin converting enzyme/neutral endopeptidase inhibitor SLV-306 (daglutril), inhibits systemic conversion of big endothelin-1 in humans. Life Sci 91(13-14):743–748
51. Parvanova A, van der Meer IM, Iliev I, Perna A, Gaspari F, Trevisan R et al (2013) Effect on blood pressure of combined inhibition of endothelin-converting enzyme and neutral endopeptidase with daglutril in patients with type 2 diabetes who have albuminuria: a randomised, crossover, double-blind, placebo-controlled trial. Lancet Diabetes Endocrinol 1(1):19–27
52. Dickstein K, De Voogd HJ, Miric MP, Willenbrock R, Mitrovic V, Pacher R et al (2004) Effect of single doses of SLV306, an inhibitor of both neutral endopeptidase and endothelin-converting enzyme, on pulmonary pressures in congestive heart failure. Am J Cardiol 94(2):237–239
53. Thone-Reinke C, Simon K, Richter CM, Godes M, Neumayer HH, Thormahlen D et al (2004) Inhibition of both neutral endopeptidase and endothelin-converting enzyme by SLV306 reduces Proteinuria and urinary albumin excretion in diabetic rats. J Cardiovasc Pharmacol 44(Suppl 1):S76–S79
54. Edelson JD, Makhlina M, Silvester KR, Vengurlekar SS, Chen X, Zhang J et al (2013) In vitro and in vivo pharmacological profile of PL-3994, a novel cyclic peptide (hept-cyclo(Cys-His-Phe-d-Ala-Gly-Arg-d-Nle-Asp-Arg-Ile-Ser-Cys)-Tyr-[Arg mimetic]-NH(2)) natriuretic peptide receptor-a agonist that is resistant to neutral endopeptidase and acts as a bronchodilator. Pulm Pharmacol Ther 26(2):229–238
55. Li Y, Sarkar O, Brochu M, Anand-Srivastava MB (2014) Natriuretic peptide receptor-C attenuates hypertension in spontaneously hypertensive rats: role of nitroxidative stress and Gi proteins. Hypertension 63(4):846–855
56. Couvineau A, Laburthe M (2012) VPAC receptors: structure, molecular pharmacology and interaction with accessory proteins. Br J Pharmacol 166(1):42–50
57. Henning RJ, Sawmiller DR (2001) Vasoactive intestinal peptide: cardiovascular effects. Cardiovasc Res 49(1):27–37
58. Free A, Brazg R, Matson M, Smith W, Chuck L, Georgopoulos L, Malatesta J, Arnold S, Kramer W, Strange P, Shi L, Gwynn J (2014) A phase 1, multi-center, randomized, double-blind, placebo controlled study to evaluate the safety/tolerability, pharmacokinetic and hemodynamic response following single ascending subcutaneous doses of PB1046 (vasomera™) in subjects with essential hypertension. Circulation 130:A19112

59. Stasch JP, Pacher P, Evgenov OV (2011) Soluble guanylate cyclase as an emerging therapeutic target in cardiopulmonary disease. Circulation 123(20):2263–2273
60. Munzel T, Daiber A, Gori T (2011) Nitrate therapy: new aspects concerning molecular action and tolerance. Circulation 123(19):2132–2144
61. Broderick KE, Alvarez L, Balasubramanian M, Belke DD, Makino A, Chan A et al (2007) Nitrosyl-cobinamide, a new and direct nitric oxide releasing drug effective in vivo. Exp Biol Med (Maywood) 232(11):1432–1440
62. Breschi MC, Calderone V, Digiacomo M, Macchia M, Martelli A, Martinotti E et al (2006) New NO-releasing pharmacodynamic hybrids of losartan and its active metabolite: design, synthesis, and biopharmacological properties. J Med Chem 49(8):2628–2639
63. Li YQ, Ji H, Zhang YH, Shi WB, Meng ZK, Chen XY et al (2007) WB1106, a novel nitric oxide-releasing derivative of Telmisartan, inhibits hypertension and improves glucose metabolism in rats. Eur J Pharmacol 577(1-3):100–108
64. Laurent S, Schlaich M, Esler M (2012) New drugs, procedures, and devices for hypertension. Lancet 380(9841):591–600
65. Townsend R, Bittar N, Rosen J, Smith W, Ramsay A, Chrysant SG et al (2011) Blood pressure effects of naproxcinod in hypertensive patients. J Clin Hypertens (Greenwich) 13(5):376–384
66. Rothermund L, Friebe A, Paul M, Koesling D, Kreutz R (2000) Acute blood pressure effects of YC-1-induced activation of soluble guanylyl cyclase in normotensive and hypertensive rats. Br J Pharmacol 130(2):205–208
67. Sharkovska Y, Kalk P, Lawrenz B, Godes M, Hoffmann LS, Wellkisch K et al (2010) Nitric oxide-independent stimulation of soluble guanylate cyclase reduces organ damage in experimental low-renin and high-renin models. J Hypertens 28(8):1666–1675
68. Ghofrani HA, Galie N, Grimminger F, Grunig E, Humbert M, Jing ZC et al (2013) Riociguat for the treatment of pulmonary arterial hypertension. N Engl J Med 369(4):330–340
69. Rich S, McLaughlin VV (2003) Endothelin receptor blockers in cardiovascular disease. Circulation 108(18):2184–2190
70. Krum H, Viskoper RJ, Lacourciere Y, Budde M, Charlon V (1998) The effect of an endothelin-receptor antagonist, bosentan, on blood pressure in patients with essential hypertension. Bosentan Hypertension Investigators. N Engl J Med 338(12):784–790
71. Bakris GL, Lindholm LH, Black HR, Krum H, Linas S, Linseman JV et al (2010) Divergent results using clinic and ambulatory blood pressures: report of a darusentan-resistant hypertension trial. Hypertension 56(5):824–830
72. Morisseau C, Hammock BD (2005) Epoxide hydrolases: mechanisms, inhibitor designs, and biological roles. Annu Rev Pharmacol Toxicol 45:311–333
73. Xu D, Li N, He Y, Timofeyev V, Lu L, Tsai HJ et al (2006) Prevention and reversal of cardiac hypertrophy by soluble epoxide hydrolase inhibitors. Proc Natl Acad Sci U S A 103(49):18733–18738
74. Spencer AG, Greasley PJ (2015) Pharmacologic inhibition of intestinal sodium uptake: a gut centric approach to sodium management. Curr Opin Nephrol Hypertens 24(5):410–416
75. Linz B, Hohl M, Reil JC, Bohm M, Linz D (2016) Inhibition of NHE3-mediated sodium absorption in the gut reduced cardiac end-organ damage without deteriorating renal function in obese spontaneously hypertensive rats. J Cardiovasc Pharmacol 67(3):225–231
76. Beliaev A, Learmonth DA, Soares-da-Silva P (2006) Synthesis and biological evaluation of novel, peripherally selective chromanyl imidazolethione-based inhibitors of dopamine beta-hydroxylase. J Med Chem 49(3):1191–1197
77. Almeida L, Nunes T, Costa R, Rocha JF, Vaz-da-Silva M, Soares-da-Silva P (2013) Etamicastat, a novel dopamine beta-hydroxylase inhibitor: tolerability, pharmacokinetics, and pharmacodynamics in patients with hypertension. Clin Ther 35(12):1983–1996
78. Helmer OM (1958) Studies on renin antibodies. Circulation 17:648–652
79. Brown MJ, Coltart J, Gunewardena K, Ritter JM, Auton TR, Glover JF (2004) Randomized double-blind placebo-controlled study of an angiotensin immunotherapeutic vaccine (PMD3117) in hypertensive subjects. Clin Sci (Lond) 107(2):167–173
80. Hong F, Quan WY, Pandey R, Yi S, Chi L, Xia LZ et al (2011) A vaccine for hypertension based on peptide AngI-R: a pilot study. Int J Cardiol 148(1):76–84

81. Tissot AC, Maurer P, Nussberger J, Sabat R, Pfister T, Ignatenko S et al (2008) Effect of immunisation against angiotensin II with CYT006-AngQb on ambulatory blood pressure: a double-blind, randomised, placebo-controlled phase IIa study. Lancet 371(9615):821–827
82. Maurer P, Bachmann MF (2010) Immunization against angiotensins for the treatment of hypertension. Clin Immunol 134(1):89–95
83. Lam GK, Hopoate-Sitake M, Adair CD, Buckalew VM, Johnson DD, Lewis DF et al (2013) Digoxin antibody fragment, antigen binding (Fab), treatment of preeclampsia in women with endogenous digitalis-like factor: a secondary analysis of the DEEP trial. Am J Obstet Gynecol 209(2):119 e111–116
84. Paidas MJ, Sibai BM, Triche EW, Frieling J, Lowry S, Group, P.-S (2013) Exploring the role of antithrombin replacement for the treatment of preeclampsia: a prospective randomized evaluation of the safety and efficacy of recombinant antithrombin in very preterm preeclampsia (PRESERVE-1). Am J Reprod Immunol 69(6):539–544
85. Manunta P, Ferrandi M, Cusi D, Ferrari P, Staessen J, Bianchi G (2016) Personalized therapy of hypertension: the past and the future. Curr Hypertens Rep 18(3):24
86. Kreutz R, Hubner N (2002) Congenic rat strains are important tools for the genetic dissection of essential hypertension. Semin Nephrol 22(2):135–147
87. Kato N, Loh M, Takeuchi F, Verweij N, Wang X, Zhang W et al (2015) Trans-ancestry genome-wide association study identifies 12 genetic loci influencing blood pressure and implicates a role for DNA methylation. Nat Genet 47(11):1282–1293
88. Staessen JA, Thijs L, Stolarz-Skrzypek K, Bacchieri A, Barton J, Espositi ED et al (2011) Main results of the ouabain and adducin for specific intervention on sodium in hypertension trial (OASIS-HT): a randomized placebo-controlled phase-2 dose-finding study of rostafuroxin. Trials 12:13
89. Tragante V, Barnes MR, Ganesh SK, Lanktree MB, Guo W, Franceschini N et al (2014) Gene-centric meta-analysis in 87,736 individuals of european ancestry identifies multiple blood-pressure-related loci. Am J Hum Genet 94(3):349–360
90. Frye SV, Arkin MR, Arrowsmith CH, Conn PJ, Glicksman MA, Hull-Ryde EA et al (2015) Tackling reproducibility in academic preclinical drug discovery. Nat Rev Drug Discov 14(11):733–734
91. Barrett JC, Dunham I, Birney E (2015) Using human genetics to make new medicines. Nat Rev Genet 16(10):561–562

Adherence to Medications in Uncontrolled Hypertension

11

Michel Burnier and Gregoire Wuerzner

Abbreviations

BP	Blood pressure
dRHTN	Drug-resistant hypertension
HTN	Hypertension

11.1 Introduction

In hypertension (HTN), lowering blood pressure (BP) to the recommended targets is the most effective way to reduce both total and cardiovascular mortality in hypertensive patients and to decrease the risk of developing cardiac, renal, and neurological complications [1–3]. Today, the clinical management of essential HTN is based essentially on the recommendation of lifestyle changes such as losing weight, eating less salt or exercising more, and on the prescription of BP-lowering drugs [1]. More recently, the development of interventional treatments such as renal denervation, baroreceptor stimulation, or the creation of an iliac arteriovenous fistula has provided additional opportunities to control BP especially in patients with drug-resistant hypertension (dRHTN) [4–6].

Whatever the therapeutic alternative proposed to control the patient's high BP, adherence is a major determinant of the success of therapy. Indeed, changes in lifestyle necessitate a long-term perseverance and persistence in order to be efficacious. Similarly, long-term adherence to drug treatments is essential to obtain the clinical

M. Burnier (✉) • G. Wuerzner
Service of Nephrology and Hypertension, Department of Medicine, Centre Hospitalier Universitaire Vaudois, Rue du Bugnon 17, Lausanne 1011, Switzerland
e-mail: michel.burnier@chuv.ch

C. Tsioufis et al. (eds.), *Interventional Therapies for Secondary and Essential Hypertension*, Updates in Hypertension and Cardiovascular Protection,
DOI 10.1007/978-3-319-34141-5_11

benefits of antihypertensive therapy even after interventional procedures. Thus, Mancia et al. have reported that the higher the percentage of clinical visits with a normal BP, the lower the incidence of clinical outcomes [7]. In addition, in a cohort of 242,594 patients aged 18 years or older, residents in the Italian Lombardy Region, who were newly treated for HTN during 2000–2001, those who continued their treatment had a 37 % reduced risk of cardiovascular outcomes when compared with those who experienced at least one episode of treatment discontinuation [8]. In patients with very low drug coverage, the risk of cardiovascular events was markedly reduced suggesting that compliance with antihypertensive therapy is crucial for the primary prevention of cardiovascular outcomes [8]. This observation is actually not specific for HTN, since similar observations have been made with other drug classes prescribed for the primary and secondary prevention of cardiovascular diseases [9].

This chapter will address several aspects of the role of drug adherence in HTN with a special emphasis on the impact of adherence in uncontrolled HTN.

11.2 Defining Adherence and Its Various Components

According to the World Health Organization, adherence is defined as the extent to which a patient's behavior – following a diet, taking medications, and executing lifestyle changes – corresponds with agreed recommendations from a healthcare provider. In 2012, a new taxonomy has been proposed following a consensus meeting [10]. According to this taxonomy, adherence to medication is the process by which patients take their medications as prescribed. Adherence can be characterized by three phases: the *initiation*, the *implementation,* and the *discontinuation. Initiation* represents the time between drug prescription and the day when the first dose is taken. *Implementation* is the extent to which a patient's actual dosing corresponds to the prescribed dosing regimen, from initiation until the last dose. Lastly, *discontinuation* represents the end of therapy when the next dose to be taken is omitted and the treatment is interrupted thereafter. One should also consider the *persistence* which is the length of time between the initiation and the last dose, which immediately precedes discontinuation and *compliance* which corresponds to the execution on a day-by-day basis. This latter includes the *taking*, i.e., is the drug taken or not, and the *timing*, i.e., is the drug taken at the right moment of the day.

Among all the various characteristics of adherence, three need to be discussed because they have a major impact on the quality of BP control in hypertension: non-initiation, non-persistence, and a poor execution [11, 12] (Fig. 11.1). Non-initiation concerns about 4–5 % of patients who never start their treatment although very often they do buy their medications. Non-persistence is definitively the greatest problem in HTN with about 30–50 % of patients ceasing their engagement with the dosing regimen on their own initiative after 1 year [13–15]. Several studies have actually demonstrated that drug persistence to most common antihypertensive ranges between 40 and 60 % at 1 year with important differences between antihypertensive classes [16–18]. Many reasons have been identified to explain this rather low

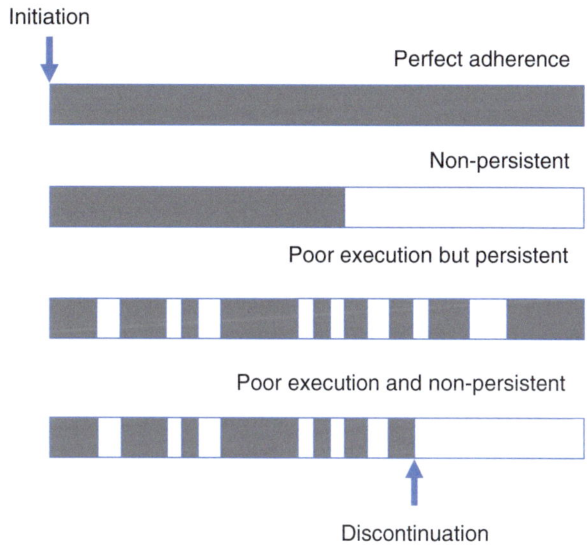

Fig. 11.1 Schematic representation of various forms of nonadherence

persistence in HTN. Among them, one could cite the incidence of short- or long-term side effects, the fact that BP remains uncontrolled, a lack of motivation, the non-affordability of drugs, and the patients' poor understanding of the reasons to treat HTN as they are asymptomatic. A poor execution of the treatment which leads to short (1–2 days) or long (up to 1 week) interruptions of drug dosing may also result in poor BP control. Lapses in implementation are typically the consequence of forgetfulness or negligence resulting in treatment interruptions. The clinical impact depends on the pharmacological characteristics of the drugs omitted. Missing one or two doses of a very long-acting drug may have no influence on BP, whereas the same length of interruption of a short acting drug may lead to an immediate increase in BP. These observations have led to the development of the concept of "forgiving drugs," i.e., drugs which can be omitted without serious consequences on the control of BP [19]. Thus, comparing three different antihypertensive drugs blocking the renin-angiotensin system (aliskiren, ramipril, and irbesartan), we have been able to show that the impact of missed doses on BP control and risk reduction depends largely on the pharmacological profile of the prescribed drugs [19].

11.3 Clinical Assessment of Drug Adherence: A Major Challenge

In all domains of science, it is difficult to solve a problem if this latter cannot be characterized and quantified correctly. In this respect, the lack of easy and reliable methods to assess drug adherence is one of the biggest problems in clinical medicine. As mentioned in a previous review, the ideal method to measure drug adherence should "provide a reliable capture, storage, analysis and communication of

Table 11.1 The four questions of the simplified Morisky questionnaire used in clinical practice

1. Do you sometimes forget to take your high blood pressure pills?
2. Have you ever cut back or stopped taking your medication without telling your doctor because you felt worse when you took it?
3. When you feel like your blood pressure is under control, do you sometimes stop taking your medicine?
4. Taking medication everyday is a real inconvenience for some people.
Do you ever feel hassled about sticking to your blood pressure treatment plan?

dosing history data in ways that make it difficult or impossible for patients or trial staff to censor or otherwise manipulate the data" [12]. Today, although no methodology really fulfills these criteria, three approaches may be considered as relatively reliable, i.e., the retrospective analysis of prescription refill records, often used in large epidemiological surveys, the analysis of chemical markers of drug exposure, and the automatic electronic monitoring of adherence. These three methods will be discussed further below.

Today, in clinical practice, the large majority of physicians estimates drug adherence using a careful interview. This approach provides a vague impression on what the patient is actually doing with his/her medications. Although it has the merit to favor a discussion between physicians and patients about adherence, it remains relatively imprecise unless patients admit that they did not initiate their treatment or that they interrupted it for reasons such as the occurrence of side effects or the fear of drug interactions. The clinical response as the reduction of heart rate on beta-blockers, the respect of medical terms, and the development of specific drug-induced side effects are often used by clinicians as indirect markers of adherence, but their adequacy of these markers remains questionable. In some countries, hypertension societies recommend to use the Morisky questionnaire or one of its simplified versions based on four questions (Table 11.1) [20]. These questionnaires have the advantage of being simple and easy to use during a consultation. However, comparisons with medication monitoring systems or plasma drug levels have shown that the Morisky questionnaire tends to overestimate the adherence probably because patients tend to forget the episodes when no medication was taken [21, 22].

When dealing with large groups of patients in clinical trials or epidemiological surveys, the most frequent methods used to monitor drug adherence are the pill count and the assessment of prescription refills. Pill count is considered the method of choice in clinical trials. Although pill count gives useful information on drug intake during a time frame, it has also a tendency to overestimate the true adherence even in clinical trials [23]. This was demonstrated in small clinical studies in which more pills were provided than actually needed for a defined time period. In these cases, adherence of 110 or 120 % could be measured suggesting either an increased intake or a discard of the pill excess. The monitoring of prescription refills is today the reference method in epidemiological surveys. This method enables to calculate the percentage of days covered by the prescribed treatment [24]. However, to obtain reliable data, it is absolutely necessary to have an adequate electronic monitoring of drug prescriptions by pharmacies or reliable registries. The major limitation of this approach is that one has no information on what patients are doing with their treatment on a day-to-day basis and, hence, one assumes that patients take their drugs adequately every day, which is certainly not the case. At last, patients may obtain their medications from different pharmacies. Therefore, it is crucial that the monitoring system covers all potential sources of medication delivery. Taken together, the various limitations of the prescription refills monitoring probably lead to an overestimation of the true patients' adherence.

Today, two methods can be considered as clinically useful because they produce reliable information on drug adherence: the electronic monitoring and the direct measurements of plasma or urine drug concentrations. Electronic monitoring of drug adherence has been used essentially in clinical trials, and few centers have introduced this approach in their clinical practice as we have been doing since two decades ago [11, 12]. The advantage of the electronic monitoring is that it provides dynamic information on adherence and the information is recorded and cannot be modified. The dynamic approach is crucial, since drug adherence is a highly *dynamic process* which can vary enormously in the same patient from one period of the year to another. This method is often criticized because it records every time the box is open and does not prove that the medication has been taken by the patient. This is actually not an issue because the most important information provided by the electronic monitoring is when the box is not opened. In this case, one can be sure that the drug was not taken. In our experience, it is extremely rare that a patient opens the pillbox every day and throws its content during months. However, knowing what patients are actually doing with their medications is very informative for physicians as it helps them to take more rational clinical decisions [25].

With the development of clinical programs on dRHTN, a new interest has emerged for the determinations of drug levels in plasma or urine [22, 26–28]. The goal of these measurements is to ascertain that patients are indeed resistant. This approach has long been limited by the difficulty to measure accurately the different antihypertensive drugs available on the market, but today, this obstacle has been surmounted with the development of new laboratory technologies such as mass spectroscopy and/or liquid chromatography. Nowadays most antihypertensive drugs can be detected with these methods, but these latter remain costly and labor intensive. The main advantage of these measurements is that they confirm that some drug was taken, but they give no information on when the medication was taken and no insight on the dosing history. Nonetheless, this approach has been found to be very useful in the diagnosis of dRHTN demonstrating a very low adherence in a large proportion of patients with apparent resistance [26–28]. Of note, this approach is often affected by the *white coat adherence* phenomenon according to which patients tend to improve their adherence during the days preceding or following a medical term [29]. In addition, one question is whether patients should be informed that blood or urine will be taken to monitor their adherence. If they are, the likelihood of a positive test will be much higher. If they are not, this might represent an ethical issue in some countries. A recent analysis based on the Markov model has suggested that therapeutic drug monitoring is cost-effective in patients with dRHTN [30]. One interesting observation made with the use of drug levels in clinical practice is that BP control improves once patients have been informed of the results [28]. This indicates once more that providing a feedback to the patients has a very positive influence [31]. Another interesting finding is that the availability of plasma drug levels enables to perform a better analysis of data collected in clinical studies as changes in BP or any other clinical results can be assessed differentially in those patients who took the drug and those who did not [32, 33].

A rarely used technique to ensure drug intake is the direct observed treatment or DOT. This method is applied for infectious diseases such as tuberculosis to be absolutely sure that drugs are taken to avoid the dissemination of the disease and/or the development of resistant strains if the treatment is incomplete. A similar approach has been used in dRHTN by some investigators [34]. This method is effective but needs time and personal and hence has some cost.

Taken together, all these data emphasize how difficult it is to assess drug adherence in clinical practice. There is definitively a great necessity of developing new tools to help physicians. Meanwhile one can only encourage physicians spending more time discussing with their patients on drug adherence.

11.4 Adherence in Hypertension

When questioned, all physicians will recognize that drug adherence is a major concern in the management of essential HTN. Surprisingly, however, when assessed in clinical studies using electronic monitoring, for example, adherence is found to be quite variable but relatively high [35, 36]. In addition, correlations between the level of adherence and the quality of BP control or the level of BP have been difficult to obtain and were, in general, weak [37, 38]. The main reason for the discrepancy between the perceived adherence and the measured adherence is certainly the measurement bias, as adherence improves as soon as it is measured. In addition, high BP values can be found in nonadherent as well as in adherent patients if the latter are insufficiently treated. However, when patients are under monitoring, BP tends to improve and to be better controlled as we observed in patients with apparent resistant hypertension. In one controlled study, monitoring adherence did not ameliorate BP but prevented changes in drug therapies. Thus, electronic monitoring drug adherence during a long period has several advantages: firstly, it provides information on how the patient is behaving with his/her medications; secondly, it generally improves BP control; and, thirdly, it may support the patient's adherence with a feedback system indicating when the past dose was taken.

With more than 20 years of experience, the use of electronic monitors such as the medication event monitoring system (MEMS) has provided a huge amount of information on the long-term behavior of hypertensive patients with many key observations for practicing physicians [11]. As already mentioned, one has realized that drug adherence is very dynamic, that patients make frequent drug holidays especially during weekends, and that they sometimes compensate drug omissions by taking more than the recommended dose during one or two days. Depending on the pharmacological characteristics of the drugs, these behaviors may have a major impact not only on BP but also on the incidence of side effects.

One question which is rarely addressed in the drug management of HTN is: what is the acceptable level of adherence that patients should achieved in order to be sure that they get the benefit of their treatment? In fact, this issue has never been addressed carefully and all authors in the field tend to consider that 80 % is the cutoff below which the patients should be considered as poorly adherent. We have observed that in patients with so-called dRHTN, BP increases significantly as soon as adherence is below 90 %. Therefore, drug adherence should be analyzed as a continuous parameter and not according to arbitrary cutoffs as often done in literature.

Despite all these observations, there is now strong evidence that a good adherence is associated with a better control of BP but also a greater reduction of the patients' cardiovascular risk and a significantly greater reduction in coronary events, in heart failure, and stroke events [8, 39–41].

11.5 When Should Adherence Be Monitored in Hypertension?

It is obvious that patients should not be bothered with an investigation of drug adherence if their BP is well controlled. Thus, adherence monitoring using any of the available methods should be envisaged whenever BP control is not achieved following the prescription of a dual therapy or more. When patients are on a monotherapy, the likelihood to normalize BP is so low (30–50) that the probability of an insufficient treatment is greater than that of nonadherence. With a dual therapy, about 60 % of hypertensive patients usually reach the BP targets. Therefore, when on a monotherapy, treatment should first be intensified and poor adherence considered in a second step.

In our opinion, physicians should ask the question of drug adherence whenever patients receiving at least two drugs remain uncontrolled, even if they do not fulfill the definition of dRHTN which is a BP > 140/90 mmHg despite a triple therapy including a diuretic, a calcium channel blocker, and a blocker of the renin-angiotensin system. In this respect, physicians should be aware of the numerous factors associated with an increased risk of poor adherence. As shown in Table 11.2, these include younger male patients, elderly subjects with cognitive impairment, depression, a complex treatment with a high pill burden, etc. [14, 42–45]. Newly treated hypertensive patients are also at higher risk of stopping their medications than patients treated for years who have accepted their treatment [16, 46]. At last, the class of antihypertensive drug chosen to initiate the therapy appears to have an important impact on long-term drug persistence [18].

The assessment of adherence becomes crucial when investigating the possible cause of treatment resistance. When BP remains high despite a heavy treatment containing several antihypertensive drugs, the logical questions are: is the patient really resistant? Or is the patient taking the medication correctly? In these clinical situations, the trend is to intensify the treatment adding a fourth or a fifth drug, and

Table 11.2 Factors associated with an increased risk of poor adherence

Age and sex (young men at higher risk)
Elderly patients with cognitive impairment
Personal and family beliefs
Asymptomatic nature of hypertension
Understanding of the benefits of treatment
Lower socioeconomic status
Cost of treatments and copayments
Severity of disease
Number of drugs and complexity of treatment
Drug tolerability (acute and long-term side effects)
Efficacy on blood pressure control
Family support
Physician-patient relationship
Depression and comorbidities

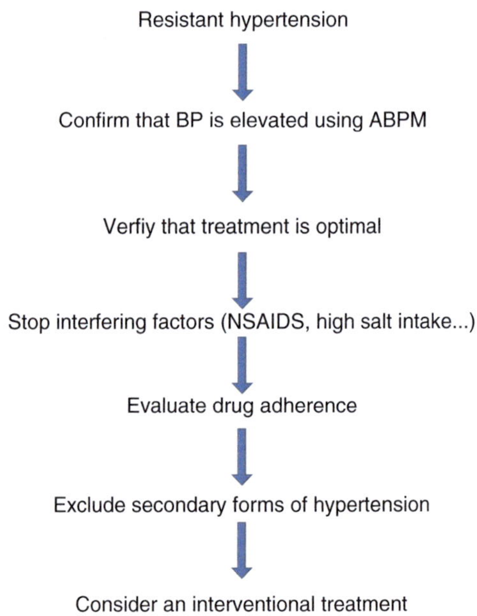

Fig. 11.2 Schematic representation of our proposed work-up of patients with resistant hypertension candidates for an interventional treatment

this strategy is actually supported by many guidelines. However, if adherence is the issue, adding new drugs is really meaningless. Recent surveys suggest that dRHTN is particularly prevalent among patients with hypertensive complications [47–49] and is simultaneously a major cause of hypertension target organ damages [50].

With the development of new therapeutic strategies for dRHTN, especially renal denervation, many studies have been conducted to better identify patients who are truly resistant to therapy and not pseudo-resistant [51]. This recent movement has actually promoted the use of ambulatory BP monitoring as well as the assessment of drug adherence [52]. In fact, according to most recommendations, these two aspects belong to the early steps of the screening of patients with dRHTN

(Fig. 11.2). Using the electronic monitoring of drug adherence, we found that 30–50 % of resistant patients had adherence problems leading to uncontrolled HTN [25, 53]. Recently, a special emphasis has been put on the use of either urinary or blood drug concentrations to verify the patient's adherence to therapy, and similar were found [26, 27, 54]. The opportunity to identify antihypertensive drugs in biological fluids has become available and affordable with the development of analytic techniques such as high-performance liquid chromatography coupled to mass spectrometry. Investigators were very surprised to find up to 50 % of total or partial nonadherence in renal denervation candidates. Interestingly nonadherence was observed in inpatients as well as in outpatients [54]. Thus, despite some major limitations discussed previously in this chapter, the demonstration of the presence or absence of the prescribed drugs in the blood or urine may sometimes be useful to identify non-adherers and might contribute to support patients in their efforts of maintaining their treatment as they offer the opportunity to address the patient's difficulties.

11.6 How to Improve Drug Adherence in Uncontrolled Hypertension?

Multiple strategies have been proposed to improve drug adherence in chronic diseases such as HTN. However, although some interventions were associated with a significant improvement of BP during a short-time period, none of them has demonstrated a major superior effect as reported in the long run in meta-analyses and Cochrane reports [55–57]. It seems that interventions should be tailored to each individual. Nevertheless, some strategies merit to be applied to every patient whatever the disease. The first is the empowerment of the patient [56]. Whatever the level of education of the patient, this latter should be clearly informed on the overall goals of therapy, on the BP targets, and on the means to achieve them with the therapy. They should also receive the adequate information on the drug side effects and on the potential complications in order to help them cope with these events. In HTN, self-measurements of BP at home have been shown to be helpful although not all patients are willing to do it. In a recent study, investigators have proposed to let the patient uptitrate the treatment to achieve BP targets. This unusual approach was found to improve BP control without major inconvenience for the patients [58].

The second effective strategy is to simplify the treatment as much as possible in order to reduce the pill burden, considering that most hypertensive patients have other concomitant diseases which need to be taken care off with oral medications. In this respect, the development of single-pill combination containing two or three active compounds is of great benefit for hypertensive patients [59, 60]. Among the numerous single-pill combinations available on the market, one should recommend those combining different long-acting drugs enabling the omission of one or two doses without any significant increase in BP. Unfortunately, in some countries, triple combinations are not reimbursed.

The use of pill organizers, recalls using telephone or emails, and rewards and behavioral interventions have all been reported to improve drug adherence and blood pressure control. However, the magnitude of their effect was found to be small. Except for pill organizers, they are also difficult to implement for a very long time period. Ideally patients with the greatest difficulty to stay on therapy should be monitored continuously. We are actually using the MEMS system in our practice to support patients, and the majority of them do appreciate the monitoring because it represents also a unique opportunity to discuss their adherence but based on data they gathered. Unfortunately, the development of the MEMS has been concentrated on clinical trials, and few centers are using them in clinical practice. Yet, it would be perfectly affordable if one considers the costs of nonadherence.

The most recent approach developed in some countries such as Canada is the multidisciplinary management of hypertensive patients with a high risk on non-persistence and uncontrolled BP [61]. The principle is to involve other healthcare professionals, for example, nurses or pharmacists, in the follow-up of hypertensive patients [62, 63]. This multidisciplinary concept has been tested and was found to be effective in improving adherence and hence clinical endpoints not only in hypertension but also in patients with heart failure or chronic kidney diseases [63, 64]. Today, this system has not been largely exported essentially because of problems of reimbursement of nurses or pharmacists and also because of the difficult collaboration between general practitioners and pharmacists. At last the cost-effectiveness of these collaborations has been questioned [62, 65].

Conclusions

In the absence of new drug development in HTN and while we are waiting the results demonstrating the efficacy and the long-term benefits of interventional treatments of HTN, physicians will have no other choice than managing HTN with the drugs available today. In this context, working on drug adherence and improving treatment persistence are the only ways to effectively improve BP control in populations and to reach the ambitious targets proposed by some countries such as Italy and France, i.e., to normalize BP in 75 % of the hypertensive population. In Canada, the implementation of the Canadian Hypertension Education Program involving pharmacists and nurses has led to an impressive increase in the percentage of hypertensive patients treated and well controlled with 68 % of patients on target [61]. This program demonstrates that it is possible to do better with what we have, as long as physicians resist to the medical inertia [66] and patients remain motivated and persist with their treatment.

References

1. ESH/ESC Task Force for the Management of Arterial Hypertension (2013) 2013 Practice guidelines for the management of arterial hypertension of the European Society of Hypertension (ESH) and the European Society of Cardiology (ESC): ESH/ESC Task Force for the Management of Arterial Hypertension. J Hypertens 31(10):1925–1938

2. James PA, Oparil S, Carter BL, Cushman WC, Dennison-Himmelfarb C, Handler J et al (2014) 2014 evidence-based guideline for the management of high blood pressure in adults: report from the panel members appointed to the Eighth Joint National Committee (JNC 8). JAMA 311(5):507–520
3. National Clinical Guideline C (2011) National Institute for Health and Clinical Excellence: Guidance. Hypertension: the clinical management of primary hypertension in adults: update of clinical guidelines 18 and 34. Royal College of Physicians (UK) National Clinical Guideline Centre, London
4. Vongpatanasin W (2014) Resistant hypertension: a review of diagnosis and management. JAMA 311(21):2216–2224
5. Victor RG (2015) Carotid baroreflex activation therapy for resistant hypertension. Nat Rev Cardiol 12(8):451–463
6. Lobo MD, Sobotka PA, Stanton A, Cockcroft JR, Sulke N, Dolan E et al (2015) Central arteriovenous anastomosis for the treatment of patients with uncontrolled hypertension (the ROX CONTROL HTN study): a randomised controlled trial. Lancet 385(9978):1634–1641
7. Mancia G, Messerli F, Bakris G, Zhou Q, Champion A, Pepine CJ (2007) Blood pressure control and improved cardiovascular outcomes in the International Verapamil SR-Trandolapril Study. Hypertension 50(2):299–305
8. Corrao G, Parodi A, Nicotra F, Zambon A, Merlino L, Cesana G et al (2011) Better compliance to antihypertensive medications reduces cardiovascular risk. J Hypertens 29(3):610–618
9. Naderi SH, Bestwick JP, Wald DS (2012) Adherence to drugs that prevent cardiovascular disease: meta-analysis on 376,162 patients. Am J Med 125(9):882–887 e1
10. Vrijens B, De Geest S, Hughes DA, Przemyslaw K, Demonceau J, Ruppar T et al (2012) A new taxonomy for describing and defining adherence to medications. Br J Clin Pharmacol 73(5):691–705
11. Blaschke TF, Osterberg L, Vrijens B, Urquhart J (2012) Adherence to medications: insights arising from studies on the unreliable link between prescribed and actual drug dosing histories. Annu Rev Pharmacol Toxicol 52:275–301
12. Burnier M, Wuerzner G, Struijker-Boudier H, Urquhart J (2013) Measuring, analyzing, and managing drug adherence in resistant hypertension. Hypertension 62(2):218–225
13. Vrijens B, Vincze G, Kristanto P, Urquhart J, Burnier M (2008) Adherence to prescribed antihypertensive drug treatments: longitudinal study of electronically compiled dosing histories. BMJ 336(7653):1114–1117
14. Qvarnstrom M, Kahan T, Kieler H, Brandt L, Hasselstrom J, Bengtsson Bostrom K et al (2013) Persistence to antihypertensive drug treatment in Swedish primary healthcare. Eur J Clin Pharmacol 69(11):1955–1964
15. Mazzaglia G, Mantovani LG, Sturkenboom MC, Filippi A, Trifiro G, Cricelli C et al (2005) Patterns of persistence with antihypertensive medications in newly diagnosed hypertensive patients in Italy: a retrospective cohort study in primary care. J Hypertens 23(11):2093–2100
16. Caro JJ, Salas M, Speckman JL, Raggio G, Jackson JD (1999) Persistence with treatment for hypertension in actual practice. CMAJ 160(1):31–37
17. Mancia G, Parodi A, Merlino L, Corrao G (2011) Heterogeneity in antihypertensive treatment discontinuation between drugs belonging to the same class. J Hypertens 29(5):1012–1018
18. Caro JJ, Speckman JL, Salas M, Raggio G, Jackson JD (1999) Effect of initial drug choice on persistence with antihypertensive therapy: the importance of actual practice data. CMAJ 160(1):41–46
19. Burnier M, Brede Y, Lowy A (2011) Impact of prolonged antihypertensive duration of action on predicted clinical outcomes in imperfectly adherent patients: comparison of aliskiren, irbesartan and ramipril. Int J Clin Pract 65(2):127–133
20. Morisky DE, Ang A, Krousel-Wood M, Ward HJ (2008) Predictive validity of a medication adherence measure in an outpatient setting. J Clin Hypertens (Greenwich) 10(5):348–354
21. Shi L, Liu J, Koleva Y, Fonseca V, Kalsekar A, Pawaskar M (2010) Concordance of adherence measurement using self-reported adherence questionnaires and medication monitoring devices. Pharmacoeconomics 28(12):1097–1107

22. Pandey A, Raza F, Velasco A, Brinker S, Ayers C, Das SR et al (2015) Comparison of Morisky Medication Adherence Scale with therapeutic drug monitoring in apparent treatment-resistant hypertension. J Am Soc Hypertens 9(6):420–426 e2
23. Lee JY, Kusek JW, Greene PG, Bernhard S, Norris K, Smith D et al (1996) Assessing medication adherence by pill count and electronic monitoring in the African American Study of Kidney Disease and Hypertension (AASK) Pilot Study. Am J Hypertens 9(8):719–725
24. Halpern MT, Khan ZM, Schmier JK, Burnier M, Caro JJ, Cramer J et al (2006) Recommendations for evaluating compliance and persistence with hypertension therapy using retrospective data. Hypertension 47(6):1039–1048
25. Burnier M, Schneider MP, Chiolero A, Stubi CL, Brunner HR (2001) Electronic compliance monitoring in resistant hypertension: the basis for rational therapeutic decisions. J Hypertens 19(2):335–341
26. Jung O, Gechter JL, Wunder C, Paulke A, Bartel C, Geiger H et al (2013) Resistant hypertension? Assessment of adherence by toxicological urine analysis. J Hypertens 31(4):766–774
27. Tomaszewski M, White C, Patel P, Masca N, Damani R, Hepworth J et al (2014) High rates of non-adherence to antihypertensive treatment revealed by high-performance liquid chromatography-tandem mass spectrometry (HP LC-MS/MS) urine analysis. Heart (British Cardiac Society) 100(11):855–861
28. Brinker S, Pandey A, Ayers C, Price A, Raheja P, Arbique D et al (2014) Therapeutic drug monitoring facilitates blood pressure control in resistant hypertension. J Am Coll Cardiol 63(8):834–835
29. Cramer JA, Scheyer RD, Mattson RH (1990) Compliance declines between clinic visits. Arch Intern Med 150(7):1509–1510
30. Chung O, Vongpatanasin W, Bonaventura K, Lotan Y, Sohns C, Haverkamp W et al (2014) Potential cost-effectiveness of therapeutic drug monitoring in patients with resistant hypertension. J Hypertens 32(12):2411–2421
31. Demonceau J, Ruppar T, Kristanto P, Hughes DA, Fargher E, Kardas P et al (2013) Identification and assessment of adherence-enhancing interventions in studies assessing medication adherence through electronically compiled drug dosing histories: a systematic literature review and meta-analysis. Drugs 73(6):545–562
32. Beaussier H, Boutouyrie P, Bobrie G, Frank M, Laurent S, Coudore F et al (2015) True antihypertensive efficacy of sequential nephron blockade in patients with resistant hypertension and confirmed medication adherence. J Hypertens 33(12):2526–2533
33. Burnier M, Wuerzner G (2015) Drug adherence monitoring in clinical trials: a necessity for a correct assessment of the efficacy and safety of antihypertensive therapies. J Hypertens 33(12):2395–2398
34. Fadl Elmula FE, Hoffmann P, Larstorp AC, Fossum E, Brekke M, Kjeldsen SE et al (2014) Adjusted drug treatment is superior to renal sympathetic denervation in patients with true treatment-resistant hypertension. Hypertension 63(5):991–999
35. Wetzels GE, Nelemans PJ, Schouten JS, Dirksen CD, van der Weijden T, Stoffers HE et al (2007) Electronic monitoring of adherence as a tool to improve blood pressure control. A randomized controlled trial. Am J Hypertens 20(2):119–125
36. Christensen A, Osterberg LG, Hansen EH (2009) Electronic monitoring of patient adherence to oral antihypertensive medical treatment: a systematic review. J Hypertens 27(8):1540–1551
37. Bramley TJ, Gerbino PP, Nightengale BS, Frech-Tamas F (2006) Relationship of blood pressure control to adherence with antihypertensive monotherapy in 13 managed care organizations. J Manag Care Pharm 12(3):239–245
38. Mallion JM, Baguet JP, Siche JP, Tremel F, de Gaudemaris R (1998) Compliance, electronic monitoring and antihypertensive drugs. J Hypertens Suppl 16(1):S75–S79
39. Perreault S, Dragomir A, Roy L, White M, Blais L, Lalonde L et al (2010) Adherence level of antihypertensive agents in coronary artery disease. Br J Clin Pharmacol 69(1):74–84

40. Perreault S, Dragomir A, White M, Lalonde L, Blais L, Berard A (2009) Better adherence to antihypertensive agents and risk reduction of chronic heart failure. J Intern Med 266(2):207–218
41. Kettani FZ, Dragomir A, Cote R, Roy L, Berard A, Blais L et al (2009) Impact of a better adherence to antihypertensive agents on cerebrovascular disease for primary prevention. Stroke 40(1):213–220
42. Iskedjian M, Einarson TR, MacKeigan LD, Shear N, Addis A, Mittmann N et al (2002) Relationship between daily dose frequency and adherence to antihypertensive pharmacotherapy: evidence from a meta-analysis. Clin Ther 24(2):302–316
43. Morris AB, Li J, Kroenke K, Bruner-England TE, Young JM, Murray MD (2006) Factors associated with drug adherence and blood pressure control in patients with hypertension. Pharmacotherapy 26(4):483–492
44. Turner BJ, Hollenbeak C, Weiner MG, Ten Have T, Roberts C (2009) Barriers to adherence and hypertension control in a racially diverse representative sample of elderly primary care patients. Pharmacoepidemiol Drug Saf 18(8):672–681
45. Neri L, Martini A, Andreucci VE, Gallieni M, Rey LA, Brancaccio D et al (2011) Regimen complexity and prescription adherence in dialysis patients. Am J Nephrol 34(1):71–76
46. Van Wijk BL, Klungel OH, Heerdink ER, de Boer A (2006) Initial non-compliance with antihypertensive monotherapy is followed by complete discontinuation of antihypertensive therapy. Pharmacoepidemiol Drug Saf 15(8):587–593
47. Smith SM, Gong Y, Handberg E, Messerli FH, Bakris GL, Ahmed A et al (2014) Predictors and outcomes of resistant hypertension among patients with coronary artery disease and hypertension. J Hypertens 32(3):635–643
48. Thomas G, Xie D, Chen HY, Anderson AH, Appel LJ, Bodana S et al (2016) Prevalence and prognostic significance of apparent treatment resistant hypertension in chronic kidney disease: report from the chronic renal insufficiency cohort study. Hypertension 67(2):387–396
49. Howard VJ, Tanner RM, Anderson A, Irvin MR, Calhoun DA, Lackland DT et al (2015) Apparent treatment-resistant hypertension among individuals with history of stroke or transient ischemic attack. Am J Med 128(7):707–714, e2
50. Muntner P, Davis BR, Cushman WC, Bangalore S, Calhoun DA, Pressel SL et al (2014) Treatment-resistant hypertension and the incidence of cardiovascular disease and end-stage renal disease: results from the Antihypertensive and Lipid-Lowering Treatment to Prevent Heart Attack Trial (ALLHAT). Hypertension 64(5):1012–1021
51. Persu A, Jin Y, Baelen M, Vink E, Verloop WL, Schmidt B et al (2014) Eligibility for renal denervation: experience at 11 European expert centers. Hypertension 63(6):1319–1325
52. Burnier M, Wuerzner G (2014) Ambulatory blood pressure and adherence monitoring: diagnosing pseudoresistant hypertension. Semin Nephrol 34(5):498–505
53. Bertholet N, Favrat B, Fallab-Stubi CL, Brunner HR, Burnier M (2000) Why objective monitoring of compliance is important in the management of hypertension. J Clin Hypertens (Greenwich) 2(4):258–262
54. Strauch B, Petrak O, Zelinka T, Rosa J, Somloova Z, Indra T et al (2013) Precise assessment of noncompliance with the antihypertensive therapy in patients with resistant hypertension using toxicological serum analysis. J Hypertens 31(12):2455–2461
55. Glynn LG, Murphy AW, Smith SM, Schroeder K, Fahey T (2010) Interventions used to improve control of blood pressure in patients with hypertension. Cochrane Database Syst Rev (3):Cd005182
56. Gwadry-Sridhar FH, Manias E, Lal L, Salas M, Hughes DA, Ratzki-Leewing A et al (2013) Impact of interventions on medication adherence and blood pressure control in patients with essential hypertension: a systematic review by the ISPOR medication adherence and persistence special interest group. Value Health 16(5):863–871
57. Ogedegbe G, Schoenthaler A (2006) A systematic review of the effects of home blood pressure monitoring on medication adherence. J Clin Hypertens (Greenwich) 8(3):174–180

58. McManus RJ, Mant J, Haque MS, Bray EP, Bryan S, Greenfield SM et al (2014) Effect of self-monitoring and medication self-titration on systolic blood pressure in hypertensive patients at high risk of cardiovascular disease: the TASMIN-SR randomized clinical trial. JAMA 312(8):799–808
59. Burnier M, Brown RE, Ong SH, Keskinaslan A, Khan ZM (2009) Issues in blood pressure control and the potential role of single-pill combination therapies. Int J Clin Pract 63(5):790–798
60. Castellano JM, Sanz G, Penalvo JL, Bansilal S, Fernandez-Ortiz A, Alvarez L et al (2014) A polypill strategy to improve adherence: results from the FOCUS (Fixed-dose Combination Drug for Secondary Cardiovascular Prevention) Project. J Am Coll Cardiol 64:2071–2082
61. McAlister FA, Feldman RD, Wyard K, Brant R, Campbell NR, Force CORT (2009) The impact of the Canadian Hypertension Education Programme in its first decade. Eur Heart J 30(12):1434–1439
62. Van Zuilen AD, Wetzels JF, Bots ML, Van Blankestijn PJ (2008) MASTERPLAN: study of the role of nurse practitioners in a multifactorial intervention to reduce cardiovascular risk in chronic kidney disease patients. J Nephrol 21(3):261–267
63. Santschi V, Chiolero A, Burnand B, Colosimo AL, Paradis G (2011) Impact of pharmacist care in the management of cardiovascular disease risk factors: a systematic review and meta-analysis of randomized trials. Arch Intern Med 171(16):1441–1453
64. Santschi V, Chiolero A, Colosimo AL, Platt RW, Taffe P, Burnier M et al (2014) Improving blood pressure control through pharmacist interventions: a meta-analysis of randomized controlled trials. J Am Heart Assoc 3(2):e000718
65. Chapman RH, Ferrufino CP, Kowal SL, Classi P, Roberts CS (2010) The cost and effectiveness of adherence-improving interventions for antihypertensive and lipid-lowering drugs*. Int J Clin Pract 64(2):169–181
66. Redon J, Coca A, Lazaro P, Aguilar MD, Cabanas M, Gil N et al (2010) Factors associated with therapeutic inertia in hypertension: validation of a predictive model. J Hypertens 28(8):1770–1777

Pathophysiology of Renal Sympathetic Denervation (RSDN)

12

Atul Pathak, Benjamin Honton, and Mel Lobo

Abbreviations

BP	Blood pressure
CGRP	Calcitonin gene-related peptide
CHF	Congestive heart failure
GFR	Glomerular filtration rate
HR	Heart rate
HTN	Hypertension
JGC	Juxtaglomerular granular cells
MSNA	Muscle sympathetic nerve activity
NOx	Nitrogen oxide
RBF	Renal blood flow
RDN	Renal denervation
SHR	Spontaneously hypertensive rats
SNA	Sympathetic nerve activity
SNS	Sympathetic nervous system
SP	Surfactant protein

A. Pathak, MD, Phd (✉) • B. Honton, MD
Department of Cardiovascular Medicine, Hypertension, Risk Factors
and Heart Failure Unit, Clinique Pasteur, Avenue de Lombez 31000, Toulouse, France
e-mail: atul.pathak@univ-tlse3.fr

M. Lobo, MD
William Harvey Research Institute, Barts NIHR Cardiovascular Biomedical Research Unit,
Queen Mary University of London, London, UK

C. Tsioufis et al. (eds.), *Interventional Therapies for Secondary and Essential Hypertension*, Updates in Hypertension and Cardiovascular Protection,
DOI 10.1007/978-3-319-34141-5_12

12.1 Introduction

Activation of the sympathetic nervous system (SNS) has been identified as a key pathophysiological feature involved in the initiation, progression but also prognosis of most cardiometabolic disorders (chronic heart failure or kidney disease, coronary heart disease, obesity, diabetes, etc.), among them hypertension (HTN). This has been established through studies recording SNS activation at systemic and local levels using different techniques to measure SNS outflow to various organs. Mechanisms leading to SNS activation are heterogeneous varying from central activation to reflex-mediated sympathoexcitation (or lack of sympathoinhibition).

The existence of a link between the autonomic nervous system and the kidney has been suspected in the middle of the nineteenth century following observations by Bernard showing that renal nerve stimulation decreased urinary flow rate while renal denervation (RDN) increased it [1] and later confirmed by Starling [2]. After 40 years the anatomic breakthrough was provided by Luciano Barajas [3] showing direct contact of the renal sympathetic nerves with the tubular segments and juxtaglomerular granular cells, making it clear that alterations in renal sympathetic nerve discharge with changes in neurotransmitter release could directly influence renal tubular transport function as well as renin secretion.

12.2 What Types of Nerves Are Linking the Kidney to the Brain?

In HTN the efferent and afferent nerves play a major role in the pathogenesis. The efferent fibres by directly interacting with the tubular, vascular or humoural part of the kidney drive HTN initiation and progression. Beyond that, the afferent fibres provide information to the central nervous system about kidney integrity and contribute to systemic SNS activation. This in turn explains why and how the kidney could play a key role in cardiometabolic diseases by systemic activation through the kidney–brain connexion of SNS activity. This chapter will focus on the SNS, but both the afferent and efferent fibres interact with other systems, such as the parasympathetic nervous system, local or systemic mediators, such as nitrogen oxide (NOx), prostaglandins, vasoactive intestinal peptide (VIP), surfactant protein (SP), etc.

12.2.1 Renal Efferent Sympathetic Nerves

In young patients with essential HTN, the use of regional norepinephrine isotope dilution methodology shows that the renal sympathetic outflow is highly activated as is the outflow to the heart [4], shown with selective cardiac norepinephrine spillover measurements, and to the skeletal muscle vasculature, demonstrated with microneurographic nerve traffic recording, but it is the renal sympathetic activation which is central to hypertension pathophysiology [5].

Anatomically, the efferent SNS fibres to the kidney, arising from the second sympathetic ganglion, form a network within the renal artery adventitia. Renal efferent innervation is targeting adrenoceptors at the level of JGC, tubular cells and renal arterial vessels. Hence, increased renal sympathetic nerve activity (SNA) leads to increased renin secretion rate via stimulation of β1-adrenoceptors on the juxtaglomerular granular cells, increased renal tubular sodium reabsorption (decreased urinary sodium excretion) via stimulation of α1B-adrenoceptors on the renal tubular epithelial cells and decreased renal blood flow (RBF) via stimulation of α1A-adrenoceptors on the renal arterial resistance vessels (Fig. 12.1).

12.2.2 Renal Afferent Sympathetic Nerves

Sensory afferent fibres away from the kidney, acting through the posterior hypothalamus, regulate sympathetic outflow to control systemic haemodynamics and reflexive sympathetic efferent activity. Two classes of renal sensory receptors have been identified: renal mechanoreceptors responding to increases in intrarenal pressure [6] and renal chemoreceptors responding to renal ischaemia and/or changes in the chemical environment of the renal interstitium [7] both contributing to the upstream signal starting from the kidney towards the brain.

The pressure-sensitive receptors in the renal pelvis are sympathoinhibitory and important in mediating renorenal reflexes. Renal mechanosensitive neurons monitor hydrostatic pressure changes within the kidney. Early studies in rats, cats and rabbits [8] showed that stretch activation of these afferent sensory nerve fibres elicits an inhibitory renorenal reflex response wherein the contralateral kidney exhibits a compensatory natriuresis and diuresis due to diminished efferent renal SNA. The renorenal reflex coordinates the excretory function of the two kidneys so as to facilitate homeostatic regulation of sodium and water balance. There is a negative feedback loop in which efferent renal SNA facilitates increases in afferent renal nerve

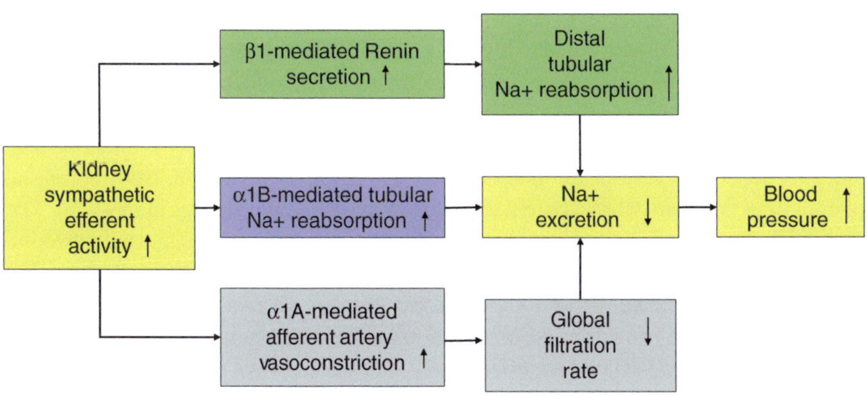

Fig. 12.1 Effect of increased kidney efferent sympathetic activity on blood pressure

activity that in turn inhibits efferent renal SNA so as to avoid excess renal sodium retention.

The nociceptive receptors or chemoreceptors, in contrast to renal mechanoreceptors, induce a sympathoexcitatory reflex in response to a renal injury. The signal is projected to the hypothalamus and increases central sympathetic outflow. Different triggers have been identified as strong activator of the SNS through this upstream pathway, among them ischaemia-induced metabolites and toxins such as urea [9]. In states of renal disease or injury, there is activation of afferent sensory nerve fibres that are excitatory, leading to increased peripheral sympathetic nerve activity, vasoconstriction and increased arterial pressure [10].

12.3 Effects of Kidney Nerves: Stimulation or Denervation?

The use of low-frequency renal nerve stimulation at low intensity induced a decrease in urinary sodium and water excretion in rat, rabbit, sheep and monkey; this was associated with an increase in renal tubular sodium and water reabsorption throughout the nephron. In the reverse mode, RDN produced an increase in urinary sodium and water excretion associated with decreases in renal tubular sodium and water reabsorption throughout the nephron, again with no change in glomerular filtration rate (GFR) or RBF.

The magnitude of renal functional responses to renal sympathetic nerve stimulation is frequency dependent. At the highest there is increased renin secretion rate and decreased urinary sodium excretion, RBF and GFR [11]. The use of reflex manoeuvres mimicking physiological changes of renal SNA produced similar results to those with renal nerve stimulation and denervation confirming the described interplay between the kidney and the autonomic nervous system. However, these studies could not exclude a confounding effect of surgery or anaesthesia. These bias were controlled by studies in trained conscious dogs in which renal sympathoexcitation and sympathoinhibition led to expected effects on natriuresis (respectively reduced and increased) abolished by cardiac and/or RDN. These changes underline the contribution of renal sympathetic innervation to maintain fluid and sodium balance but also blood pressure (BP) regulation or oedema formation in various clinically relevant models of rats (spontaneously hypertensive rats (SHR), congestive heart failure (CHF), nephrotic syndrome).

Similarly stimulation of afferent nerves has been associated to sympathoexcitatory response, but results are more conflicting. Chemical irritation, from intrarenal phenol injection, can act as a potent stimulus in experimental studies in rats [12]. The nociceptive renal afferents have been implicated in generating increased systemic sympathetic activity in drug-resistant essential hypertension and chronic kidney disease. However selective disruption of afferent fibres leads to a reduction of BP and/or SNS activity only in some experimental model. Similarly blocking the effects of SP or calcitonin gene-related peptide (CGRP) does not always reduce BP in different experimental model of hypertension. Hence, most of evidence strongly suggests the role of efferent sympathetic fibres in the pathophysiology of hypertension while the role of afferent fibres is more controversial. However, it should also be noted that not all experimental forms of hypertension are ameliorated by RDN; RDN does not affect the development of hypertension in the Dahl NaCl-sensitive rat [13] or in canine hypertension induced by chronic NOS inhibition [14]. Finally, the efferent renal sympathetic nerve fibres are predominantly unmyelinated small fibres with conduction velocities <2 m/s. However, the finding that the distribution of rat renal nerve fibre diameters showed a bimodal distribution suggested a certain degree of heterogeneity. Anatomic studies of neurovascular contacts in the kidney disclosed different ultrastructural types of sympathetic axons, again supporting heterogeneity. Additional neurophysiological and renal functional studies support the existence of functionally specific renal sympathetic nerve fibres for specific tasks. This suggests that not all efferent fibres are sympathoexcitatory leading to expected vasoconstriction and BP effect [15].

Beyond this direct interaction of the kidney and the brain through afferent and efferent fibres, other systems are also influencing this relationship. Thus, the aortic and carotid sinus baroreceptors play differential roles in the control of heart rate, but they contribute similarly to the control of kidney sympathetic nerve activity [16]. Other mediators such as prostaglandins or NOx modulate the effect of efferent sympathetic outflow to the kidney as do antihypertensive drugs.

12.4 Kidney–Nerve Interaction: Role of Denervation in Hypertension

The role of afferent and efferent kidney fibres in the pathogenesis of HTN is underlined by experimental and clinical dates suggesting their role in sympathoexcitation. In hypertensive models, there is a regional activation of the sympathetic tone at the kidney level. Activation of the renin–angiotensin system, arterial vasoconstriction and sodium reabsorption all lead to the initiation, maintenance and progression of hypertension and related disease. Hence, the renal nerves provide the critical link between increased central sympathetic outflow and impairment of renal excretory function that leads to chronic HTN [9, 10]. This has led to the development of various approaches to disrupt these nerves by the use of pharmacological or non-pharmacological tools (selective and non-selective denervation using surgery or alternative approaches). Most of the studies where RDN is reported to reduce BP in different forms of experimental HTN were conducted in rodents but without any consistent finding [17, 18] due to the experimental design, method of BP measurement, etc. The only exception are studies conducted in SHR, known to have elevated kidney sympathetic activity [19]; however, RDN has minimal effect on BP when animals display target organ damage or more advanced stages of HTN. In dogs, the classical model of HTN (disease induced by Goldblatt clip or by infusion of angiotensin/aldosterone) is not associated with an increased activity of the SNS tone. The only exception is high-fat diet-induced HTN where there is evidence of a BP-lowering effect following RDN [20]. These experimental studies indicate that the renal nerves do not contribute to all forms of HTN, but that they do play a critical role in chronically increasing arterial pressure when sympathetic nerve trafficking to the kidney is elevated.

In humans, the seminal papers by Smithwick and Thompson [21] about surgical sympathectomy studies conducted in hypertensive patients in the middle of the twentieth century suggest that this procedure reduces BP but also improved mortality and survival rates. However the severity of HTN was attenuated in only about half of the 1,266 patients analysed.

Taken together, these observations indicate that RDN as developed through catheter-based approach could be of interest not only to reduce BP but also to reduce sympathetic tone. This procedural approach is more selective than surgery however cannot target independently afferent and/or efferent fibres. Expected effect of RDN is reduction in sympathetic tone both at systemic and local levels though conflicting results have been published. Hence, the first paper by Schlaich showed reduction in muscle sympathetic nerve activity (MSNA) in a case report confirmed by reduction in both MSNA [22] and single nerve activity [23] in a larger sample; others have shown no effect on MSNA [24]. This is related to the experimental design of the study and the type plus location of measurement of SNS activity (kidney spillover versus MSNA or cardiac sympathetic nerve activity). The discrepancy of the results also suggests that reinnervation may occur. Studies of central and renal changes post denervation are required to understand the causes of the prolonged or lack of hypotensive response to catheter-based RDN in human hypertension [25]. Beyond SNS modulation, RDN also increases sodium excretion [26] and does not modify blood flow to the kidney, thus contributing to the BP-lowering effect.

12.5 Perspective–Conclusion

The pleiotropic sympathetic innervation also underlines collateral benefits of RDN beyond BP and in different type of patients known to have elevated sympathetic tone. Hence, enhancement of insulin sensitivity in patient with type 2 diabetes or metabolic syndrome, reduction of apnoea–hypopnea index in patient with obstructive sleep apnoea or less arrhythmia in patient at risk are some of the additional effects linked to sympathomodulation driven by RDN. Finally, this technique, again through reduction of the sympathetic drive to organs, has been associated to favourable cardiac remodelling and functional effect in heart failure patient or on nephrological parameters in patient with chronic kidney disease. These effects remain to be confirmed but underline the role of RDN on the pathophysiology of most sympathetic-driven diseases [27].

References

1. Bernard C Leçons sur les Propriétés Physiologiques et les Altérations Pathologiques des Liquides de l'Organisme, vol. 2. Paris: Bailliere; 1859.
2. Starling EH. The chemical control of the body. Harvey lectures 1907–1908. New York: JB Lippincott Co.; 1909.

3. Muller J, Barajas L. Electron microscopic and histochemical evidence for a tubular innervation in the renal cortex of the monkey. J Ultrastruct Res. 1972;41(5):533–49.
4. Esler M, Jennings G, Lambert G, Meredith I, Horne M, Eisenhofer G. Overflow of catecholamine neurotransmitters to the circulation: source, fate, and functions. Physiol Rev. 1990; 70(4):963–85.
5. Esler M, Lambert E, Schlaich M. Point: chronic activation of the sympathetic nervous system is the dominant contributor to systemic hypertension. J Appl Physiol (Bethesda, Md: 1985). 2010;109(6):1996–8; discussion 2016. doi:10.1152/japplphysiol.00182.2010.
6. Kopp UC, Olson LA, DiBona GF. Renorenal reflex responses to mechano- and chemoreceptor stimulation in the dog and rat. Am J Physiol. 1984;246(1 Pt 2):F67–77.
7. Recordati GM, Moss NG, Genovesi S, Rogenes PR. Renal receptors in the rat sensitive to chemical alterations of their environment. Circ Res. 1980;46(3):395–405.
8. Nijima A. Afferent discharges from arterial mechanoreceptors in the kidney of the rabbit. J Physiol. 1971;219(2):477–85.
9. Esler M. Renal denervation for hypertension: observations and predictions of a founder. Eur Heart J. 2014;35(18):1178–85. doi:10.1093/eurheartj/ehu091.
10. Grassi G, Mark A, Esler M. The sympathetic nervous system alterations in human hypertension. Circ Res. 2015;116(6):976–90. doi:10.1161/circresaha.116.303604.
11. DiBona GF, Sawin LL. Effect of renal denervation on dynamic autoregulation of renal blood flow. Am J Physiol Renal Physiol. 2004;286(6):F1209–18. doi:10.1152/ajprenal.00010.2004.
12. Campese VM, Kogosov E, Koss M. Renal afferent denervation prevents the progression of renal disease in the renal ablation model of chronic renal failure in the rat. Am J Kidney Dis: the official journal of the National Kidney Foundation. 1995;26(5):861–5.
13. Wyss JM, Sripairojthikoon W, Oparil S. Failure of renal denervation to attenuate hypertension in Dahl NaCl-sensitive rats. Can J Physiol Pharmacol. 1987;65(12):2428–32.
14. Granger J, Novak J, Schnackenberg C, Williams S, Reinhart GA. Role of renal nerves in mediating the hypertensive effects of nitric oxide synthesis inhibition. Hypertension. 1996;27 (3 Pt 2):613–8.
15. DiBona GF. Physiology in perspective: the wisdom of the body. Neural control of the kidney. Am J Physiol Regul Integr Comp Physiol. 2005;289(3):R633–41. doi:10.1152/ajpregu.00258.2005.
16. Ishii K, Idesako M, Matsukawa K. Differential contribution of aortic and carotid sinus baroreflexes to control of heart rate and renal sympathetic nerve activity. J Physiol Sci: JPS. 2015;65(5):471–80. doi:10.1007/s12576-015-0387-2.
17. Kline RL. Renal nerves and experimental hypertension: evidence and controversy. Can J Physiol Pharmacol. 1987;65(8):1540–7.
18. Kline RL, Mercer PF. Functional reinnervation and development of supersensitivity to NE after renal denervation in rats. Am J Physiol. 1980;238(5):R353–8.
19. Norman Jr RA, Dzielak DJ. Role of renal nerves in onset and maintenance of spontaneous hypertension. Am J Physiol. 1982;243(2):H284–8.
20. Lohmeier TE, Iliescu R, Liu B, Henegar JR, Maric-Bilkan C, Irwin ED. Systemic and renal-specific sympathoinhibition in obesity hypertension. Hypertension. 2012;59(2):331–8. doi:10.1161/hypertensionaha.111.185074.
21. Smithwick RH, Thompson JE. Splanchnicectomy for essential hypertension; results in 1,266 cases. JAMA. 1953;152(16):1501–4.
22. Hering D, Marusic P, Walton AS, Lambert EA, Krum H, Narkiewicz K, Lambert GW, Esler MD, Schlaich MP. Sustained sympathetic and blood pressure reduction 1 year after renal denervation in patients with resistant hypertension. Hypertension. 2014;64(1):118–24. doi:10.1161/hypertensionaha.113.03098.
23. Hering D, Lambert EA, Marusic P, Walton AS, Krum H, Lambert GW, Esler MD, Schlaich MP. Substantial reduction in single sympathetic nerve firing after renal denervation in patients with resistant hypertension. Hypertension. 2013;61(2):457–64. doi:10.1161/hypertensionaha.111.00194.
24. Tank J, Heusser K, Brinkmann J, Schmidt BM, Menne J, Bauersachs J, Haller H, Diedrich A, Jordan J. Spike rate of multi-unit muscle sympathetic nerve fibers after catheter-based renal nerve ablation. J Am Soc Hypertens: JASH. 2015;9(10):794–801. doi:10.1016/j.jash.2015.07.012.

25. Booth LC, Nishi EE, Yao ST, Ramchandra R, Lambert GW, Schlaich MP, May CN. Reinnervation following catheter-based radio-frequency renal denervation. Exp Physiol. 2015;100(5):485–90. doi:10.1113/expphysiol.2014.079871.
26. Poss J, Ewen S, Schmieder RE, Muhler S, Vonend O, Ott C, Linz D, Geisel J, Rump LC, Schlaich M, Bohm M, Mahfoud F. Effects of renal sympathetic denervation on urinary sodium excretion in patients with resistant hypertension. Clin Res Cardiol Off J German Cardiac Soc. 2015;104(8):672–8. doi:10.1007/s00392-015-0832-5.
27. McArdle MJ, deGoma EM, Cohen DL, Townsend RR, Wilensky RL, Giri J. Beyond blood pressure: percutaneous renal denervation for the management of sympathetic hyperactivity and associated disease states. J Am Heart Assoc. 2016;4(3):001415. doi:10.1161/jaha.114.001415.

13 Renal Denervation: A Historical Perspective

Vasilios Papademetriou, Michael Doumas, Costas Tsioufis, and Venkatesh K. Raman

Abbreviations

AF	Atrial fibrillation
BP	Blood pressure
dRHTN	Drug-resistant hypertension
GFR	Glomerular filtration rate
HF	Heart failure
NEPI	Norepinephrine
RDN	Renal denervation
RF	Radiofrequency
SHR	Spontaneously hypertensive rats
SNS	Sympathetic nervous system
WKY	Wistar Kyoto

V. Papademetriou, MD (✉)
Veteran Affairs Medical Center and Georgetown University,
50 Irving Street, NW, Washington, DC 20422, USA
e-mail: vpapademetriou@va.gov

M. Doumas
Veteran Affairs Medical Center and George Washington University, Washington, DC, USA

Aristotle University, Thessaloniki, Greece

C. Tsioufis
1st Cardiology Clinic, National and Kapodistrian University of Athens,
Hippokration Hospital, Athens, Greece

V.K. Raman
MedStar Heart & Vascular Institute, MedStar Georgetown University Hospital,
Washington, DC, USA

C. Tsioufis et al. (eds.), *Interventional Therapies for Secondary and Essential Hypertension*, Updates in Hypertension and Cardiovascular Protection,
DOI 10.1007/978-3-319-34141-5_13

13.1 Introduction

The role of the sympathetic nervous system (SNS) in the development of hypertension and in particular of resistant hypertension has long been recognized. A great deal of work has been done attempting to explore potential interventions to interrupt the sympathetic influence on systemic vasculature and target organs. Renal denervation (RDN) is not a new technique, and it does not address a newly discovered concept. Surgical RDN was applied almost 150 years ago in an attempt to treat a variety of disorders including renal pain, proteinuria, and severe or malignant hypertension. In animal models surgical RDN was utilized to totally resect and interrupt sympathetic fibers. Renal nerves were resected with a scalpel bilaterally, and the renal arteries were painted with phenol to totally eradicate all sympathetic fibers. Indeed surgical renal denervation resulted in up to 99 % reduction of renal norepinephrine.

Device-based RDN was invented only recently in an attempt to disrupt the sympathetic fibers coursing in the adventitia of the renal arteries. Early studies provided impressive results in patients with dRHTN and in patients suffering from diseases associated with sympathetic overactivity. However, the negative results of Symplicity HTN-3, the largest and only sham control study, abated enthusiasm and put the whole field of RDN into a hibernation state. In this article we'll briefly review the history of renal denervation and the preclinical scientific evidence that lead us to believe that renal denervation is a viable option for treatment and control of resistant hypertension.

13.2 Historical Perspective

13.2.1 Animal Models

The important role of renal SNS was first described more than a century and a half ago. Claude Bernard described that unilateral stimulation of the splanchnic nerves resulted in sodium and fluid retention by the ipsilateral kidney, whereas unilateral section of the splanchnic nerve was accompanied by enhanced ipsilateral diuresis [1]. In 1889, after meticulous experiments on dogs, Bradford [2] reported that stimulation of dorsal and splanchnic nerves causes changes in blood pressure (BP) and kidney size measured by plethysmography. Whether BP increased or decreased depended on the anatomic area stimulated, as well as the electric impulse frequency, but outcomes were consistent and reproducible.

Since then it became apparent that kidneys act both as generators and recipients of sympathetic signals. Sympathetic afferent fibers originate from the kidneys and travel to the central nervous system, where, after processing, coordinated by the nucleus tractus solitarius of the midbrain, they regulate sympathetic outflow and promote SNS overactivity in response to renal injury [3, 4]. On the other hand, renal efferent sympathetic nerves originate from the brain, travel through the spinal cord, reach the kidney from the second sympathetic ganglia, course through the adventitia of the renal arteries, and innervate the peripheral segments in the renal cortex ending in glomerular arterioles where they can affect renal function. Overactivity of the efferent sympathetic fibers results in enhanced renin release, increased sodium and water absorption, and reduced renal blood flow and glomerular filtration rate [5]. It seems that both the afferent and efferent fibers contribute to the development and persistence of hypertension. By the 1980s it was well established that kidneys are important sensory organs with abundant baroreceptors and chemoreceptors and significant afferent innervation. In 1987, Webb and Brody [6] published results from a thesis in which they addressed signal trafficking via the afferent sympathetic fibers in a rat model. Through extensive instrumentation and careful monitoring, they demonstrated that electric stimulation of afferent sympathetic fibers can reduce BP in a dose-dependent manner. They also demonstrated that BP responses could be abolished by spinal transection and interruption of the efferent sympathetic fibers coursing through the spine. Subsequently, in a controlled study, Campese and Kogosov [7] showed that resection of the afferent renal nerves through ventral rhizotomy can prevent activation of the noradrenergic neurons in the hypothalamus and can prevent the development of hypertension in rats with chronic renal insufficiency.

Later, through elaborate research, it was shown that efferent renal nerve stimulation results in vasoconstriction of the renal vasculature [8]. Sympathetic nerve endings directly release norepinephrine on renal epithelial cells and can cause a 30–40 % increase in sodium and water reabsorption via α–1 adrenergic receptors even before any hemodynamic changes could be detected [9, 10]. In 1981, Osborn et al. [11] demonstrated that low frequency stimulation of the renal nerve in dogs can directly mediate renin secretion via β-1 adrenergic receptors. In other experiments, surgical renal denervation has been shown to affect hypertension. In deoxycorticosterone acetate-treated miniature swine with established hypertension, O'Hagan et al. [12] demonstrated that RDN results in immense natriuresis and BP reduction. Similarly, Huang et al. [13] in a hyperinsulinemia-induced hypertension model demonstrated that renal denervation can prevent hypertension development if done early or can normalize BP after hypertension is established. Changes in tissue norepinephrine (NEPI) followed the same patterns.

In many experimental models, acute increases in SNS activity produced disproportionately greater vasoconstriction in the renal vascular bed than what occurs in most other vascular beds. Increased SNS activity has been implicated in the pathogenesis of 11-Deoxycorticosterone (DOCA)-salt hypertension in the rat and attenuation of renal sympathetic tone has been shown to delay the development of this form of hypertension.

Katholi et al. [14] performed RDN in 5-week-old uninephrectomized male Sprague-Dawley rats 1 week before beginning DOCA-salt treatment and compared them to sham-operated rats. Systolic blood pressure was measured using the tail cuff method. In 32 sham-operated rats systolic BP was significantly ($p<0.05$) elevated above control by day 5 (115 ± 3 vs 128 ± 3 mmHg) of DOCA-salt administration and continued to rise, reaching a plateau by day 21 (192 ± 5 mmHg). In contrast, DOCA-salt administration in 32 renal denervated rats did not result in a significant elevation of BP above control until day 17 (121 ± 3 vs 135 ± 3 mmHg, $p < 0.05$). During the first 2 weeks of DOCA-salt treatment, fractional urinary sodium excretion was significantly greater ($p < 0.05$) in renal denervated rats than in sham animals. During the 3rd week of DOCA-salt administration, renal denervated rats had a rapid rise in BP and a fall in fractional urinary sodium excretion to the level of the sham-operated animals. Coincident with the development of hypertension was a threefold increase in renal norepinephrine content ($p < 0.01$), suggesting reinnervation. The authors concluded that increased renal sympathetic tone in the DOCA-salt rat facilitates sodium retention and is necessary for the development of the hypertension. The authors also concluded that re-innervation may occur in this model [14].

Other studies have also emphasized the role of high-sodium diet in conjunction with sympathetic overactivity for hypertension development. Greenberg et al. [15] studied the effects of low- and high-sodium diet in spontaneously hypertensive rats (SHR) and Wistar Kyoto (WKY) rats with or without RDN. RDN was performed surgically using a dissecting microscope, and all visible renal nerves were resected from renal arteries, veins, and ureters. The pedicle was then painted with phenol to destroy any remaining fibers. RDN was effective in only denervated animals going from low- to high-sodium diet, whereas it was ineffective in denervated SHRs going from high to low sodium diet. Renal denervation was not effective in WKY rats. These data indicated that renal denervation is effective only in strains characterized by sympathetic overactivity and only under conditions of high-sodium diet. In other experiments Katholi et al. studied the effects of renal denervation in the one-kidney, one-clip Sprague-Dawley rat model [16]. Two weeks after nephrectomy and clipping of the remaining kidney, BP increased to >200 mmHg in this model. Renal denervation or unclipping of the renal artery on day 14 resulted in impressive BP reduction, whereas sham procedure had no effect. These experiments demonstrate the importance of renal ischemia and sympathetic overactivity in the development of hypertension.

13.3 Renal Denervation in Humans

Neurosurgical treatment of hypertension was independently suggested by researchers in 1923 [17]. Adson, however, was the first to perform surgical sympathectomy for the treatment of malignant hypertension in 1925 [18]. During the following years and in the 1930s, Peet in Ann Arbor, Page and Heuer in New York, and Adson, Craig, and Brown from the Mayo Clinic operated and reported on a series of patients all experiencing malignant hypertension [19]. At the same time, renal decapsulation, which was considered a form of sympathectomy by disrupting the fibers between the capsule and the renal cortex, was being performed to treat unexplained hematuria and perinephritis. Sen [20] reported a significant but not permanent decrease in BP in 85 subjects who underwent decapsulation between 1925 and 1935. Surgical denervation of the kidneys alone was first performed in humans by Papin and Ambard [21] in 1924 in an attempt to relieve intractable pain originating from the kidney. The first case of bilateral sympathetic denervation of the kidney to treat severe essential hypertension was presented in 1934 by Page and Heuer [22]. The patient was a 25-year-old woman who reported easy fatigability and had severe headaches and BP in the range of 208/140 mmHg. The patient underwent surgical staged, bilateral renal sympathectomy with no clinically meaningful effect on BP after follow-up for 5 months. However, the case established that the procedure was safe and had no negative effect on renal function. In 1935, Page and Heuer [23] reported bilateral renal denervation in five patients with chronic and progressive nephritis, which resulted in no change in renal clearance or concentrating ability of the kidney but caused diminished proteinuria and a decrease in BP that lasted for months in the majority of those patients, but returned toward baseline in most patients. Because of these early unsatisfactory results, surgical RDN gave way to the more radical sympathectomy procedure, the surgical removal of splanchnic nerves (splanchnicectomy), which showed dramatic results in the majority of patients with malignant hypertension. Peet published series and case reports of patients with malignant hypertension responding in a dramatic way to supradiaphragmatic splanchnicectomy [24]. Since then and for the subsequent 2 decades, surgical sympathectomy (thoracolumbar splanchnicectomy) became the procedure of choice for patients with severe/malignant hypertension not responding to diet or to then-limited pharmacologic therapy. Between 1938 and 1947, Smithwick and Thompson [25] published results from 3500 patients with severe/malignant hypertension. Of those, 2400 patients underwent thoracolumbar splanchnicectomy, and the rest were followed on a medical regimen. Of those, 1266 patients had splanchnicectomy, and 467 patients on medical therapy had a follow-up of 5–14 years and were included in the final analysis. At 5 years of follow-up, all-cause mortality was 19 % in the surgical series and 54 % in the medically treated patients. Of the surgically treated patients, only 45 % demonstrated substantial BP reduction, but mortality benefits were realized across the board. Peet et al. [26] reported 51.4 % significant BP reduction and 3.4 % operative mortality in 350 patients with severe/malignant hypertension. However, the use of surgical sympathectomy was abandoned during the second half of the twentieth century, mainly because of high surgical mortality and periprocedural complications. The operation was associated with significant perioperative mortality (3–11 %), and the adverse effects were intolerable. Pronounced postural hypotension limiting daily activities, impotence, bowel abnormalities, and hyper- and hypohidrosis were the most frequent problems. In the mid-1950s the first oral antihypertensive medication became available for the treatment of hypertension, and for the first time a well-tolerated regimen could be given long term [27]. Pharmacologic therapy helped treat many patients with severe hypertension, and the number of patients progressing to accelerated/malignant stage gradually diminished [28], thus settling the issue for the next 5 decades. Very few patients not responding to pharmacologic therapy have been referred for splanchnicectomy since then.

However, during this time a great deal of research has been pursued to uncover and better understand the role of the SNS and, in particular, of the renal sympathetic nerves in the development and maintenance of hypertension [29]. As described above a wealth of experimental data point toward an important role of SNS overactivity for the development and persistence of hypertension [30]. Excessive SNS activity is also involved in a variety of other conditions such as the metabolic syndrome, obesity, structural and functional myocardial alterations [31], and several other disease states, including congestive heart failure, chronic kidney disease, polycystic ovary syndrome, obstructive sleep apnea, and cirrhosis [32–36].

13.4 Catheter-Based Renal Denervation

Renal sympathetic denervation has been performed, through the years, both in experimental models and in humans by surgical exposure of renal nerves. The renal nerves were interrupted or resected using mostly a surgical scalpel, although later electrocautery, cryoablation, and thermal radiofrequency (RF) ablation have also been used. With progress in technology and the advent of transcatheter techniques, it was natural to progress to transvascular methods to interrupt nerve integrity. Catheter-based RF ablation techniques have been used in electrophysiology for more than two decades to ablate accessory pathways and abnormal cardiac structures in patients with Wolff-Parkinson-White syndrome or supraventricular and ventricular arrhythmia. In 1999, a series of experiments completed at the University of Oklahoma using a basket catheter demonstrated that it was possible to stimulate and ablate autonomic nerves on the outside of blood vessels. Notably, Schauerte et al. used an innovative approach to stimulate [37] and ablate [38] the vagal nerve to treat patients with vagally mediated atrial fibrillation (AF). RF energy was applied transvascularly to ablate the vagal nerve. The currently used technique for catheter-based renal nerve ablation uses a very similar concept. Patients with drug resistant hypertension (dRHTN) have increased sympathetic outflow. The early Symplicity studies and many more that followed [39–45] used RF-based thermal energy to ablate and interrupt the renal sympathetic fibers. The disadvantage of the transcatheter techniques in humans is the inability to assess the effect of renal nerve stimulation in the laboratory and thus inability to intelligently place the tip of the ablating catheter and achieve complete RDN. Rational and results from these studies will be described in other chapters. Weaknesses and deficiencies of the transcatheter techniques have been discussed elsewhere [46, 47]. Here we'll describe in brief animal research that developed following the publication of Symplicity HTN-3 [48], which was a randomized sham-controlled study that failed to meet its primary efficacy end point.

A number of explanations have been offered to provide insight into the disappointing results of the trial, including attenuation of the placebo effect with sham-treated controls, a circumscribed role for SNS activity in some hypertensives, lack of intraprocedural measures (for vessel wall contact or for nerve destruction), and limited understanding of neurovascular anatomy resulting in clinical failure. Efficacy of the single, monopolar RF catheter was predicated on relatively circumscribed radial density and uniform longitudinal distribution of efferent sympathetic nerves along the renal artery and within the penetration depth of energy delivery achievable by the system. Fortunately, subsequent pathology studies in swine and in humans have better characterized the morphologic substrate for

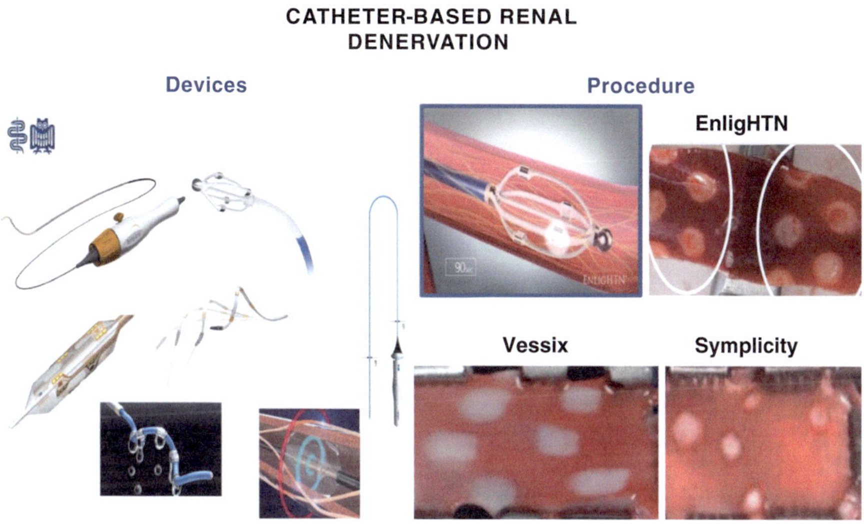

Fig. 13.1 Renal denervation devices and patterns of lesions induced by thermal energy (radiofrequency)

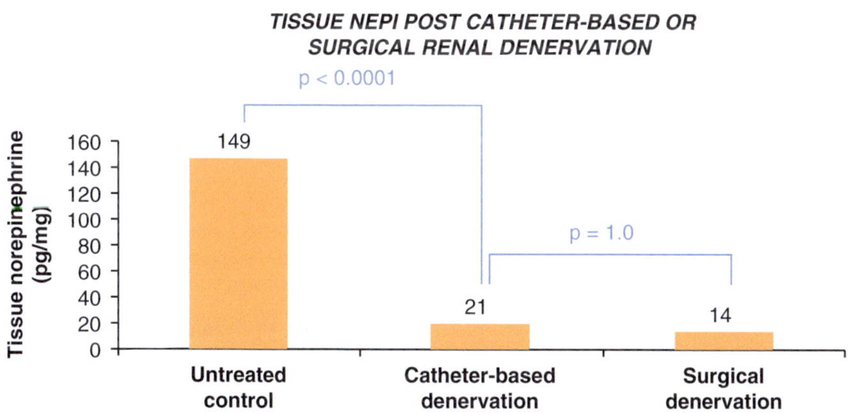

Fig. 13.2 Tissue NEPI reduction with either surgical denervation or catheter-based renal denervation. Effect should be similar under optimal conditions

treatment that should focus efforts to realize an effective transcatheter approach that recapitulates but defines surgical therapy. Lesion distribution with different approved devices is shown in Fig. 13.1 demonstrates lesion distribution with different approved devices. Optimal lesion placement should be circumferential, covering the whole circumference of the renal artery and achieve depth that affects most of the sympathetic fibers. In doing so the catheter-based renal denervation should result in tissue NEPI reduction similar to surgical renal denervation (about 90 % reduction) (Fig. 13.2).

Tellez and colleagues studied perirenal nerve distribution and density in juvenile Yorkshire mini pigs [49]. Renal arteries were segmented at intervals along their lengths from aorto-ostium to the first bifurcation (15–27 mm) and divided into proximal, mid, and distal portions. Sections were examined radially to depths of 10 mm, at least twice that of an earlier description from human autopsy subjects [50]. Unlike those descriptions that 90 % of fibers were confined within a 2 mm radius of the renal artery lumen, Tellez and team discovered only about half of the total nerves along the main renal arteries were found up to a radial depth of 2.5 mm from the lumen. Roughly one-fifth of fibers were located at depths greater than 5 mm. The highest nerve counts were in the proximal vessel which accounted for about 45 % of the total. Additionally, there were a consistently larger number of fibers coursing along the right compared to the left renal artery with the difference most apparent in the proximal segment. The analysis revealed a marked predominance of sympathetic efferent compared to sensory afferent fibers. A more recent human autopsy series corroborated the complexity of renal nerve distribution. Sakakura [51] and colleagues examined several 100 sections of 40 arteries from 20 subjects, extending from ostium to beyond the renal artery bifurcation. They also observed the maximal mean number of nerves in the proximal and mid-vessel segments with circumferential distribution highest in the ventral and lowest in the dorsal segments. Fifty percent of nerves were found more than 2.44 mm from the lumen-wall interface with one-quarter beyond 4.28 mm. These investigators also pointed out that tissue shrinkage with formalin fixation might approach 20 %, suggesting even greater circumferential depth needed for therapeutic targeting. This has implications particularly for radiofrequency ablation, generally limited to penetration depths of 3–4 mm, risking incomplete or insufficient denervation to achieve therapeutic effects. Furthermore, the concern for thermal injury causing "restenosis" has led to avoidance of a planar circumferential delivery system (i.e., loop or ring electrode of renal artery diameter), but this risks another failure mode if unable to target based upon observed distributions (i.e., higher density in ventral segments near the ostium).

Systematic characterization of nerve microanatomy was extended in another study of Yorkshire mini pigs by Tzafriri et al. [52]. Control animals served to describe longtitudinal and circumferential nerve distributions in comparison to the smaller group treated with bilateral RF ablation using a Biosense Webster (Diamond Bar, California) prototype multielectrode catheter. Treated animals were euthanized at Day 7 for tissue analysis. Nerves and ganglia were quantified at several points along the renal artery from ostium to 6 mm and by circumferential quadrant to radial depths of more than 10 mm from the lumen-wall interface. Identifying areas of ablation by coagulative or necrotic changes, the percentage of affected nerves and ganglia were calculated in treated sections. As a biomarker of the effectiveness of sympathetic interruption, renal parenchymal NEPI levels were measured and related to affected neural networks. A higher density of nerves and ganglia were found at the ostium compared to 6 mm inside but at greater distance with median radial depths of 6.3 mm and 2.0 mm, respectively. Significant circumferential variability in distribution was also noted, particularly near the ostium, with a preponderance in the superior and anterior segments. Remarkably, only one out of eight treated arteries was associated with a significant reduction in tissue NEPI levels. Although a larger ablation depth and area were achieved at the ostium in this artery, fewer than one-third of nerves were affected due to their greater distance from the lumen at this location. At 6 mm, however, all four quadrants were encompassed by treatment with nearly 100 % of nerves affected despite significantly smaller ablation depth and area. The authors were able to demonstrate a monotonic dependence of NEPI levels on fraction of affected nerves and estimated an approximately 50 % reduction to achieve a threshold effect. While the clinical approach to RF denervation has emphasized treatment at or near the renal artery ostium, these preclinical and clinical findings suggest more complete transcatheter denervation may be possible in distal arterial segments where nerves are closer to the lumen.

Demonstration of the physiological sequelae following effective RF denervation was provided in a well-described obese, hypertensive dog model [53]. Animals were maintained on a high-fat, high-sodium diet with a gain of 55–60 % in body weight and exhibited cardiovascular, renal, and metabolic changes similar to those in obese humans. An expandable basket catheter with four electrodes (EnligHTN catheter, St Jude Medical) was used to perform denervation with analysis at 8 weeks. Just under half of the nerves exhibited injury, primarily within 3.5 mm from the lumen-wall interface. Cortical NEPI levels fell 42 % and correlated with the observed reduction in mean arterial pressure of 9 mmHg. Importantly, there was no change in glomerular filtration rate (GFR) or other parameters of renal physiology. Similarly, Mahfoud and colleagues used the next-generation Medtronic Spyral RDN system comprised of a helical, quadripolar catheter to study RF dose and location in mini pigs [54]. The authors effected unilateral RDN, using the contralateral kidney as control, with groups comprised of increasing lesion numbers and/or extension beyond the bifurcation into each branch of the renal artery. Average lesion depth was observed at about 3.5 mm. Analysis at 1 week post-RDN showed that NEPI levels and cortical axon area were significantly reduced. There was not a clear dose–response relationship, although the largest reduction occurred following lesions in each branch artery as compared to treatment in the main artery alone.

The studies described above have several limitations, including the relatively short-term endpoints at 1–3 months, which leave unanswered questions about durability. Booth and colleagues' recently published study provides some insights into potential failure modes [55]. Normotensive sheep were divided into control, acute, 5.5-month, and 11-month groups. The Symplicity Flex catheter (Medtronic), as in clinical trials, was used to deliver lesions in an approximated helical configuration. Characteristic increase in mean arterial pressure and decreases in renal blood flow (RBF) and renal vascular conductance were observed following renal nerve stimulation in the control group. One week post-procedure, the acute group showed no response to renal nerve stimulation; however, animals at 5.5 and 11 months demonstrated a similar pattern to the control group with an increase in mean arterial pressure and decrease in RBF. Additionally, NEPI levels were markedly reduced in the acute group but increased at 5.5 months and were effectively at baseline in the 11-month group. Histology showed widespread smaller nerve branches in the later time point groups.

Immunohistochemistry revealed an initial marked decrease in tyrosine hydroxylase levels but return to baseline at the later time points. Taken together, these histopathologic and clinical data confirm nerve regeneration in an intermediate time frame with near complete restoration of physiologic responses at 11 months.

Many of the existing systems use some form of energy delivery for thermal injury to achieve renal nerve destruction. As described above in these preclinical studies, variability in nerve depth and circumferential distribution, as well as subsequent regeneration, may all limit the effectiveness of these platforms. To address these potential shortcomings, Fischell and colleagues used a novel 3-needle delivery device (Peregrine System, Ablative Solutions Inc., Kalamazoo, MI), which has been FDA-approved via a 510(K) mechanism, for perivascular injection and drug delivery. The system is comprised of a catheter with three guide tubes separated by 120° from each other and housing 30-gauge equivalent needles that are actuated up to 3.5 mm beyond into the adventitial space following vessel wall contact. Choosing alcohol as a potent neurolytic, they demonstrated the feasibility of this approach in mini pigs and at 2 weeks showed a dose–response of ethanol volumes of 0.15, 0.3, and 0.6 mL and reduction in (NEPI) levels of 54, 78, and 88 % [56]. In an important follow-up paper that also included first-in-man treatment for refractory/resistant hypertension, they extended findings to 3 months, observing the same dose–response relationship with the two higher volumes from the initial study [57]. Perhaps most importantly, they found circumferential and deep nerve injury to depths of 13.4 mm. An inflammatory response was absent, and there was no evidence of generalized fibrosis, showing a relative sparing of non-nerve tissue. The injury appeared permanent with perineural sheath damage that would prevent regeneration and, perhaps, permit a durable response to therapy. Of note the early results in humans demonstrated impressive BP reduction and discontinuation of medicine in most patients.

Conclusion

The role of renal nerve sympathetic function in blood pressure (BP) homeostasis has been firmly established from animal experiments dating back to the nineteenth century through therapeutic surgical interruption in the 1920s. Although extremely effective, the more radical thoracolumbar sympathectomy was relatively short-lived due to intolerable side effects. The advent of percutaneous coronary intervention in the late 1970s evolved into catheter-based treatment throughout the cardiovascular system and more recently has opened up the possibility of a nonsurgical approach to hypertension. Successes in refractory hypertension with catheter RF renal denervation in the early Symplicity HTN-1 and HTN-2 trials prompted great enthusiasm and plans to extend therapy to the broader hypertensive population with attendant public health implications. Unfortunately, the randomized, sham-controlled Symplicity HTN-3 trial failed to meet its primary efficacy endpoint, casting doubt upon the future of the field. Subsequent preclinical and clinical studies provide insight into nerve density and distribution that may rationalize platform development. Thus reaching fibers up to 10 mm in depth or treating distally and into the branches may be important in order to achieve adequate renal denervation.

While BP reduction may depend upon impacting a certain percentage of the renal sympathetic network (>50 % of fibers), a system interrupting nerves to significant, circumferential depths by mechanisms that render damage permanent may realize the promise of interventional hypertension treatment.

References

1. Bernard C (1859) Lecons sur les proprietes physiologiques et les alterations pathologiques des liquides de l'organisme. Bailliere, Paris 2:170–191
2. Bradford JR (1889) The innervation of the renal blood vessels. J Physiol 10:358–432, 18
3. DiBona GF, Esler M (2010) Translational medicine: the antihypertensive effect of renal denervation. Am J Physiol Regul Integr Comp Physiol 298:R245–R253
4. Campese VM, Ku E, Park J (2011) Sympathetic renal innervation and resistant hypertension. Int J Hypertens 2011:814354
5. DiBona GF (2005) Physiology in perspective: the wisdom of the body–neural control of the kidney. Am J Physiol Regul Integr Comp Physiol 289:R633–R641
6. Webb RL, Brody MJ (1987) Functional identification of the central projections of afferent renal nerves. Clin Exp Hypertens A 9(Suppl 1):47–57
7. Campese VM, Kogosov E (1995) Renal afferent denervation prevents hypertension in rats with chronic renal failure. Hypertension 25(4 pt 2):878–882
8. Malpas SC, Evans RG (1998) Do different levels and patterns of sympathetic activation all provoke renal vasoconstriction? J Auton Nerv Syst 69:72–82
9. DiBona GF, Sawin LL (1982) Effect of renal nerve stimulation on NaCl and H2O transport in Henle's loop of the rat. Am J Physiol 243:F576–F580
10. Smyth DD, Umemura S, Pettinger WA (1985) Renal nerve stimulation causes alpha 1-adrenoceptor-mediated sodium retention but not alpha 2-adrenoceptor antagonism of vasopressin. Circ Res 57:304–311
11. Osborn JL, DiBona GF, Thames MD (1981) Beta-1 receptor mediation of renin secretion elicited by low-frequency renal nerve stimulation. J Pharmacol Exp Ther 216:265–269
12. O'Hagan KP, Thomas GD, Zambraski EJ (1990) Renal denervation decreases blood pressure in DOCA-treated miniature swine with established hypertension. Am J Hypertens 3:62–64
13. Huang WC, Fang TC, Cheng JT (1998) Renal denervation prevents and reverses hyperinsulinemia-induced hypertension in rats. Hypertension 32:249–254
14. Katholi RE, ALLEN J, Naftilan AJ, Oparil S (1980) Importance of renal sympathetic tone in the development of DOCA-salt hypertension in the rat. Hypertension 2:266–273
15. Greenberg SG, Enders C, Osborn JL (1993) Renal nerves affect rate of achieving sodium balance in spontaneously hypertensive rats. Hypertension 22:1–8
16. Katholi RE, Wimnetrnitz SR, Oparil S (1982) Decrease in peripheral sympathetic nervous activity system activity following renal denervation or unclipping in the one-kidney one-clip Goldblatt hypertensive rat. J Clin Inv 69:55–62
17. Author unknown (1947) Neurosurgical treatment, indications and results (chapter 7, methods of operation). J Intern Med 127:72–76
18. Adson AW, McCraig W, Brown GE (1936) Surgery in its relation to hypertension. Surg Gynecol Obstet 62:314–331
19. Weiss E (1939) Recent advances in the pathogenesis and treatment of hypertension, a review. Psychosom Med 1:180–198
20. Sen SK (1936) Some observations on decapsulation and denervation of the kidney. Brit J Urol 8:319–328
21. Papin E, Ambard L (1924) Resection of the nerves of the kidney for nephralgia and small hydronephroses. J Urol 11:337–349

22. Page IH, Heuer GJ (1935) The effect of renal denervation on the level of arterial blood pressure and renal function in essential hypertension. J Clin Invest 14:27–30
23. Page IH, Heuer GJ (1935) The effect of renal denervation on patients suffering from nephritis. J Clin Invest 14:443–458
24. Peet MM (1948) Hypertension and its surgical treatment by supradiaphragmatic splanchnicectomy. Am J Surg LXXV:48–68
25. Smithwick RH, Thompson JE (1953) Splanchnicectomy for essential hypertension; results in 1,266 cases. J Am Med Assoc 152:1501–1504
26. Peet MM, Woods WW, Braden S (1940) The surgical treatment of hypertension. JAMA 115:1875–1885
27. Freis ED, Wanko A, Wilson IM, Parrish AE (1958) Treatment of essential hypertension with chlorothiazide (diuril); its use alone and combined with other antihypertensive agents. J Am Med Assoc 166:137–140
28. VA Cooperative Study Group (1967) Effects of treatment on morbidity in hypertension. Results in patients with diastolic blood pressures averaging 115 through 129 mm Hg. JAMA 202:1028–1034
29. Wallin BG, Charkoudian N (2007) Sympathetic neural control of integrated cardiovascular function: insights from measurement of human sympathetic nerve activity. Muscle Nerve 36:595–614
30. Grassi G, Seravalle G, Quarti-Trevano F (2010) The 'neuroadrenergic hypothesis' in hypertension: current evidence. Exp Physiol 95:581–586
31. Fisher JP, Young CN, Fadel PJ (2009) Central sympathetic overactivity: maladies and mechanisms. Auton Neurosci 148:5–15
32. Floras JS (2009) Sympathetic nervous system activation in human heart failure: clinical implications of an updated model. J Am Coll Cardiol 54:375–385
33. Grassi G, Quarti-Trevano F, Seravalle G, Arenare F, Volpe M, Furiani S, Dell'Oro R, Mancia G (2011) Early sympathetic activation in the initial clinical stages of chronic renal failure. Hypertension 57:846–851
34. Sverrisdóttir YB, Mogren T, Kataoka J, Janson PO, Stener-Victorin E (2008) Is polycystic ovary syndrome associated with high sympathetic nerve activity and size at birth? Am J Physiol Endocrinol Metab 294:E576–E581
35. Prabhakar NR, Kumar GK (2010) Mechanisms of sympathetic activation and blood pressure elevation by intermittent hypoxia. Respir Physiol Neurobiol 174:156–161
36. Stadlbauer V, Stadlbauer VP, Wright GA, Banaji M, Mukhopadhya A, Mookerjee RP, Mookerjee R, Moore K, Jalan R (2008) Relationship between activation of the sympathetic nervous system and renal blood flow autoregulation in cirrhosis. Gastroenterology 134:111–119
37. Schauerte P, Scherlag BJ, Scherlag MA, Goli S, Jackman WM, Lazzara R (1999) Ventricular rate control during atrial fibrillation by cardiac parasympathetic nerve stimulation: a transvenous approach. J Am Coll Cardiol 34:2043–2050
38. Schauerte P, Scherlag BJ, Pitha J, Scherlag MA, Reynolds D, Lazzara R, Jackman WM (2000) Catheter ablation of cardiac autonomic nerves for prevention of vagal atrial fibrillation. Circulation 102(22):2774–2780
39. Krum H, Schlaich M, Whitbourn R, Sobotka PA, Sadowski J, Bartus K, Kapelak B, Walton A, Sievert H, Thambar S, Abraham WT, Esler M (2009) Catheter-based renal sympathetic denervation for resistant hypertension: a multicentre safety and proof-of-principle cohort study. Lancet 373:1275–1281
40. Symplicity HTN-2 Investigators (2010) Renal sympathetic denervation in patients with treatment-resistant hypertension (the symplicity HTN-2 trial): a randomised controlled trial. Lancet 376:1903–1909
41. Brinkmann J, Heusser K, Schmidt BM, Menne J, Klein G, Bauersachs J, Haller H, Sweep FC, Diedrich A, Jordan J, Tank J (2012) Catheter-based renal nerve ablation and centrally generated sympathetic activity in difficult- to-control hypertensive patients: prospective case series. Hypertension 60:1485–1490, 58

42. Mahfoud F, Böhm M, Rump LC, Vonend O, Schmieder RE, Kintscher U (2013) Catheter-based renal nerve ablation and centrally generated sympathetic activity in difficult-to-control hypertensive patients: prospective case series. Hypertension 61:e17, 59
43. Schlaich M, Hering D, Lambert G, Lambert E, Esler M (2013) Blood pressure and sympathetic nervous system response to renal denervation. Hypertension 61:e13
44. Tsioufis C, Papademetriou V, Tsiachris D, Dimitriadis K, Kasiakogias A, Kordalis A, Antonakis V, Kefala A, Thomopoulos C, Kallikazaros I, Lau EO, Stefanadis C (2014) Drug-resistant hypertensive patients responding to multielectrode renal denervation exhibit improved heart rate dynamics and reduced arrhythmia burden. J Hum Hypertens 28(10):587–593. doi:10.1038/jhh
45. Papademetriou V, Tsioufis CP, Sinhal A, Chew DP, Meredith IT, Malaiapan Y, Worthley MI, Worthley SG (2014) Catheter-based renal denervation for resistant hypertension: 12-month results of the EnligHTN I first-in-human study using a multielectrode ablation system. Hypertension 64(3):565–572
46. Papademetriou V, Rashidi AA, Tsioufis C, Doumas M (2014) Renal nerve ablation for resistant hypertension: how did we get here, present status, and future directions. Circulation 129(13):1440–1451
47. Papademetriou V, Tsioufis C, Doumas M (2014) Renal denervation and symplicity HTN-3: "Dubium Sapientiae Initium" (doubt is the beginning of wisdom). Circ Res 115(2):211–214. doi:10.1161/CIRCRESAHA.115.304099. No abstract available
48. Bhatt DL, Kandzari DE, O'Neill WW, D'Agostino R, Flack JM, Katzen BT, Leon MB, Liu M, Mauri L, Negoita M, Cohen SA, Oparil S, Rocha-Singh K, Townsend RR, Bakris GL (2014) SYMPLICITY HTN-3 investigators. A controlled trial of renal denervation for resistant hypertension. N Engl J Med 370(15):1393–1401
49. Tellez A, Rousselle S, Palmieri T et al (2013) Renal artery nerve distribution and density in the porcine model: biologic implications for the development of radiofrequency ablation therapies. Transl Res 162:381–389
50. Atherton DS, Deep NL, Mendelsohn FO (2012) Micro-anatomy of the renal sympathetic nervous system: a human postmortem Histologic study. Clin Anat 25:628–633
51. Sakakura K, Ladic E, Cheng Q, Otsuka F, Yahagi K, Fowler DR, Kolodgie FK, Virmani R, Joner M (2014) Anatomic assessment of sympathetic peri-arterial renal nerves in man. JACC 64:635–643
52. Tzafriri AR, Mahfoud F, John H. Keating JH, Peter M, Markham PM, Spognardi A, Wong G, Fuimaono K, Böhm M, Edelman ER (2014) Innervation patterns may limit response to endovascular renal denervation. J Am Coll Cardiol 64(11):1079–1087.
53. Henegar JR, Yongxing Zhang Y, RamaDR, Cary Hata C, Michael E, Hall ME, Hall JE (2014) Catheter-Based radiorefrequency renal denervation lowers blood pressure in obese hypertensive dogs. Am J Hypertens 27(10):1285–1292
54. Mahfoud F, Tunev S, Ewen S, Cremers B, Ruwart J, Schulz-Jander D, Linz D, Davies J, Kandzari DE, Whitbourn R, Bohm M, Melder RJ (2015) Impact of lesion placement on efficacy and safety of catheter-based radiofrequency renal denervation. J Am Coll Cardiol 66:1766–1775
55. Booth LC, Nishi EE, Yao ST, Ramchandra R, Lambert GW, Schlaich MP, May CN (2015) Reinnervation of renal afferent and efferent nerves at 5.5 and 11 months after catheter-based radiofrequency renal denervation in sheep. Hypertention 65:393–400
56. Fischell TA, Vega F, Raju N, Johnson ET, Kent DK, Ragland RR, Fischell DR, Almany SL, Ghazarossian VE (2013) Ethanol-mediated perivascular renal sympathetic denervation: preclinical validation of safety and efficacy in a porcine model. EuroIntervention 9:140–147
57. Fischell TA, Fischell DR, Ghazarossian VE, Vega F, Ebner A (2015) Next generation renal denervation: chemical "perivascular" renal denervation with alcohol using a novel drug infusion catheter. Cardiovasc Revasc Med 16:221–227

Procedural Aspects of Renal Sympathetic Denervation

14

Ina Zivanovic, Sebastian Ewen, Michael Böhm,
and Felix Mahfoud

Abbreviations

BP	Blood pressure
HTN	Hypertension
RDN	Renal denervation

14.1 Introduction

Renal sympathetic denervation (RDN) is a minimally invasive, percutaneous, endovascular procedure for the transluminal disruption of efferent and afferent renal sympathetic nerve fibers, most commonly utilized for the treatment of severe resistant hypertension. Energy has to be delivered to the area where nerve fibers are located while simultaneously preserving the renal arterial wall. Ablation with radiofrequency energy is the most frequently utilized technique, while alternative methods include ultrasound and chemical ablation. As RDN is still, to a great degree, a black box procedure, technique, and detailed knowledge of renal neurovascular anatomy are required for effective ablation.

I. Zivanovic • S. Ewen • M. Böhm • F. Mahfoud, MD, FESC (✉)
Universitätsklinikum des Saarlandes, Klinik für Innere Medizin III,
Kardiologie, Angiologie und Internistische Intensivmedizin, Kirrberger Str.,
Homburg/Saar, DE 66424, Germany
e-mail: felix.mahfoud@uks.eu

C. Tsioufis et al. (eds.), *Interventional Therapies for Secondary and Essential Hypertension*, Updates in Hypertension and Cardiovascular Protection,
DOI 10.1007/978-3-319-34141-5_14

14.2 Optimal Sites for RDN

14.2.1 Renal Vascular Characteristics

In the majority of patients, renal arteries originate from the aorta between the upper L1 and lower L2 margin, just below the superior mesenteric artery, most commonly at the level of the intervertebral disk (Fig. 14.1) [1, 2]. Both arteries exit the aorta perpendicularly. The left renal artery originates more posterolaterally and travels posterior to the left renal vein. Renal artery variations are present in 17–37 % and include prehilar branching as well as extra renal arteries, leading either to the hilum (accessory artery) or the pole (polar artery) of the kidney [1]. There are also variations in the origins of the gonadal and inferior suprarenal arteries [3]. The latter, particularly important for the supply of the adrenal gland, most often originates from the proximal part of the main renal artery and should be avoided during RDN [3, 4].

14.2.2 Locating Sympathetic Nerves

The postganglionic efferent renal sympathetic nerves travel from the thoracolumbar sympathetic trunk and ganglia mainly through the outer adventitial and peri-adventitial tissue [5]. Afferent sympathetic nerves transmit impulses centrally [6]. It was initially postulated a 2–4 mm ablation depth could reach the majority of the sympathetic fibers. An analysis of nine human renal arteries found 90.5 % of all nerves to be within a 2 mm interval from the lumen, distributed relatively evenly around the renal artery circumference, and the number of nerves increasing distally [7]. A later study on porcine models revealed only 45 % of nerves were located within 2 mm from the arterial wall [6]. The greatest nerve counts were

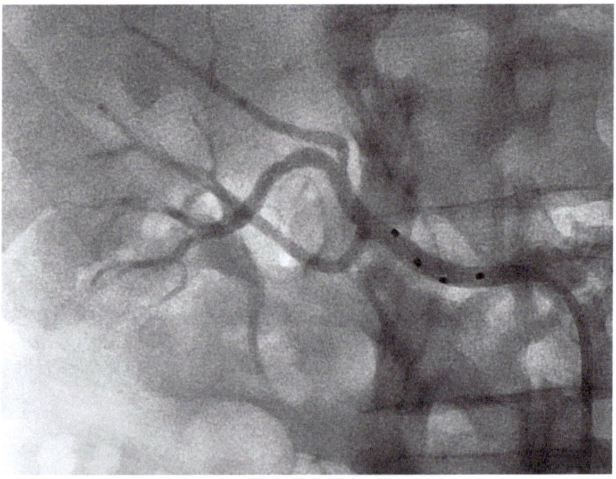

Fig. 14.1 Renal angiogram during a renal denervation procedure

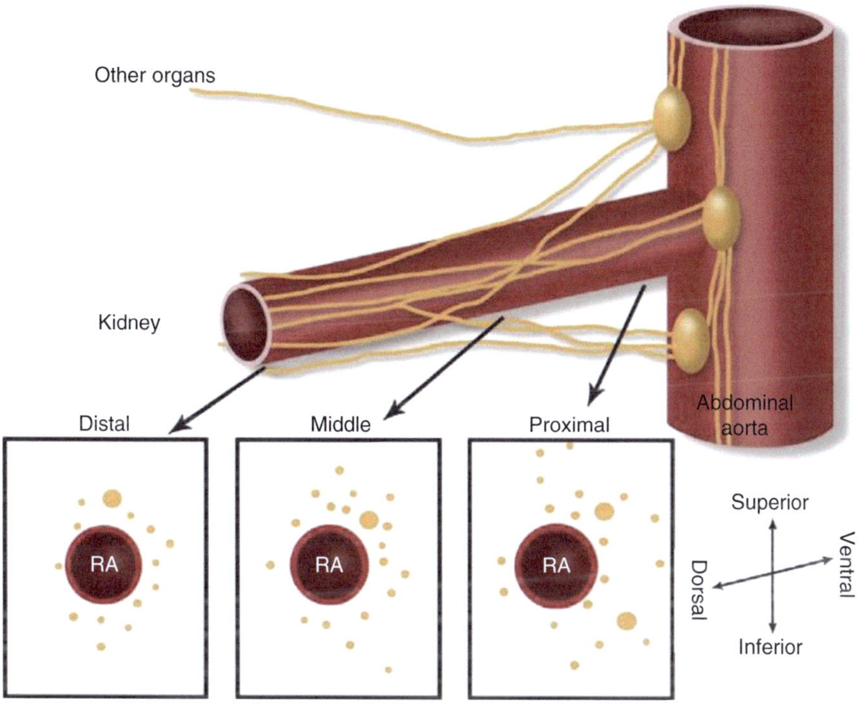

Fig. 14.2 Diagram of the renal artery with periarterial nerve distribution [8]

found proximally; the bundles, however, were progressing closer to the wall distally. Afferent nerves were scarcer compared to efferent nerves.

Finally, Sakakura et al. studied 20 patients with 10.329 individual nerves, confirming that the path of the sympathetic plexus in relation to the renal artery is not parallel nor are the fibers evenly distributed along the artery's circumference [8, 9] (Fig. 14.2). The number of nerves was greatest in the proximal (39.6 ± 16.7 per section) and middle (39.9 ± 13.9 per section) renal artery segments, but the mean distance from the lumen was also highest proximally (3.40 ± 0.78 mm) as compared to the middle (3.10 ± 0.69 mm) or distal segment (2.60 ± 0.77 mm) [8]. In the distal segment, the nerves were fewer (33.6 ± 13.1 per section), however converged on the renal artery. At a 3 mm distance from the lumen, the cumulative percentile of nerves was approximately 50 % in the proximal and middle segments and 75 % in the distal segment (Fig. 14.3) [9]. The circumferential distribution was greatest ventrally (11.0 ± 3.5 per section) and lowest dorsally (6.2 ± 3.0 per section) (Fig. 14.3) [8, 9]. Afferent fibers, which were lower in number, converged toward the proximal segment. Sympathetic nerves also surrounded the accessory artery. No significant differences between hypertensive and non-hypertensive subjects were noted.

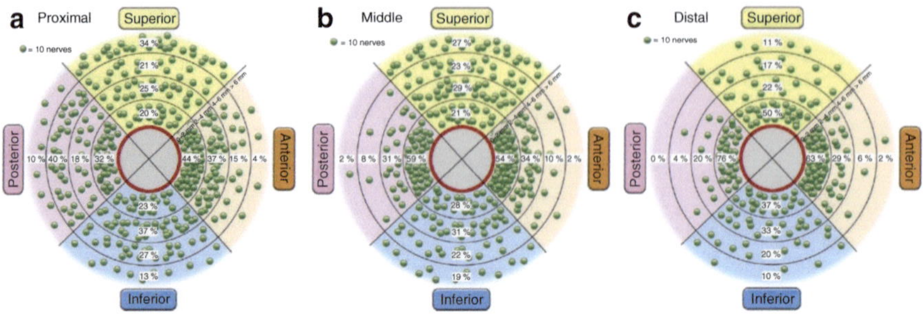

Fig. 14.3 Periarterial distribution of sympathetic nerves [9]. Distribution of nerves stratified according to the total number (each green dot represents ten nerves), relative number as percent per segment, and distance from the lumen in relative (**a**) proximal, (**b**) middle, and (**c**) distal location

14.2.3 Lesion Sites for Increased Efficacy

With the data on sympathetic nerve location at hand, it was still unclear whether ablations would be more effective proximally, where efferent and afferent nerve density is greater, or distally, where the nerves run closer to the lumen. Recently, the impact of denervation patterns on renal norepinephrine concentration and axon density was studied in porcine models (Fig. 14.4) [10]. The study revealed that four, eight, or twelve ablations within the main artery all produced a significant effect without a significant dose–response relationship. Treatment of the branch arteries or the distal main artery, however, reduced the variability of the response and yielded greater reductions in renal norepinephrine concentration. When comparing treatment sites, lesions in branch arteries (the V pattern group) resulted in greater reductions in cortical norepinephrine concentrations and axon density compared to the main artery (the I pattern group), while the effect was greatest after treating both the branches and the main artery (the Y pattern group). The combination treatment effect also showed the lowest variability as well as durability at 28 days post treatment. A second cycle of combined treatment (the Y2 pattern group) did not improve its effectiveness, however, and remained superior to non-combination treatments. Furthermore, the experience-based recommendation that one ablation should be made superiorly, as close as possible to the main renal artery ostium, has been disputed. A study by Tzafriri et al. revealed ablations 6 mm or more from the aorta affected up to 85 % of nerves, while ablations up to 5 mm from the ostium only affected up to 40 % [11].

The second question at hand is which quadrants should be ablated. Variable renal nerve anatomy supports the notion of asymmetric nerve targeting along the artery circumference. In an analysis of response predictors in the Symplicity HTN-3 trial, blood pressure reduction correlated highly with the presence of four-quadrant ablations and the number of ablation attempts [12]. While the protocol indicated the delivery of at least one superior, one inferior, and two anterior/posterior ablations within a main artery, this was implemented in only a quarter of patients. Although several contributing factors for not reaching its primary end points have been suggested by the authors, lesion placement may play a highly important role. A recent

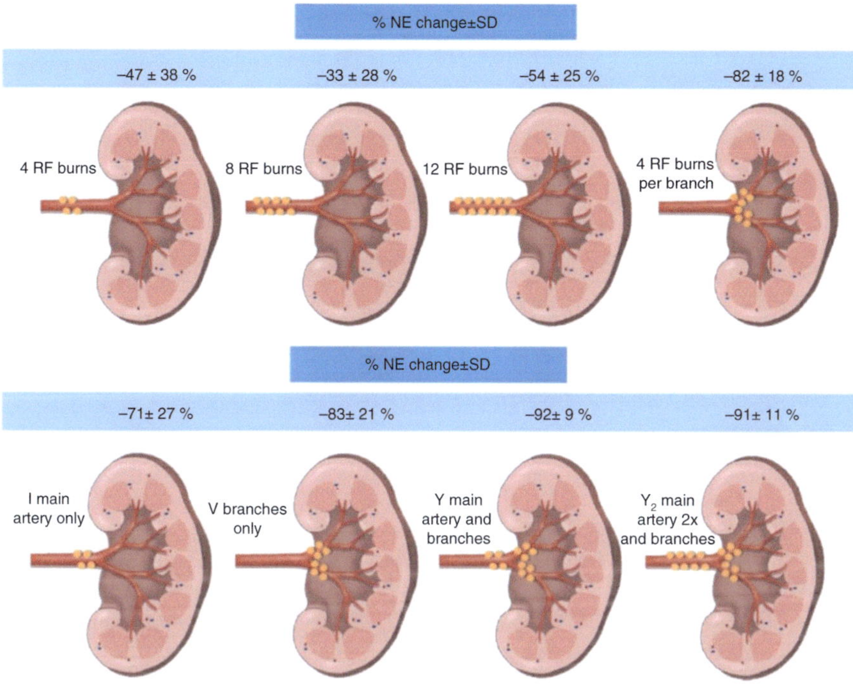

Fig. 14.4 Renal cortical norepinephrine concentration change in response to increasing numbers of lesions in the main artery and treatment of branch arteries (*top*) and in response to targeted treatment of the distal main artery or branches (*bottom*) [10]. Percentage reduction = (mean control NE – test sample NE)/mean control × 100. *NE* norepinephrine concentration, *RF* radiofrequency

study by Rosa et al. also noted greater blood pressure changes in the group of patients who received four or more ablations [13].

RDN has previously been avoided in the accessory renal arteries. An observational study showed blood pressure lowering can be achieved effectively through dominant-vessel treatment [14]. A prospective study which followed, however, found the treatment was less successful in patients with accessory arteries and that the effect doubled when they were ablated as well [15].

Studies to date suggest RDN may be most effective when treating the main artery and its branches, as well as the accessory artery (given it is present and of a sufficient diameter), with asymmetric four-quadrant ablation. These notions are being tested in the currently ongoing Symplicity HTN trials and will shape pivotal clinical trials which are to follow [16].

14.3 Modalities and Systems for RDN

Currently available systems for renal denervation utilize radiofrequency energy, ultrasound energy, and chemical ablation (Table 14.1).

Table 14.1 Catheter types for renal denervation

Catheter	Electrode	Lesion	Form	Cooling	Energy delivery time	Max power	Guide size	Over the wire	Clinical studies	Depiction
Radiofrequency ablation										
Symplicity™ flex (medtronic)	Single unipolar	Operator dependent	Single electrode (2 mm)	Blood	120 s	8 W	6 Fr	No	Symplicity HTN-1 (completed) Symplicity HTN-2 (completed) Symplicity HTN-3 (follow-up) Symplicity HTN-4 (ongoing)	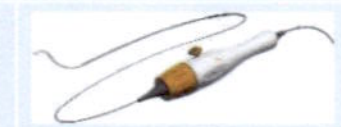
Iberis™ (terumo)	Single unipolar	Operator dependent	Single electrode	Blood	120 s	8 W	4 Fr	No	ALLEGRO-HTN	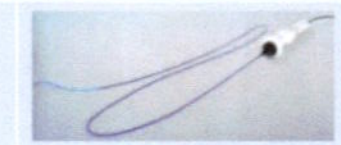
Symplicity™ spyral (medtronic)	Multiple (4) unipolar	Helical	Spiral	Blood	60 s	8 W	6 Fr	Yes	SymplicitySpyral feasibility study (completed) Spyral HTN OFF MED (recruiting) Spyral HTN ON MED (recruiting)	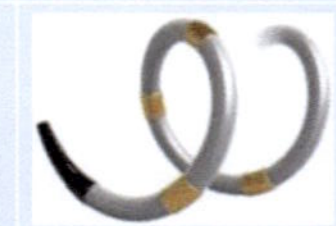
EnligHTN™ (St Jude)	Multiple (4) unipolar	Helical	Basket, 16/18 mm	Blood	60 s	6 W	8 Fr	No	EnligHTN I (completed) EnligHTN II (recruiting) EnligHTN III (completed) EnligHTNment	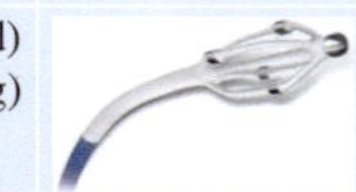
Vessix™ (Boston scientific)	Multiple (4–8) bipolar	Helical	Balloon, 4/5/6/7 mm	None	30 s	1 W	7–8 Fr	Yes	REDUCE-HTN (completed) REDUCE HTN: REINFORCE (recruiting)	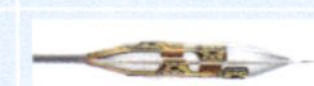

OneShot™ (covidien)	Spiral electrode, irrigation	Helical	Balloon	Open saline irrigation	120 s	25 W	7–9 Fr	Yes	RAPID (completed) RAPID II (withdrawn)	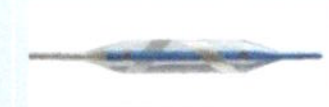
ThermoCool® (biosense webster)[a]	Single unipolar/ multiple (5)	Operator dependent/ helical	Helical platform	Open saline irrigation	N/A	15–24 W	6–7 Fr	Yes	RENABLATE (completed) RENABLATE II (completed) SWAN HT (ongoing) SAVE (terminated) RELIEF (completed)	N/A
Chilli II® (Boston scientific)[a]	Single unipolar	Operator dependent	Single electrode (4 mm)	Closed irrigation	120 s	50 W	7 Fr	N/A	SAVE (terminated)	N/A
Ultrasound ablation										
Paradise® (Recor)	Multi-directional ultrasound transducer	Circum ferential	Balloon, 5/6/7/8 mm	Closed irrigation	10 s	30 W	6 Fr	No	REALISE (ongoing) ACHIEVE (recruiting) RADIANCE (not yet recruiting)	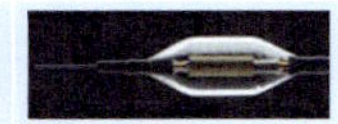
TIVUS™ (cardiosonic)	Uni-/ multidirectional ultrasound transducer	Operator dependent/ circum ferential	Catheter	None	40 s	12 W	6 Fr	Yes	TIVUS II (ongoing) TROPHY (not yet recruiting)	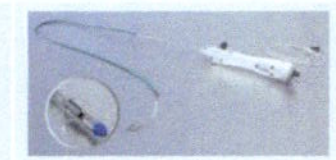
SurroundSound™ (Kona medical)[a]	Externalultrasound energy source								WAVE I, II, III (completed) WAVE IV (recruiting)	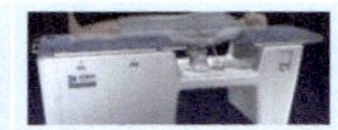
Chemical ablation										
Peregrine system™ (ablative solutions)	None	Circum ferential	Needle infusion catheter	None	Delivery of 0.6 ml dehydrated alcohol per renal artery			N/A	The peregrine study (ongoing) Postmarket study (recruiting)	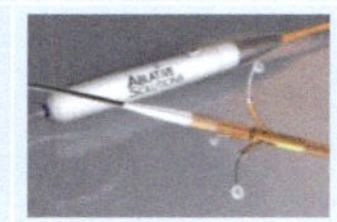

[a]ThermoCool®, Chilli II® and Surround Sound™ are investigational devices and not yet approved for sale

N/A not available

14.3.1 Radiofrequency Ablation

Radiofrequency ablation is the most commonly used modality with the greatest variety of available systems and clinical data. Systems were initially unipolar such as Symplicity™ Flex and Iberis™, requiring two minutes for a single ablation and their lesions being operator dependent [17–19]. Without a means to assess for successful renal nerve ablation during the procedure, this was problematic, as several factors influence a formation of a lesion: good wall contact with tissue and interface temperature, power delivery, the impedance of target tissue, as well as the size of the electrode [12, 20]. Considered together with the data on renal nerve anatomy, this led to the development of multiple-ablation systems with helically or circumferentially distributed electrodes. It not only shortens procedure time, but, more importantly, enables good wall contact and automatic four-quadrant ablation without operator dependence. Examples include Symplicity™ Spyral in a spiral, EnligHTN™ in a basket, and Vessix™ in a balloon form, all with asymmetrically distributed ablation points [16, 21]. OneShot™, on the other hand, uses only one helically shaped electrode. Radiofrequency catheters create lesions up to 2–4 mm deep [20]. Ablation times for one four-quadrant ablation range from 30 to 120 s and catheter sizes from 6 to 8 Fr. Some catheters, such as OneShot™, also feature an additional cooling system for the protection of renal artery endothelium, while the shape of Symplicity™ Spyral and EnligHTN™ enables cooling through blood flow in the renal arteries.

14.3.2 Ultrasound Ablation

In contrast to other modalities, ultrasound ablation does not require contact with the arterial wall. It is utilized in systems such as Paradise® and TIVUS™. Ultrasound waves generate heat in the surrounding tissue, which is then transmitted to adjacent tissue [22]. The Paradise® catheter incorporates a multidirectional circumferential ultrasound transducer, encased in a balloon with internal cooling, thereby preserving arterial wall integrity [22]. The 6 Fr device offers different balloon sizes and only takes ten seconds for a circumferential ablation. Although the circumferential pattern could theoretically pose a threat of developing stenosis, studies so far have proven the system's safety. Furthermore, ultrasound RDN is not limited to intravascular procedures. Surround Sound™, an investigational device, enables the extracorporeal delivery of ultrasound energy [23].

14.3.3 Chemical Ablation

Chemical ablation requires the contact of a neurolytic substance with sympathetic nerves. The Peregrine System™ is an infusion catheter with three microneedles positioned radially with 120° separation. Injecting dehydrated alcohol with the Peregrine System™ enables circumferential denervation up to 13.5 mm deep at target sites with a short procedural time [24]. Studies so far have confirmed the procedure's safety, while it also seems promising for treating regions not possible with radiofrequency energy; however, further trials are necessary to enable an accurate comparison.

14.4 Prior to Procedure

14.4.1 Confirming Resistant Hypertension

Prior to procedure, it should be confirmed that the patient is suffering from severe resistant HTN with an office systolic blood pressure (BP) ≥160 mmHg (≥150 mmHg in patients with diabetes type 2) in spite of treatment with three or more antihypertensive drugs including a diuretic, in adequate doses [25]. Thorough history and physical, correct office BP measurement, ambulatory BP monitoring, and additional testing should be performed to rule out failure to comply to medication intake, contributing lifestyle factors and drugs (e.g., nonsteroidal anti-inflammatory drugs), pseudo-resistance (e.g., the white coat effect) as well as secondary causes of HTN such as renal artery stenosis, hyperthyroidism, hyperaldosteronism, pheochromocytoma, Cushing's syndrome, and obstructive sleep apnea syndrome (Fig. 14.5) [25, 26]. Work-up should be conducted by an HTN specialist or an HTN (excellence) center team, while the final assessment should be done by a multidisciplinary, specialized RDN team [26, 27].

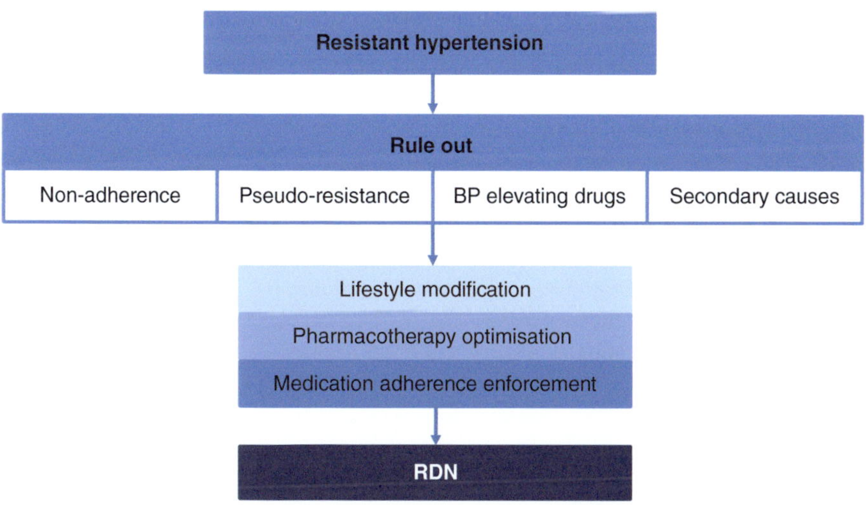

Fig. 14.5 Approach to patients with resistant hypertension [25, 26]. *BP* blood pressure, *RDN* renal sympathetic denervation

14.4.2 Kidney Function

Studies have confirmed the safety of RDN in patients with an estimated glomerular filtration rate (eGFR) ≥45 ml/min/1.73 m^2, calculated by the Modification of Diet in Renal Disease (MDRD) formula [13, 17–19, 21, 26, 28, 29]. More recently, the DENERHTN study included patients with an eGFR above 40 ml/min/1.73 m^2 [30], while a pilot study by Ott et al. suggests RDN could slow or even halt the decline of renal function in patients with chronic kidney disease at stages 3 and 4 [31]. RDN has also been successfully applied to treat resistant HTN in patients with solitary kidneys [32].

14.4.3 Age, Comorbidities, and Special Conditions

RDN is currently recommended for patients aged 18–80 years who have been included in trials so far [13, 17–19, 21, 28–30]. The decision to treat patients within 3 months after a myocardial infarction, unstable angina pectoris, or a cerebrovascular accident should be made by a multidisciplinary team, as these patients have been excluded from studies to date [13, 17–19, 21, 28–30]. Apart from radiation risks, there is no data on risks and benefits of RDN in pregnancy, since pregnant women, women nursing, or women planning to become pregnant have also been excluded from clinical trials [13, 17–19, 21, 28–30]. In women of childbearing potential, a pregnancy test is advised prior to procedure.

14.4.4 Imaging

To ensure the safety and efficiency of RDN, appropriate renal vascular anatomy must be confirmed. Preferred imaging methods include renal duplex ultrasound, magnetic resonance angiography, and computed tomography [1, 33]. Morphological renal artery criteria for RDN, although differing slightly between RDN methods, include the following [4]:

1. Main renal artery diameter of 4–8 mm
2. Main renal artery length prior to branching ≥20 mm
3. Main renal artery stenosis ≤50 %
4. Identification of existing accessory and polar arteries
5. Treatment possibility >5 mm from:
   (a) Atheroma
   (b) Calcification
   (c) Aneurysm
   (d) Fibromuscular dysplasia
   (e) Renal artery stent, in which case treatment must be possible distally [34, 35]

14.4.5 Prevention of Contrast Nephropathy

Preparation for RDN includes the prevention of contrast nephropathy by temporarily withholding potentially nephrotoxic drugs such as nonsteroidal anti-inflammatory drugs, metformin, and high-dose diuretics 48 h prior to procedure, as well as pre-hydrating the patient. Pre-hydration may be oral or intravenous in cases of significantly reduced renal function. Some centers even offer the option of carbon dioxide angiography. Antihypertensive therapy, as well as treatment for associated comorbidities, such as statins and acetylsalicylic acid, should be continued.

14.5 Renal Denervation

14.5.1 Patient Preparation

To prevent aspiration of gastric contents, the patient should be in a fasting state. Patient preparation consists of groin (or arm) sterilization, ground pad placement (depending on the catheter), and the setting up of monitoring including ECG, intra-arterial BP, and oxygen saturation.

14.5.2 Periprocedural Medication

Anticoagulation is required because RDN might induce thrombus formation [36]. To obtain an activated clotting time greater than 250 s, an intravenous heparin bolus of 3,000–5,000 units should be administered and appropriately titrated [4]. Additionally, studies recommend initiating a 4-week antiplatelet treatment with 100–500 mg of acetylsalicylic acid or, alternatively, 300–600 mg of clopidogrel, although without clear support by evidence. Nitroglycerine should be injected into the main renal artery to prevent spasm. Because RDN is a relatively short procedure, general anesthesia is normally not required. Some countries, however, may require the presence of an anesthesiologist. Analgesics and sedatives are mandatory to control the pain from nociceptor stimulation during ablation. Recommendations consist of:

- Sedation with midazolam 2.5 mg i.v. and an additional 1–1.5 mg bolus before ablation, which can be repeated up to 10–15 mg in total
- Analgesia with fentanyl (0.05–1 mg i.v. with an equivalent bolus before ablation), morphine (5 mg i.v. and a 2–3 mg bolus before ablation), or remifentanil (continuous infusion)
- Oxygen flow of 2–6 l/min

Medication protocols during the procedure vary from center to center.

14.5.3 Angiography

Initially, a 6–9 Fr sheath is introduced into the femoral artery, followed by an aortography to confirm eligibility for RDN and select the guiding catheter [4]. The renal double curve (RDC1) is recommended, but the internal mammary artery (IMA)-shaped catheter is more appropriate for low take-off angles and an inferiorly directed ostium. The 20–30 % left anterior oblique view is recommended for imaging the renal artery origins and the anterior–posterior view for imaging the course. A nonionic contrast in 1:1 or 1:2 dilution should be used for the renal arteriogram.

14.5.4 Renal Denervation Procedure

While the majority of catheters utilize a femoral approach, the Iberis™ system also enables a radial approach. The systems' sizes and characteristics are presented in Table 14.1. The ablation catheter should pass the renal artery ostium under fluoroscopy to prevent disengagement when inserting the ablation device. Treatment should be done in a distal-to-proximal fashion while avoiding double treatment of already treated sites. Proper electrode contact with the vessel wall is important for radiofrequency ablations [24]. It can be assessed using fluoroscopy and the detection of appropriate impedance readings. An effective and safe ablation takes place between 60 and 80 °C with a gradual impedance decline of 5–20 %. Rapid decline might signal loss of contact or cloth formation, which may cause an automatic termination of ablation in some generators.

14.5.5 System-Specific Steps

14.5.5.1 Single-Electrode Systems

Once the Symplicity™ Flex denervation catheter is positioned, the denervation catheter tip has to be deflected, pulling the lever on the handle. A stable impedance (220–320 ± 5 Ω) is required prior to ablation, as it indicates proper contact with the arterial wall. RDN should begin in an appropriately sized branch artery and continued proximally. The catheter tip should be pulled and rotated to perform four-quadrant ablations with ≥5 mm distances between lesions.

The Iberis™ system may be applied femorally or radially. The later requires a longer, 135 cm multipurpose catheter (Climber™, Terumo Corp.). After the insertion of hydrophilic coated 0.035 inch guide wire, the latter is exchanged for Iberis™. The following procedure is similar to Symplicity™ Flex. There is no cooling mechanism and the generated temperature is up to 70 °C.

14.5.5.2 Multielectrode Systems

The Symplicity™ Spyral catheter is advanced and removed over a 0.014 inch guide wire, distal to the renal artery hilum. It takes on its spiral shape when the wire is pulled back. Wall contact must be confirmed similarly to Symplicity™ Flex.

Simultaneous four-quadrant ablations should include appropriate branches and the main artery. If the main renal artery length is >20 mm, two ablations can be implemented with a slight rotation in between.

The EnligHTN™ basket must be collapsed when moving and expanded for positioning. Before ablation, a check for wall contact must be conducted. The ablation is then undertaken simultaneously with four electrodes in a fashion similar to Symplicity™ Spyral.

14.5.5.3 The Paradise® Ultrasound System

The Paradise® catheter is advanced and placed just proximal to the renal artery bifurcation and, if the balloon is not occlusive, it is changed to the next largest catheter size. The transducer should be in the center of the balloon and in parallel with the artery before treating. While flushing with cooling solution, the catheter is automatically inflated to 2 atm, and the ultrasound energy is emitted circumferentially for 30 s. After initial energy delivery, the balloon catheter is automatically deflated, pulled back about 10 mm, and checked for balloon occlusion of the artery using contrast injection.

14.5.5.4 Concluding RDN

After administering ablations, the renal angiogram should be repeated to check for dissections, stenosis, or vasospasm. Ablation notches, discrete beady irregularities, are normal phenomena due to intimal edema and spasm, which disappear within a few hours [19]. Hemostasis at the puncture site can be achieved using manual compression or closure devices. The patient is then moved to a recovery unit. Post-procedural intravenous hydration for the prevention of contrast nephropathy is recommended for patients at risk.

14.6 Follow-Up

Blood pressure changes in the following months are monitored during follow-up visits in the RDN center as well as in the general practitioner's clinic. Antihypertensive drugs should be adjusted according to blood pressure, preferably additionally assessed through ambulatory BP monitoring. Additionally, patient compliance should be enforced, and patients should be advised not to change drug regimens themselves.

14.7 Centers for Renal Denervation

An RDN center should include a hypertension excellence center with an HTN specialist and a multidisciplinary team. It should perform a minimal number of 25 RDN procedures per year and have the capabilities to treat potential complications (i.e., percutaneous renal stenting). Renal duplex ultrasound, magnetic resonance angiography, and/or computed tomography angiography should be available.

14.8 Renal Nerve Stimulation

Due to a lack of intra-procedural markers of efficacy, RDN remains a procedure, determined by anatomy. Studies, however, suggest optimal lesion sites could be determined by sympathetic nerve stimulation, triggering a response in blood pressure and heart rate [37]. Similarly, RDN efficacy could be assessed intra-procedurally by restimulating these areas after ablation and observing a dampened response.

Conclusion

RDN represents an important therapy option for resistant HTN when pharmacological treatments are exhausted. Within the last 2 years, crucial advancements have been made in the field of RDN. In addition to several studies confirming the procedure's safety and efficiency, expanding knowledge on sympathetic nerve anatomy and effective lesion placement, the development of new ablation systems, and beginnings of intra-procedural assessment have contributed to RDN gradually ceasing to be a black box procedure.

References

1. Ozkan U, Oguzkurt L, Tercan F, Kizilkilic O, Koc Z, Koca N (2006) Renal artery origins and variations: angiographic evaluation of 855 consecutive patients. Diagn Interv Radiol 12(4):183–186
2. Turba UC, Uflacker R, Bozlar U, Hagspiel KD (2009) Normal renal arterial anatomy assessed by multidetector CT angiography: are there differences between men and women? Clin Anat 22(2):236–242. doi:10.1002/ca.20748
3. Manso JC, DiDio LJ (2000) Anatomical variations of the human suprarenal arteries. Ann Anat 182(5):483–488. doi:10.1016/S0940-9602(00)80064-3
4. Tsioufis C, Mahfoud F, Mancia G, Redon J, Damascelli B, Zeller T, Schmieder RE (2014) What the interventionalist should know about renal denervation in hypertensive patients: a position paper by the ESH WG on the interventional treatment of hypertension. EuroIntervention 9(9):1027–1035. doi:10.4244/EIJV9I9A175
5. Esler M (2015) The sympathetic nervous system in hypertension: back to the future? Curr Hypertens Rep 17(2):11. doi:10.1007/s11906-014-0519-8
6. Tellez A, Rousselle S, Palmieri T, Rate WR, Wicks J, Degrange A, Hyon CM, Gongora CA, Hart R, Grundy W, Kaluza GL, Granada JF (2013) Renal artery nerve distribution and density in the porcine model: biologic implications for the development of radiofrequency ablation therapies. Transl Res 162(6):381–389. doi:10.1016/j.trsl.2013.07.002
7. Atherton DS, Deep NL, Mendelsohn FO (2012) Micro-anatomy of the renal sympathetic nervous system: a human postmortem histologic study. Clin Anat 25(5):628–633. doi:10.1002/ca.21280
8. Sakakura K, Ladich E, Cheng Q, Otsuka F, Yahagi K, Fowler DR, Kolodgie FD, Virmani R, Joner M (2014) Anatomic assessment of sympathetic peri-arterial renal nerves in man. J Am Coll Cardiol 64(7):635–643. doi:10.1016/j.jacc.2014.03.059
9. Mahfoud F, Edelman ER, Böhm M (2014) Catheter-based renal denervation is no simple matter: lessons to be learned from our anatomy? J Am Coll Cardiol 64(7):644–646. doi:10.1016/j.jacc.2014.05.037
10. Mahfoud F, Tunev S, Ewen S, Cremers B, Ruwart J, Schulz-Jander D, Linz D, Davies J, Kandzari DE, Whitbourn R, Böhm M, Melder RJ (2015) Impact of lesion placement on

efficacy and safety of catheter-based radiofrequency renal denervation. J Am Coll Cardiol 66(16):1766–1775. doi:10.1016/j.jacc.2015.08.018
11. Tzafriri AR, Mahfoud F, Keating JH, Markham PM, Spognardi A, Wong G, Fuimaono K, Böhm M, Edelman ER (2014) Innervation patterns may limit response to endovascular renal denervation. J Am Coll Cardiol 64(11):1079–1087. doi:10.1016/j.jacc.2014.07.937
12. Kandzari DE, Bhatt DL, Brar S, Devireddy CM, Esler M, Fahy M, Flack JM, Katzen BT, Lea J, Lee DP, Leon MB, Ma A, Massaro J, Mauri L, Oparil S et al (2015) Predictors of blood pressure response in the SYMPLICITY HTN-3 trial. Eur Heart J 36(4):219–227. doi:10.1093/eurheartj/ehu441
13. Rosa J, Widimsky P, Tousek P, Petrak O, Curila K, Waldauf P, Bednar F, Zelinka T, Holaj R, Strauch B, Somloova Z, Taborsky M, Vaclavik J, Kocianova E, Branny M et al (2015) Randomized comparison of renal denervation versus intensified pharmacotherapy including spironolactone in true-resistant hypertension: six-month results from the Prague-15 study. Hypertension 65(2):407–413. doi:10.1161/HYPERTENSIONAHA.114.04019
14. Schmid A, Ditting T, Sobotka PA, Veelken R, Schmieder RE, Uder M, Ott C (2013) Does renal artery supply indicate treatment success of renal denervation? Cardiovasc Intervent Radiol 36(4):987–991. doi:10.1007/s00270-013-0652-9
15. Id D, Kaltenbach B, Bertog SC, Hornung M, Hofmann I, Vaskelyte L, Sievert H (2013) Does the presence of accessory renal arteries affect the efficacy of renal denervation? JACC Cardiovasc Interv 6(10):1085–1091. doi:10.1016/j.jcin.2013.06.007
16. Kandzari DE, Kario K, Mahfoud F, Cohen SA, Pilcher G, Pocock S, Townsend R, Weber MA, Böhm M (2016) The SPYRAL HTN global clinical trial program: rationale and design for studies of renal denervation in the absence (SPYRAL HTN OFF-MED) and presence (SPYRAL HTN ON-MED) of antihypertensive medications. Am Heart J 171(1):82–91. doi:10.1016/j.ahj.2015.08.021
17. Krum H, Schlaich M, Whitbourn R, Sobotka PA, Sadowski J, Bartus K, Kapelak B, Walton A, Sievert H, Thambar S, Abraham WT, Esler M (2009) Catheter-based renal sympathetic denervation for resistant hypertension: a multicentre safety and proof-of-principle cohort study. Lancet 373(9671):1275–1281. doi:10.1016/S0140-6736(09)60566-3
18. Esler MD, Krum H, Sobotka PA, Schlaich MP, Schmieder RE, Böhm M (2010) Renal sympathetic denervation in patients with treatment-resistant hypertension (the symplicity HTN-2 trial): a randomised controlled trial. Lancet 376(9756):1903–1909. doi:10.1016/S0140-6736(10)62039-9
19. Bhatt DL, Kandzari DE, O'Neill WW, D'Agostino R, Flack JM, Katzen BT, Leon MB, Liu M, Mauri L, Negoita M, Cohen SA, Oparil S, Rocha-Singh K, Townsend RR, Bakris GL et al (2014) A controlled trial of renal denervation for resistant hypertension. N Engl J Med 370(15):1393–1401. doi:10.1056/NEJMoa1402670
20. Patel HC, Dhillon PS, Mahfoud F, Lindsay AC, Hayward C, Ernst S, Lyon AR, Rosen SD, di Mario C (2014) The biophysics of renal sympathetic denervation using radiofrequency energy. Clin Res Cardiol 103(5):337–344. doi:10.1007/s00392-013-0618-6
21. Worthley SG, Tsioufis CP, Worthley MI, Sinhal A, Chew DP, Meredith IT, Malaiapan Y, Papademetriou V (2013) Safety and efficacy of a multi-electrode renal sympathetic denervation system in resistant hypertension: the EnligHTN I trial. Eur Heart J 34(28):2132–2140. doi:10.1093/eurheartj/eht197
22. Pathak A, Coleman L, Roth A, Stanley J, Bailey L, Markham P, Ewen S, Morel C, Despas F, Honton B, Senard JM, Fajadet J, Mahfoud F (2015) Renal sympathetic nerve denervation using intraluminal ultrasound within a cooling balloon preserves the arterial wall and reduces sympathetic nerve activity. EuroIntervention 11(4):477–484. doi:10.4244/EIJV11I4A96
23. Gertner M, Crura F, Zhang J (2015) Renal denervation using externally delivered focused ultrasound: summary of clinical experience to date and validation of supporting computational simulations. J Ther Ultrasound 3(Suppl 1):O68. doi:10.1186/2050-5736-3-S1-O68
24. Fischell TA, Fischell DR, Ghazarossian VE, Vega F, Ebner A (2015) Next generation renal denervation: chemical "perivascular" renal denervation with alcohol using a novel drug infusion catheter. Cardiovasc Revasc Med 16(4):221–227. doi:10.1016/j.carrev.2015.04.008
25. Schlaich MP, Schmieder RE, Bakris G, Blankestijn PJ, Böhm M, Campese VM, Francis DP, Grassi G, Hering D, Katholi R, Kjeldsen S, Krum H, Mahfoud F, Mancia G, Messerli FH et al (2013)

International expert consensus statement: percutaneous transluminal renal denervation for the treatment of resistant hypertension. J Am Coll Cardiol 62(22):2031–2045. doi:10.1016/j.jacc.2013.08.1616

26. Mancia G, Fagard R, Narkiewicz K, Redon J, Zanchetti A, Böhm M, Christiaens T, Cifkova R, De Backer G, Dominiczak A, Galderisi M, Grobbee DE, Jaarsma T, Kirchhof P, Kjeldsen SE et al (2013) 2013 ESH/ESC guidelines for the management of arterial hypertension: the Task Force for the Management of Arterial Hypertension of the European Society of Hypertension (ESH) and of the European Society of Cardiology (ESC). Eur Heart J 34(28):2159–2219. doi:10.1093/eurheartj/eht151
27. Persu A, Jin Y, Baelen M, Vink E, Verloop WL, Schmidt B, Blicher MK, Severino F, Wuerzner G, Taylor A, Pechere-Bertschi A, Jokhaji F, Fadl Elmula FE, Rosa J, Czarnecka D et al (2014) Eligibility for renal denervation: experience at 11 European expert centers. Hypertension 63(6):1319–1325. doi:10.1161/HYPERTENSIONAHA.114.03194
28. Böhm M, Mahfoud F, Ukena C, Hoppe UC, Narkiewicz K, Negoita M, Ruilope L, Schlaich MP, Schmieder RE, Whitbourn R, Williams B, Zeymer U, Zirlik A, Mancia G, Investigators GSR (2015) First report of the Global SYMPLICITY Registry on the effect of renal artery denervation in patients with uncontrolled hypertension. Hypertension 65(4):766–774. doi:10.1161/HYPERTENSIONAHA.114.05010
29. Desch S, Okon T, Heinemann D, Kulle K, Rohnert K, Sonnabend M, Petzold M, Muller U, Schuler G, Eitel I, Thiele H, Lurz P (2015) Randomized sham-controlled trial of renal sympathetic denervation in mild resistant hypertension. Hypertension 65(6):1202–1208. doi:10.1161/HYPERTENSIONAHA.115.05283
30. Azizi M, Sapoval M, Gosse P, Monge M, Bobrie G, Delsart P, Midulla M, Mounier-Vehier C, Courand PY, Lantelme P, Denolle T, Dourmap-Collas C, Trillaud H, Pereira H, Plouin PF et al (2015) Optimum and stepped care standardised antihypertensive treatment with or without renal denervation for resistant hypertension (DENERHTN): a multicentre, open-label, randomised controlled trial. Lancet 385(9981):1957–1965. doi:10.1016/S0140-6736(14)61942-5
31. Ott C, Mahfoud F, Schmid A, Toennes SW, Ewen S, Ditting T, Veelken R, Ukena C, Uder M, Böhm M, Schmieder RE (2015) Renal denervation preserves renal function in patients with chronic kidney disease and resistant hypertension. J Hypertens 33(6):1261–1266. doi:10.1097/HJH.0000000000000556
32. Ribichini F, Ferrara A, Pighi M, Pesarini G, Gambaro A, Valvo E, Lupo A, Vassanelli C (2014) Single-side renal sympathetic denervation to treat malignant refractory hypertension in a solitary kidney patient. J Nephrol. doi:10.1007/s40620-014-0059-y
33. Rountas C, Vlychou M, Vassiou K, Liakopoulos V, Kapsalaki E, Koukoulis G, Fezoulidis IV, Stefanidis I (2007) Imaging modalities for renal artery stenosis in suspected renovascular hypertension: prospective intraindividual comparison of color Doppler US, CT angiography, GD-enhanced MR angiography, and digital substraction angiography. Ren Fail 29(3):295–302. doi:10.1080/08860220601166305
34. Mahfoud F, Tunev S, Ruwart J, Schulz-Jander D, Cremers B, Linz D, Zeller T, Bhatt DL, Rocha-Singh K, Böhm M, Melder RJ (2014) Efficacy and safety of catheter-based radiofrequency renal denervation in stented renal arteries. Circ Cardiovasc Interv 7(6):813–820. doi:10.1161/CIRCINTERVENTIONS.114.001506
35. Ziegler AK, Franke J, Bertog SC (2013) Renal denervation in a patient with prior renal artery stenting. Catheter Cardiovasc Interv 81(2):342–345. doi:10.1002/ccd.24507
36. Templin C, Jaguszewski M, Ghadri JR, Sudano I, Gaehwiler R, Hellermann JP, Schoenenberger-Berzins R, Landmesser U, Erne P, Noll G, Luscher TF (2013) Vascular lesions induced by renal nerve ablation as assessed by optical coherence tomography: pre- and post-procedural comparison with the Simplicity catheter system and the EnligHTN multi-electrode renal denervation catheter. Eur Heart J 34(28):2141–2148, 2148b. doi:10.1093/eurheartj/eht141
37. Chinushi M, Izumi D, Iijima K, Suzuki K, Furushima H, Saitoh O, Furuta Y, Aizawa Y, Iwafuchi M (2013) Blood pressure and autonomic responses to electrical stimulation of the renal arterial nerves before and after ablation of the renal artery. Hypertension 61(2):450–456. doi:10.1161/HYPERTENSIONAHA.111.00095

Safety of Renal Denervation

15

Costas Thomopoulos, Alexandros Kasiakogias, Ioannis Kallikazaros, and Costas Tsioufis

Abbreviations

BP	Blood pressure
CT	Computed tomography
dRHT	Drug-resistant hypertension
eGFR	Estimated glomerular filtration rate
HTN	Hypertension
MR	Magnetic resonance
OCT	Optical coherence tomography
RDN	Renal denervation

15.1 Introduction

Even though surgical splanchnicectomy was an effective procedure that reduced blood pressure (BP) in a substantial amount of patients with malignant hypertension (HTN), it was accompanied by significant side effects, the most prominent being postural hypotension. This is not the case for renal denervation (RDN) that is a focused and far less radical nerve ablation procedure. Indeed, it has been variably shown to be a safe treatment with rare periprocedural and longer-term side effects.

Safety data for RDN come from a few experimental studies, mostly uncontrolled safety (and efficacy) trials of the various RDN systems, some controlled studies and the

C. Thomopoulos, MD, PhD • A. Kasiakogias, MD, PhD • I. Kallikazaros, MD, PhD
First Cardiology Clinic, University of Athens, Hippokration Hospital, Athens, Greece

C. Tsioufis, MD, PhD (✉)
1st Cardiology Clinic, National and Kapodistrian University of Athens, Hippokration Hospital, Athens, Greece
e-mail: ktsioufis@gmail.com

C. Tsioufis et al. (eds.), *Interventional Therapies for Secondary and Essential Hypertension*, Updates in Hypertension and Cardiovascular Protection,
DOI 10.1007/978-3-319-34141-5_15

ever growing registries (Table 15.1). It is true that the greatest bulk of evidence comes from studies using the Symplicity catheter, yet current safety results seem comparable among different RDN systems. On the other hand, most trials have a duration of 6 months. Currently, only the Symplicity HTN-1 and two studies have reported a follow-up period of up to 3 years and unfortunately not on the respective entire initial cohorts.

Main safety endpoints in RDN studies may be classified in two categories: (a) peri-procedural events mainly represented by access site complications (e.g. haematomas and aneurysms) and renal events (e.g. renal artery dissection or perforation, renal artery embolism and infarction) and (b) longer-term events associated with development of symptomatic hypotension, hypertensive emergencies, deterioration of renal function or development of stenoses. Of note, an event inherent to the procedure is diffuse visceral pain during energy delivery that is easily managed with sedation and analgesia, while intraprocedural vagally mediated bradycardia is treated with atropine.

15.2 An Overview of Preclinical and Laboratory Data

In a preclinical study by Rippy MK et al., seven domestic swines underwent RDN with the Symplicity catheter system, while renal angiography was performed before, right after and 6 months after the procedure [7]. Histological examinations of the renal vessels as well as gross and microscopic examination of the kidneys and urinary system were also performed to assess for relevant abnormalities. Regarding renal nerve injury, principal findings were fibrosis, nerve fascicle replacement with fibrous connective tissue and modest thickening of the epineurium and perineurium. Other structural findings included fibrosis of up to 25 % of the total media and underlying adventitia, with mild rupture of the external elastic lamina and without changes on the smooth muscular layer. There were no angiographic or histological evidence of renal artery stenosis. The kidney and urinary bladder presented no device-related abnormalities.

In another study, Steigerwald K et al. treated seven domestic female pigs with RDN using the Symplicity catheter in order to elucidate morphological changes in the vessel wall [8]. The protocol included blood analyses, quantitative renal angiography, optical coherence tomography (OCT) imaging and histopathology including immunostaining for nerve fascicles and neovascularisation. No signs of kidney failure were identified. Acutely after RDN, circumscribed transmural injury far into the adventitia fatty tissue was noted. There was thrombus formation due to local loss of the endothelial monolayer as well as cellular swelling and connective tissue coagulation within the medial and adventitial layer reflected on local notches. Ten days after RDN, the luminar surface was re-endothelialised, but scar tissue formation of the media and transmural fibrosis, adventitial inflammation and reduction in nerve fascicle quantity and size were observed. The study raised the question whether acute yet local thrombus formation may lead to thrombotic closure of the artery as well as thrombotic embolisation. Focal scar formation could also predispose to renal artery aneurysm or dissection especially in atherosclerotic vessels. Nevertheless, both the Steigerwald K et al. and the Rippy MK et al. studies show that a partial return to normal anatomy may be expected at least 6 months post-RDN.

Table 15.1 Safety profile of renal denervation in major reports

	Symplicity HTN-1 [1]	Symplicity HTN-2 [2]	Symplicity HTN-3 [3]	EnligHTN 1 [4]	Reduce-HTN [5]	Global Symplicity Registry [6]
Number of centres, *n*	19	24	88	4	23	134
Number of patients at baseline, *n*	153	52	364	46	146	998
Number of patients for final safety analysis, *n*	88	70[a]	364	46	146	998 (718)
Device	Symplicity	Symplicity	Symplicity	EnligHTN	Vessix	Symplicity
Months of follow-up, *n*	36	36	6	24	6	6
Renal imaging, method for screening during follow-up	Duplex or CT or MRI	Duplex or CT or MRI	Duplex	Duplex (24 months) and CT (6 months)	Duplex	Not mandatory
Complications at insertion site, *n*	3	1	–	8	5	4
Periprocedural renal artery complication, *n*	1	1	–	12 (all vasospasms)	1	2
Hypotension, *n*	3	2	–	1	0	–
Hypertensive emergency, *n*	13	14	9	1	1	5
Renal artery stenosis >70 % or in need of stenting during follow-up, *n*	2	0	1	1	2	1
Significant worsening of renal function during follow-up, *n*	1	2	5	1	15	5
eGFR at baseline, ml/min/1.73 m^2	83.6 ± 19.7	77 ± 19	72.8 ± 15.7	84.7 ± 18	83.9 ± 24.1	76.2 (60–92)
eGFR at follow-up, ml/min/1.73 m^2	74.3 ± 28.0	77 ± 18	70.6 ± 17.4	76.4 ± 25.3	82.9 ± 23.7	74.4 (57–89)

Safety data are derived from the publications of the respective studies, are based on the respective methods of reporting and should not be used for comparisons among studies

A dash (–) denotes unavailable exact data in the manuscripts

eGFR estimated glomerular filtration rate

[a]Total number of patients including the crossover group

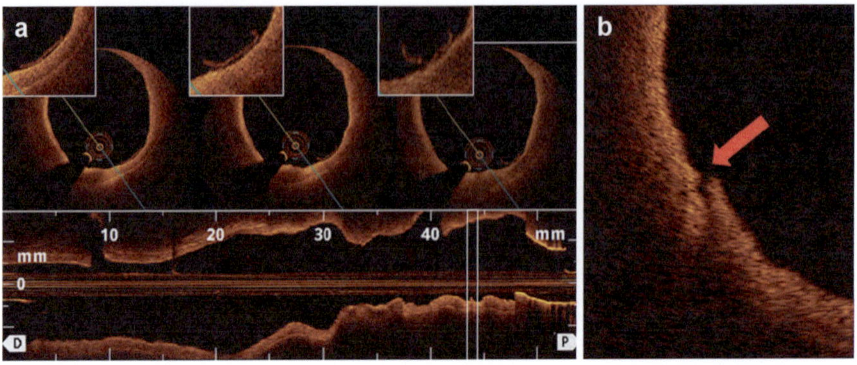

Fig. 15.1 Dissections after RDN as shown by optical coherence tomography. Endothelial detachments (**a**, *white box*) and vessel wall dissections (**b**, *red arrow*) (Reproduced from Templin et al. [9])

In order to better understand the renal vascular changes of RDN in humans, Templin C et al. studied using OCT the renal arteries of 16 patients with drug-resistant hypertension (dRHT) on single antiplatelet therapy that underwent the procedure with the use of either the Symplicity or the EnligHTN catheter [9]. Endothelial-intimal oedema was found in 96 % of cases after RDN, and thrombus formation (more prevalent with the EnligHTN catheter) was a frequent finding. Other findings included diffuse renal artery spasm, as well as an arterial dissection with the Symplicity catheter and endothelial and intimal disruptions with the EnligHTN catheter (Fig. 15.1). Also, a "pearl-of-string" pattern identified with OCT was attributed to the mechanical stress by the ablation catheter. Overall, such findings may not have a clear clinical relevance but signify the need for use of antiplatelet therapy in patients undergoing the procedure.

It has been proposed that endovascular ultrasound-based RDN combined with a cooling balloon preserves the integrity of the arterial wall while providing effective ablation. In an experimental study, ten normotensive pigs underwent RDN with the use of the Paradise system [10]. Acutely, renal artery staining showed viable tissue consistent with preservation of the arterial medial layer. Histology showed no endothelial injury and minimal to no injury to the media of the renal arterial wall at seven days. Renal nerves were ablated circumferentially, and there was a significant reduction in kidney norepinephrine.

15.3 Safety Data from Principal Trials

15.3.1 The Symplicity HTN-1 and HTN-2 Studies

In the proof-of-principle uncontrolled Symplicity HTN-1 trial, the safety evaluation protocol included physical examination, basic blood chemistry and anatomic assessment of renal vasculature by renal angiography before, immediately after and 14–30 days (in 18 patients) after the procedure and magnetic resonance (MR) angiography 6 months after the procedure (in 14 patients) [11]. Angiography showed focal renal artery irregularities right after radiofrequency energy delivery that were attributed to minor spasm or oedema and were not flow-limiting. One out of the 45 patients had renal dissection upon placement of the catheter and thus needed stenting, while another had a pseudoaneurysm treated with antibiotics and analgesics. Short-term angiograms and 6-month MR angiograms did not show any irregularities at the sites of treatment. Renal function, available in 25 patients at both baseline and the 6-month follow-up, was stable.

In the 153 patients that were included in the extended Symplicity HTN-1 registry, a total of three patients all treated with an 8F guide developed a pseudoaneurysm that was managed conservatively [12]. Renal artery imaging with MR angiography, computed tomographic (CT) angiography or duplex at 6 months (in 81 patients) did not show any new stenosis, but there was one case of progression of a pre-existing proximal stenosis away from the energy application sites that was successfully stented. Other events included flank pain, transient dizziness and pitting oedema as well as two deaths considered unrelated to the procedure. The final 3-year report of the study, on 88 patients, documented a new 80 % stenosis of the right renal artery in need of stenting at 24 months, as well as in total 4 hypotensive episodes, 13 hypertensive episodes and 3 deaths [1]. The estimated glomerular filtration rate (eGFR) decreased from 83.6 ml/min/m^2 at baseline to 74.3 ml/min/m^2 at 36 months.

In the randomised Symplicity HTN-2 trial on 106 patients, apart from laboratory tests (serum creatinine, cystatin C, urine albumin), the protocol included imaging of kidneys at baseline and 6 months, mainly by renal duplex ultrasound and if needed by CT or MR angiography [13]. Safety endpoints included a reduction of eGFR > 25 % or new stenosis >60 % confirmed by angiogram at 6 months and a composite cardiovascular endpoint. Only minor periprocedural events were noted including one pseudoaneurysm, one case of symptomatic hypotension in need of reduction of drugs, one urinary tract infection (UTI), a case of paraesthesia and a case of back pain that were resolved after 1 month. Seven patients had intraprocedural bradycardia requiring atropine. At 6 months, imaging in 43 patients (of which by CT/MR angiography in ten patients) showed a possible progression of a previous atherosclerotic lesion not located at an ablation site, which required no intervention. After the initial 6-month follow-up, a renal artery dissection prior to catheter insertion requiring stenting was noted in the crossover group. Up to 1 year, there were a total of nine hypertensive events and two hypotensive events requiring hospitalisation [14]. Between 12 and 36 months of follow-up and out of a total of 70 patients that underwent RDN, there were only a few hypertensive and hypotensive events as well as three deaths unrelated to the procedure [2]. Renal function was stable in both intervention and control groups at 6 months and no change in mean eGFR was recorded at the 36-month follow-up.

15.3.2 The Symplicity HTN-3 Study

In the first single-blind, randomised sham-controlled study of the efficacy and safety of RDN using the Symplicity catheter in 535 patients with dRHT (with increased cardiovascular risk compared to the previous Symplicity trials), the primary safety endpoint was a composite of major events (set as death from any cause, end-stage renal disease, an embolic event resulting in end-organ damage, renal artery or other vascular complications or hypertensive crisis within 30 days or new renal artery stenosis of more than 70 % within 6 months) [3]. The overall number of adverse events was very low, and no significant differences were noted between groups. Rates of major adverse events did not significantly differ between the denervation group (1.4 %) and the control group (0.6 %). The documented access path complication rate of 0.3 % was rather low and may be attributed to the special care used for study patients. In clinical routine, an average complication rate would be expected to be at about 1.3 % [15]. Kidney function did not differ between groups at any time point. Regarding an increase in creatinine by 50 % compared to baseline, it was observed in 5 cases out of 352 (1.4 %) in the RDN group and in 1 case out of 171 (0.6 %) in the control group.

15.3.3 The EnligHTN I Study

The prospective multicentre EnligHTN I trial was the first-in-human trial that assessed the safety of the multielectrode EnligHTN catheter on 46 patients with dRHT [4]. An independent Clinical Event Committee adjudicated all adverse effects. Renal function was followed with eGFR, cystatin C and urine albumin excretion. Renal artery anatomy was assessed with duplex ultrasonography and CT angiography. The first report did not document any serious vascular access site or renal artery vascular adverse events during the procedure (i.e. renal artery dissections, aneurysms or significant vasospasm). Minor periprocedural events were rare, resolved without further sequelae and included non-flow-limiting vasospasms, vascular access site haematomas, hypotension and vasovagal episodes, bradycardia, transient haematuria, pain and nausea. Computed tomographic angiography at 6 months showed asymptomatic worsening of pre-existing renal artery stenosis in two patients. In one subject, the stenotic lesion progressed to 75 % at about 10 months and was treated with stent implantation [16]. Yet, at the 18-month follow-up and with a poor BP response, a new angiogram was performed revealing a new stenotic lesion of 70 % extending from the distal part of the stent that was again treated with a new stent. Up to 24 months of follow-up, a trend for a decrease in renal function was observed with eGFR decreasing from 84.7 ml/min/m^2 at baseline to 76.4 ml/min/m^2 at 2 years [17]. However, albumin to creatinine ratio showed a favourable decrease during follow-up.

15.3.4 The RAPID Study

The RAPID trial enrolled 50 patients and was a safety and efficacy study of the now debunk OneShot balloon RDN system that was suggested to have a favourable profile with respect to vasospasm, oedema or intraluminal thrombus formation [18]. With respect to acute procedural safety, there were no serious adverse events related to groin and vascular access complications or renal artery injury. Up to 12 months, three events were reported, namely, infection at access site due to use of a closure device, paraesthesia of the right groin and renal artery stenosis. Imaging at 6 months revealed a non-haemodynamically significant stenosis of the left renal artery that was within the treatment area.

15.3.5 The REDUCE-HTN Study

In the REDUCE-HTN study, 146 patients with dRHT underwent RDN by the Vessix balloon multielectrode bipolar catheter [5]. Kidney function was monitored with eGFR and kidney anatomy with renal ultrasound (in 123 patients) at 6 months. Only a mild procedural vessel dissection was reported. Within the first month, the few serious events that were recorded and resolved included two access site infections, one access site pseudoaneurysm, one femoral artery thrombus and one haematoma. Within 6 months, there was one case of hypertensive emergency and no cases of orthostatic hypotension. Mean eGFR remained stable at 6 months, but there were 15 cases of eGFR reduction >25 %, two of which presenting as medication-related acute renal failure. Imaging revealed progression to more than 60 % of pre-existing mild renal artery stenosis in four patients.

15.4 Safety Data from Registries and Meta-analyses

In an initial report of the real-world ALSTER BP registry of 93 patients that underwent RDN with the Symplicity catheter, renal function was stable during the 6-month follow-up [19]. One renal artery dissection prior to insertion of the ablation catheter was recorded. There was one case of a small kidney infarct potentially associated with a thrombus at the ablation sites, even though the patient was on dual antiplatelet therapy.

The single-centre Heidelberg registry followed for 12 months a total of 63 patients that underwent RDN with the Symplicity catheter [20]. The registry included patients with fibromuscular dysplasia, unilateral renal artery stenting and single kidneys. Three patients presented vascular access complications (two aneurysms and one acute arterial occlusion due to use of a closure device requiring surgery). Renal function remained stable during follow-up. Renal duplex available in 15 patients at 6 months did not show any significant pathology.

In the open-label, multicentre Global SYMPLICITY Registry, data for the first 1,000 enrolled patients at 6 months are available [6]. Even though underreporting of adverse events may have been possible, there were only six periprocedural adverse events related to the procedure, including four vascular access site complications (0.34 %) and two renal artery dissections that were stented. Other events included five hospitalisations for hypertensive emergency (0.5 %), six for atrial fibrillation (0.6 %), seven strokes (0.7 %), four hospitalisations for new onset heart failure (0.4 %), seven myocardial infarctions (0.7 %) and two cases of new onset end-stage kidney disease (0.2 %) that were considered unrelated to the procedure.

A systematic review of 12 studies of RDN with five different catheters on 506 patients reported a total of five procedural complications (<1 %) including one renal artery dissection and four pseudoaneurysms at the site of arterial puncture (all from the initial Symplicity registry) [21]. In another meta-analysis of nine studies on 1096 patients, adverse events were rare and were represented mainly by femoral access site complications, while renal function was preserved during the respective follow-ups [22]. In a recent meta-analysis by the European Network Coordinating Research on Renal Denervation (ENCOReD) Consortium of seven randomised trials of RDN with the Symplicity catheter, a total of 985 patients were studied that had been randomised to either RDN ($n=588$) or control ($n=397$) [23]. Major adverse events were documented in 56 RDN patients and 29 controls (9.9 % and 7.4 %, respectively, $p=0.20$). The pooled estimate of renal function assessed with eGFR over 6 months did not differ between groups.

15.5 Special Issues

15.5.1 Autonomic Dysfunction

Data collected so far show that a disturbance of the normal autonomic balance may have been an issue for surgical denervation but not for RDN. Intraprocedural bradycardia may be considered only as an acute effect of RDN, since regulation of BP as well as chronotropic competence is well preserved after the procedure. Furthermore, cases of impressive BP decreases have been reported by most investigators, yet no concern has risen regarding any debilitating effect that would not resolve with a decrease in drugs. Similarly, orthostatic hypotension has been a rather rare adverse event of RDN as documented in various patient series. This subject has been specifically studied in 36 patients that underwent tilt-table testing before and 3 months after RDN [24]. Change in systolic BP and heart rate after tilting as well as total number of (pre-) syncope was not influenced by the procedure. Nevertheless, it is unclear whether the irreversible denervation of kidneys may affect circulatory homeostasis in cases of extreme stress or in patients with, e.g. diabetes-induced autonomic neuropathy.

15.5.2 Renal Artery Stenosis

It has been feared that application of radiofrequency thermal energy may cause structural damage and subsequently renal artery stenosis, similar to what was seen in pulmonary vein ablation [25] and currently remains a concern among experts. In the various cohorts, renal artery stenosis has been unequivocally a rare complication (<5 %). However, assessment of renal artery anatomy has varied widely in terms of standardisation and frequency (especially after the 6-month follow-up), and imaging of renal arteries during follow-up has ranged from the simple Doppler ultrasound to the more sensitive and specific CT and MR scans. In any case, slowly developing changes in vascular wall morphology are hard to detect. In a study by Lambert T et al., incidence of significant renal artery stenosis 6 months after RDN with the Symplicity catheter was assessed in 76 patients via MR (87 %) or CT (13 %) angiography [26]. In this series, there were only two cases of new nonsignificant stenosis.

A series of case reports have documented the development of unilateral or bilateral significant renal artery stenosis, mostly in patients with a high atherosclerotic risk [27–38]. These events were documented as early as 2 months and as late as 2 years after RDN and usually associated with a relapse of high BP or deterioration of renal function or repeated pulmonary oedemas. The proposed mechanisms include radiofrequency energy-induced tissue injury, cell proliferation, neointimal stenotic lesions and fibrosis. Less likely causes are catheter-induced mechanical injury or a new atherosclerotic lesion. It has been proposed that an abnormal vascular response after application of energy such as a transient spasm may itself predict late arterial disease [39]. Accordingly, it has been speculated that in patients with atheromatous plaques or calcifications of renal arteries, delivery of energy near a diseased vessel may trigger an augmented tissue response and damage, and this is particularly relevant for cases of worsening of pre-existing stenosis.

The extent of vascular damage may be affected by a series of factors including catheter design, use of an irrigation system, applied temperature and sites of ablation. It is still unclear which RDN system would be associated with smaller renal artery damage. A study investigated the anatomical impact of balloon-based systems (Paradise, OneShot and Vessix) compared to nonballoon-based systems (Symplicity and EnligHTN) in 25 patients with dRHT with angiography, intravascular ultrasound and OCT [40]. Vascular injury in the form of dissection, thrombus or oedema and of a varying extent was observed with all systems. Balloon-based RDN was associated with greater longitudinal extent of dissection, while nonballoon-based RDN was associated with greater thrombus area. Acutely, a significant reduction in lumen size was observed only in nonballoon RDN. By OCT, dissection was seen in 14 arteries (32.6 %), and frames with dissection were higher in balloon-based systems, in which dissections were associated with a higher balloon/artery ratio, thus underlining the importance of careful balloon size selection.

Interestingly, there have been a few reports of RDN in patients that had previously undergone renal artery stenting [41–44]. Energy was preferred to be delivered 5 mm distally to the placed stent, and the authors reported significant BP reductions and preserved renal anatomy (assessed by renal duplex) and renal function as late as 24 months post-procedure. A preclinical study in porcine models with renal stents did not document thrombus formation or histological changes in the kidneys but clarified that ablation within the stent, unlike distally to the stent, does not produce significant nerve ablation [44].

Current contraindications for RDN include previous renal artery interventions and renal artery stenosis > 50 %, while energy delivery on atherosclerotic lesions should be avoided. The few reports that incriminate RDN for development of renal artery stenosis underline the importance of careful documentation of such events in RDN studies and running registries. A careful selection of the correct RDN catheter size (at least in the case of balloon-based devices) and the use of antiplatelet therapy to limit the risk of dissection and thrombus formation respectively are advised.

15.5.3 Kidney Function

Development of acute or chronic renal damage has been one of the initial concerns regarding RDN, as a potential result of loss of autoregulatory mechanisms [45]. Accordingly, even though kidney disease is typically associated with sympathetic overactivity, patients with significant chronic kidney disease (eGFR < 45 ml/min/m^2) have traditionally been excluded from RDN trials. However, in practically all studies, RDN has not been associated with significant deterioration of kidney function either acutely or in the mid- to long-term, at least, well beyond what is expected in patients of high cardiovascular risk by definition and with the progression of age. It is thus considered reassuring that overall a relatively stable renal function during follow-up has been documented in uncontrolled studies and registries as well as controlled studies.

The effect of RDN on renal function has been specifically investigated in 100 patients (88 of which underwent RDN with the Symplicity catheter and 12 served as controls) via blood chemistry, urine albumin and renal duplex ultrasound [46]. Mean eGFR and cystatin C remained unchanged during a 6-month follow-up, but the number of patients with microalbuminuria or macroalbuminuria decreased. Renal resistive index was also stably reduced at the 3-month and 6-month follow-up visits. In another study of 62 patients, who underwent RDN, there were no changes in the early biomarker neutrophil gelatinase-associated lipocalin and kidney injury molecule over the first 48 h or at a 3-month follow-up [47]. The eGFR and creatinine levels did not significantly change as well, and this was also observed in eight patients that had an eGFR of <45 ml/min/m^2.

On the other hand, in the 36-month report of the Symplicity HTN-1 registry, eGFR was shown to have decreased by 9.3 ml/min/1.73 m^2, significantly more compared to other hypertension trials that included patients of high cardiovascular risk. Albeit smaller decrease in eGFR was shown in the 24-month report of the EnligHTN 1 trial. This decrease in eGFR as well as the recording of a few cases with more than a 25 % drop in renal function among trials may have been due to chronically uncontrolled HTN and the use of drugs such as diuretics, renin-angiotensin inhibitors and aldosterone antagonists. Again, careful long-term observation of patients undergoing RDN in large registries will provide a clearer picture of renal behaviour.

References

1. Krum H, Schlaich MP, Sobotka PA, Böhm M, Mahfoud F, Rocha-Singh K et al (2014) Percutaneous renal denervation in patients with treatment-resistant hypertension: final 3-year report of the Symplicity HTN-1 study. Lancet 383:622–629
2. Esler MD, Böhm M, Sievert H, Rump CL, Schmieder RE, Krum H et al (2014) Catheter-based renal denervation for treatment of patients with treatment-resistant hypertension: 36 month results from the SYMPLICITY HTN-2 randomized clinical trial. Eur Heart J 35:1752–1759
3. Bhatt DL, Kandzari DE, O'Neill WW, D'Agostino R, Flack JM, Katzen BT et al (2014) A controlled trial of renal denervation for resistant hypertension. N Engl J Med 370: 1393–1401

4. Worthley SG, Tsioufis CP, Worthley MI, Sinhal A, Chew DP, Meredith IT et al (2013) Safety and efficacy of a multi-electrode renal sympathetic denervation system in resistant hypertension: the EnligHTN I trial. Eur Heart J 34:2132–2140
5. Sievert H, Schofer J, Ormiston J, Hoppe UC, Meredith IT, Walters DL et al (2015) Renal denervation with a percutaneous bipolar radiofrequency balloon catheter in patients with resistant hypertension: 6-month results from the REDUCE-HTN clinical study. EuroIntervention 10:1213–1220
6. Böhm M, Mahfoud F, Ukena C, Hoppe UC, Narkiewicz K, Negoita M, et al; GSR Investigators (2015) First report of the Global SYMPLICITY Registry on the effect of renal artery denervation in patients with uncontrolled hypertension. Hypertension 65:766–774
7. Rippy MK, Zarins D, Barman NC, Wu A, Duncan KL, Zarins CK (2011) Catheter-based renal sympathetic denervation: chronic preclinical evidence for renal artery safety. Clin Res Cardiol 100:1095–1101
8. Steigerwald K, Titova A, Malle C, Kennerknecht E, Jilek C, Hausleiter J et al (2012) Morphological assessment of renal arteries after radiofrequency catheter-based sympathetic denervation in a porcine model. J Hypertens 30:2230–2239
9. Templin C, Jaguszewski M, Ghadri JR, Sudano I, Gaehwiler R, Hellermann JP et al (2013) Vascular lesions induced by renal nerve ablation as assessed by optical coherence tomography: pre- and post-procedural comparison with the Simplicity catheter system and the EnligHTN multi-electrode renal denervation catheter. Eur Heart J 34:2141–2148, 2148b
10. Pathak A, Coleman L, Roth A, Stanley J, Bailey L, Markham P et al (2015) Renal sympathetic nerve denervation using intraluminal ultrasound within a cooling balloon preserves the arterial wall and reduces sympathetic nerve activity. EuroIntervention 11:477–484
11. Krum H, Schlaich M, Whitbourn R, Sobotka PA, Sadowski J, Bartus K et al (2009) Catheter-based renal sympathetic denervation for resistant hypertension: a multicentre safety and proof-of-principle cohort study. Lancet 373:1275–1281
12. Symplicity HTN-1 Investigators (2011) Catheter-based renal sympathetic denervation for resistant hypertension: durability of blood pressure reduction out to 24 months. Hypertension 57:911–917
13. Esler MD, Krum H, Sobotka PA, Schlaich MP, Schmieder RE, Böhm M (2010) Renal sympathetic denervation in patients with treatment-resistant hypertension (The Symplicity HTN-2 Trial): a randomised controlled trial. Lancet 376:1903–1909
14. Esler MD, Krum H, Schlaich M, Schmieder RE, Böhm M, Sobotka PA, Symplicity HTN-2 Investigators (2012) Renal sympathetic denervation for treatment of drug-resistant hypertension: one-year results from the Symplicity HTN-2 randomized, controlled trial. Circulation 126:2976–2982
15. Applegate RJ, Sacrinty MT, Kutcher MA, Kahl FR, Gandhi SK, Santos RM et al (2008) Trends in vascular complications after diagnostic cardiac catheterization and percutaneous coronary intervention via the femoral artery, 1998 to 2007. J Am Coll Cardiol Intv 1:317–326
16. Papademetriou V, Tsioufis CP, Sinhal A, Chew DP, Meredith IT, Malaiapan Y et al (2014) Catheter-based renal denervation for resistant hypertension: 12-month results of the EnligHTN I first-in-human study using a multielectrode ablation system. Hypertension 64:565–572
17. Tsioufis CP, Papademetriou V, Dimitriadis KS, Kasiakogias A, Tsiachris D, Worthley MI et al (2015) Catheter-based renal denervation for resistant hypertension: twenty-four month results of the EnligHTN I first-in-human study using a multi-electrode ablation system. Int J Cardiol 201:345–350
18. Verheye S, Ormiston J, Bergmann MW, Sievert H, Schwindt A, Werner N et al (2015) Twelve-month results of the rapid renal sympathetic denervation for resistant hypertension using the OneShotTM ablation system (RAPID) study. EuroIntervention 10:1221–1229
19. Kaiser L, Beister T, Wiese A, von Wedel J, Meincke F, Kreidel F et al (2014) Results of the ALSTER BP real-world registry on renal denervation employing the Symplicity system. EuroIntervention 10:157–165
20. Vogel B, Kirchberger M, Zeier M, Stoll F, Meder B, Saure D et al (2014) Renal sympathetic denervation therapy in the real world: results from the Heidelberg registry. Clin Res Cardiol 103:117–124

21. Davis MI, Filion KB, Zhang D, Eisenberg MJ, Afilalo J, Schiffrin EL et al (2013) Effectiveness of renal denervation therapy for resistant hypertension: a systematic review and meta-analysis. J Am Coll Cardiol 62:231–241
22. Sun D, Li C, Li M, Liu J, Wen S (2015) Renal denervation vs pharmacotherapy for resistant hypertension: a meta-analysis. J Clin Hypertens (Greenwich). doi:10.1111/jch.12742
23. FadlElmula FE, Jin Y, Yang WY, Thijs L, Lu YC, Larstorp AC, Persu A, et al; European Network Coordinating Research On Renal Denervation (ENCOReD) Consortium (2015) Meta-analysis of randomized controlled trials of renal denervation in treatment-resistant hypertension. Blood Press 24:263–274
24. Lenski M, Mahfoud F, Razouk A, Ukena C, Lenski D, Barth C et al (2013) Orthostatic function after renal sympathetic denervation in patients with resistant hypertension. Int J Cardiol 169:418–424
25. Cappato R, Calkins H, Chen SA, Davies W, Iesaka Y, Kalman J et al (2005) Worldwide survey on the methods, efficacy, and safety of catheter ablation for human atrial fibrillation. Circulation 111:1100–1105
26. Lambert T, Nahler A, Reiter C, Schwarz S, Gammer V, Blessberger H et al (2015) Frequency of renal artery stenosis after renal denervation in patients with resistant arterial hypertension. Am J Cardiol 115:1545–1548
27. Vonend O, Antoch G, Rump LC, Blondin D (2012) Secondary rise in blood pressure after renal denervation. Lancet 380:778
28. Kaltenbach B, Id D, Franke JC, Sievert H, Hennersdorf M, Maier J et al (2012) Renal artery stenosis after renal sympathetic denervation. J Am Coll Cardiol 60:2694–2695
29. Cordeanu ME, Gaertner S, Bronner F, Jahn C, Prinz E, Hannedouche T et al (2014) Neointimal thickening resulting in artery stenosis following renal sympathetic denervation. Int J Cardiol 177:e117–e119
30. Versaci F, Trivisonno A, Olivieri C, Caranci F, Brunese L, Prati F (2014) Late renal artery stenosis after renal denervation: is it the tip of the iceberg? Int J Cardiol 172:e507–e508
31. JaénÁguila F, Mediavilla Garcia JD, Navarro EM, Vargas Hitos JA, Fernandez-Torres C (2014) Bilateral renal artery stenosis after renal denervation. Hypertension 63:e126–e127
32. Chandra AP, Marron CD, Puckridge P, Spark JI (2015) Severe bilateral renal artery stenosis after transluminal radiofrequency ablation of renal sympathetic nerve plexus. J Vasc Surg 62:222–225
33. Bacaksiz A, Uyarel H, Jafarov P, Kucukbuzcu S (2014) Iatrogenic renal artery stenosis after renal sympathetic denervation. Int J Cardiol 172:e389–e390
34. Bhamra-Ariza P, Rao S, Muller DW (2014) Renal artery stenosis following renal percutaneous denervation. Catheter Cardiovasc Interv 84:1180–1183
35. Pucci G, Battista F, Lazzari L, Dominici M, Boschetti E, Schillaci G (2014) Progression of renal artery stenosis after renal denervation. Impact on 24-hour blood pressure. Circ J 78:767–768
36. Raman B, Pathik B, Bridgman C (2014) Recurrent pulmonary oedema after percutaneous radiofrequency renal denervation. Int J Cardiol 174:e42–e43
37. Celik IE, Acar B, Kurtul A, Murat SN (2015) De novo renal artery stenosis after renal sympathetic denervation. J Clin Hypertens (Greenwich) 17:242–243
38. Koppelstaetter C, Kerschbaum J, Lenzhofer M, Glodny B, Esterhammer R, Frick M et al (2015) Distal renal artery stenosis after percutaneous renal denervation leading to renal impairment but normotension. J Clin Hypertens (Greenwich) 17:162–164
39. Versaci F, Trivisonno A, Olivieri C, Magri G, Caranci F, Prati F (2014) Is an abnormal vascular response after renal sympathetic denervation predictive of permanent damage? An unusual case of late renal artery stenosis after energy delivery. J Endovasc Ther 21:191–196
40. Karanasos A, Van Mieghem N, Bergmann MW, Hartman E, Ligthart J, van der Heide E et al (2015) Multimodality intra-arterial imaging assessment of the vascular trauma induced by balloon-based and nonballoon-based renal denervation systems. Circ Cardiovasc Interv 8(7):e002474

41. Ziegler AK, Franke J, Bertog SC (2013) Renal denervation in a patient with prior renal artery stenting. Catheter Cardiovasc Interv 81:342–345
42. Berra E, Rabbia F, Rossato D, Covella M, Totaro S, Chiara F et al (2014) Renal sympathetic denervation in a previously stented renal artery. J Clin Hypertens (Greenwich) 16:238–239
43. Bausback Y, Friedenberger J, Hertting K, Werner M, Branzan D, Freitas B et al (2014) Renal denervation for hypertension refractory to renal artery stenting. J Endovasc Ther 21:181–190
44. Mahfoud F, Tunev S, Ruwart J, Schulz-Jander D, Cremers B, Linz D et al (2014) Efficacy and safety of catheter-based radiofrequency renal denervation in stented renal arteries. Circ Cardiovasc Interv 7:813–820
45. Petidis K, Anyfanti P, Doumas M (2011) Renal sympathetic denervation: renal function concerns. Hypertension 58(4):e19
46. Dörr O, Liebetrau C, Möllmann H, Achenbach S, Sedding D, Szardien S et al (2013) Renal sympathetic denervation does not aggravate functional or structural renal damage. J Am Coll Cardiol 61:479–480
47. Mahfoud F, Cremers B, Janker J, Link B, Vonend O, Ukena C et al (2012) Renal hemodynamics and renal function after catheter-based renal sympathetic denervation in patients with resistant hypertension. Hypertension 60:419–424

Efficacy of Renal Denervation on Blood Pressure Reduction

16

Costas Tsioufis and Dimitrios Tousoulis

Abbreviations

BP	Blood pressure
dRHTN	Drug-resistant HTN
HTN	Hypertension
RDN	Renal denervation
SHR	Spontaneously hypertensive rats
SNS	Sympathetic nervous system
SSAHT	Standardized stepped-care antihypertensive treatment

16.1 Introduction

The modulation of the increased sympathetic nervous system (SNS) activity for the treatment of high blood pressure (BP) was applied at the first half of the twentieth century for the management of malignant hypertension (HTN), a disease with a 5-year mortality rate in over 50 % of cases [1]. Surgical sympathectomy, called thoracolumbar splanchnicectomy, was effective not only in reducing high BP (with a meaningful BP reduction in about two-thirds of patients undergoing the procedure) but also in reversing target organ damage and reducing mortality. The use of surgical sympathectomy was abandoned during the second half of the twentieth century, not only due to significant perioperative mortality (3–5 %) and operation-associated adverse effects but also due to the development of several antihypertensive drugs

C. Tsioufis (✉) • D. Tousoulis
1st Cardiology Clinic, National and Kapodistrian University of Athens, Hippokration Hospital, Athens, Greece
e-mail: ktsioufis@gmail.com

C. Tsioufis et al. (eds.), *Interventional Therapies for Secondary and Essential Hypertension*, Updates in Hypertension and Cardiovascular Protection,
DOI 10.1007/978-3-319-34141-5_16

that were effective in reducing high BP in the majority of patients along with a favorable safety profile with fewer and better tolerated adverse events.

The well-established reciprocal relationship between the HTN, the kidneys, and the SNS activity was matched with recent technologic advancements permitting the transcatheter injury of renal sympathetic fibers, in an attempt to better address an unmet need in the management of patients with drug-resistant HTN (dRHTN) [2–6]. The latter is defined as the failure to achieve BP control despite the use of three or more antihypertensive drugs, including a diuretic, in maximal tolerated doses [6]. Observational and randomized trials, including the sham-controlled HTN-3 trial, proved that renal denervation (RDN) is a safe procedure, but its efficacy in BP control in patients with dRHTN is still debatable [4, 7–14]. The present chapter firstly provides a short overview of all RDN trials (preclinical studies, early observational clinical studies, randomized trials with control group and blinded studies with sham ablation arm, and registries) and secondly highlights the potential reasons explaining the discrepancy in the BP reduction post RDN as well as the current status of RDN.

16.2 Preclinical Data

In various experimental forms of HTN (Table 16.1), complete RDN (in the vast majority of cases, the technique employed produced a combined surgical-pharmacological disruption of the entire renal nerve population, both afferent and efferent) delays the development of HTN or attenuates the magnitude of the increase of BP [2, 15]. In several of the models, the effect of complete RDN in hypertensive process was associated with changes in renal function characteristic of decreases in efferent renal sympathetic nerve activity. For example, in spontaneously hypertensive rats (SHR), the effect of complete RDN to delay the development of the HTN was associated with an increase in the fraction of the ingested sodium excreted in the urine (denervation natriuresis, more negative sodium balance), and the subsequent development of the HTN was paralleled by a return of renal tissue norepinephrine content toward normal (evidence of renal reinnervation) and a decrease in the fraction of the ingested sodium excreted in the urine (more positive sodium balance) [2]. This effect of complete RDN to ameliorate HTN is not due to afferent RDN as

Table 16.1 Main models of experimental hypertension in which renal denervation prevents or delays the development of hypertension

Spontaneously hypertensive rat
New Zealand spontaneously hypertensive rat
Goldblatt, one kidney, one clip (rat)
Goldblatt, two kidneys, one clip (rat)
Aortic coarctation (dog)
Aortic nerve transection (rat)
DOCA-NaCl (rat)
DOCA (pig)
Obesity hypertension (dog)

selective afferent denervation by dorsal rhizotomy (T_8-L_1) had no effect on the development of HTN in SHR. In the dog obesity model of hypertension, prior RDN profoundly decreased the magnitude of the subsequent HTN (an approximate 80 % reduction in the BP rise) in association with large decrease in sodium retention (an approximate 45 % reduction). Despite the above uniform effect of complete RDN on the development of HTN in such a diverse group of experimental forms of hypertension, it should be noted that RDN does not affect the development of HTN in the Dahl NaCl-sensitive rat or in the canine HTN induced by chronic NOS inhibition [2]. Additionally, the issue of whether the effect of complete RDN is mediated by interruption of afferent or efferent renal nerve activity has been studied by more direct techniques involving selective interruption in the afferent renal pathways. Thoracolumbar dorsal rhizotomy to produce selective afferent RDN attenuated the severity of hypertension in rats with one-kidney, one-clip, and two-kidney one-clip Goldblatt hypertension and in dogs with chronic aortic coarctation HTN but not in SHR. With the use of intrathecal capsaicin administration to deplete substance P and calcitonin gene-related peptide from primary afferent neurons in the dorsal horn of the thoracolumbar spinal cord, the HTN of Goldblatt one-kidney, one-wrap rats was enhanced, while that of DOCA NaCl rats was unaffected. The effect of selective afferent RDN is mediated by a central feedback mechanism involving a reduction in hypothalamic norepinephrine stores that results in a decrease in peripheral SNS activity, thereby reducing BP. These results indicate that afferent renal nerves are important modulators of central integrative centers involved in the regulation of the peripheral SNS activity contributing to HTN. Renorenal reflexes, which are mediated by both renal mechanoreceptors and chemoreceptors with contribution in the coordination of renal excretory activity between the two kidneys, are abnormal in SHR. This abnormality is related to the effect of arterial pressure on the kidney, since the abnormality is not present in young hypertensive SHR or in treated SHR who are normotensive.

16.3 Proof-of-Concept Studies

The first RDN proof-of-concept and safety study (Symplicity 1), published in 2009 in *The Lancet* included 45 patients with severe dRHTN (i.e., systolic office BP>160 mmHg, three antihypertensive drugs including one diuretic) who underwent bilateral RDN with the use of a single-electrode radiofrequency ablation catheter inserted through the femoral artery (Symplicity flex), while five patients with inappropriate renal artery anatomy for RDN served as controls (Table 16.2) [4]. Blood pressure was gradually and impressively reduced during the follow-up period of the study, reaching a 27/17 mmHg drop at 1-year post-procedure, while no serious safety issues came up. In a small subset of ten patients, renal noradrenaline spillover was reduced by 46 %, documenting that the procedure results in partial RDN. Although these results were uncontrolled and unblinded, and should have been assessed with caution, the study created a lot of enthusiasm. Many companies with different RDN ablation systems (either using radiofrequency or ultrasound or

Table 16.2 Published observational RDN studies: effects on blood pressure

	HTN-1	HTN-1	HTN-1	EnligHTN I	Reduce-HTN	Rapid trial
First author/year of publication (follow-up)	Krum [4]/2009/ (6 months)	Symplicity HTN Investigators [50]/2011/ (24 months)	Krum [16]/2013/ (36 months)	Worthley [7]/2013/ (6 months)/ Papademetriou [17]/2014/ (12 months) Tsioufis [18]/2015/ (24 months)	Sievert [8]/2015/ (6 months)	Verheye [11]/2015/ (6 months)
NCT	00483808, 00664638	00483808, 00664638	00483808, 00664638, 00753285	01438229	015411865	01520506
n	45	153	88	46	146	50
Age (years)	58 ± 9	57 ± 11	57 ± 11	60 ± 10	58 ± 10	63 ± 9.5
Office BP at baseline (mmHg)	177 ± 20/101 ± 15	176 ± 17/98 ± 15	175 ± 16/98 ± 14	176/96	182 ± 18/100 ± 14	181 ± 20/95 ± 15
Heart rate (bpm)	72 ± 11	NA	NA	71	72 ± 14	NA
Number of baseline antihypertensive medications	4.7 ± 1.5	5 ± 1.4	5 ± 1.7	4.1 ± 0.5	5.3 ± 1.9	5.1 ± 1.7
Changes in office SBP at 6/12/24/36 months (mmHg)	−22/NA/NA/NA	−25/−26/32/NA	−26/−27/−30/−32	−26/−27/−29/NA	−25/NA/NA/NA	−20/−22/NA/NA
Changes in office DBP at 6/12/24/36 months (mmHg)	−11/NA/NA/NA	−11/−14/14/NA	−11/−12/−13/−14	−10/−11/−13/NA	−10/NA/NA/NA	−8/−8/NA/NA
24-h BP at baseline (mmHg)	NA	NA	NA	150/83	153/87.5	154/87.7

Changes in 24-h SBP at 6/12/36 months (mmHg)	NA	NA	NA	−10/−7/−13/NA	−8.4/NA/NA/NA	−11/−9/NA/NA
Changes in 24-h DBP at 6/12/36 months(mmHg)	NA	NA	NA	−6/−4/−7/NA	−5.9/NA/NA/NA	−6/−5/NA/NA
RDN device	Symplicity	Symplicity	Symplicity	EnligHTN ™	Vessix system	OneShot™

NA not available

chemical ablation) planned new observational studies and called for randomized trials. Moreover, at 36 months post RDN, office BP fell further and the rate of controlled (<140 mmHg) or at least to some extent controlled patients (140–159 mmHg) nearly reached 50 and 85 %, respectively [16].

EnligHTN I was the first-in-human, prospective, multicenter study designed to assess the safety and efficacy of multielectrode radiofrequency ablation system (EnligHTN™) that can deliver lesions with a predetermined pattern in 46 patients with dRHTN [7]. Renal sympathetic denervation, using the EnligHTN™ multielectrode catheter, provided a rapid and significant office, ambulatory, and home BP reduction that was sustained through a follow-up period of 6, 12, and 24 months of the entire studied population of 46 patients with dRHTN [17, 18].

Few other studies (Reduce-HTN, RAPID) were able to confirm the BP-lowering effect of RDN (ranging between 20–30 mmHg systolic and 7–15 mmHg diastolic) in patients with dRHTN using different energy modalities and catheters [8, 11]. Overall, the inclusion and exclusion criteria as well as the results were in line with the abovementioned Symplicity trials.

16.4 Randomized Controlled Studies

Four randomized controlled RDN trials provided controversial results regarding the efficacy of RDN on BP reduction: two studies were in favor of RDN (HTN-2 and the DENER study) [9, 13], one study was neutral (the Prague-15) [10], and one study was negative (the Oslo study) [12] (Table 16.3).

In the first prospective, randomized clinical trial of RDN (*Symplicity* 2) also published in *The Lancet* only 1 year after Symplicity 1, 106 patients with dRHTN were randomly assigned either to RDN by using the Symplicity catheter (Medtronic) ($n=52$ patients) or continuation of previous administered antihypertensive medication ($n=54$ patients) [9]. At 6 months post RDN, the primary end point was met: office BP was significantly reduced by 32/12 mmHg, while there was no significant difference in the BP of the control group (change of only 1/0 mmHg). The percentage of responders, defined as a fall in systolic BP by 10 mmHg, was 85 % in the RDN group and 35 % in the controlled treated with medication. However, it was noted that the study was not blinded and not appropriately controlled, since no BP reduction was observed in the control group, which is highly unusual and subject to bias. Regarding the long-term follow-up data of Symplicity HTN-2, after 6 months, 37 control subjects crossed over to RDN, and 40 subjects from the original RDN group and 30 from the crossover group were followed up for 3 years. The systolic and diastolic BP reduction at 36 months for the initial RDN group was −33/−14 mmHg, starting from baseline BP 178/97 mmHg. In the crossover group, baseline BP increased throughout the first 6-month (waiting) period to 191/100 mmHg, but dropped by −33 mmHg at 36-month follow-up visit [19]. In summary, RDN resulted in a sustained lowering of BP during 3 years in a selected population of subjects with severe dRHTN without serious safety concerns (Table 16.4).

Table 16.3 Published randomized RDN controlled studies: effects on blood pressure

	HTN-2	OSLO RDN	Prague-15	DENERHTN
NCT	00888433	01673516	01560312	01570777
First author/year of publication	Esler [9]/2010	Elmula [12]/2014	Rosa [10]/2015	Azizi [13]/2015
Comparator (RDN vs. control)	RDN plus previous antihypertensive treatment vs. previous antihypertensive treatment	RDN plus previous antihypertensive treatment vs. clinically adjusted drug therapy by using the HOTMAN System	RDN plus optimal antihypertensive therapy vs. intensified pharmacological treatment including spironolactone (if tolerated and not contraindicated)	RDN plus an SSAHT vs. an SSAHT guided by home BP
Entire study population (n) (RDN vs. control)	106 (52 vs. 54)	19 (9 vs. 10)	106 (52 vs. 54)	106 (53 vs. 53)
Age (years)	58	60	58	55
Confirmation of dRHTN with ABPM	No	Yes	Yes	Yes
Number of antihypertensive medications at baseline (RDN vs. control)	5.2 vs. 5.3	5.1 vs. 5	5.1 vs. 5.4	The same SSAHT
Baseline office BP (mmHg) (RDN vs. control)	178/97 vs. 178/98	156/91 vs. 160/89	159/92 vs. 155/89	159/93 vs. 155/91
Baseline 24-h BP (mmHg) (RDN vs. control)	NA	151/89 vs. 149/85	149/86 vs. 147/84	151/90 vs. 146/88
Baseline daytime SBP (mmHg) (RDN vs. control)	NA	152 vs. 152	152 vs. 150	155 vs. 151
Changes in office SBP (mmHg) (RDN vs. control)	−32 vs. +1	−8 vs. −28	−12.4 vs. −14.3	−15.1 vs. −9.5
Δ in changes in office SBP between groups (mmHg) (RDN vs. control)	−33	+20	−5.8	−5.6
Changes in office diastolic BP (mmHg) (RDN vs. control)	−12 vs. 0	−2 vs. −11	−7 vs. −7	−9 vs. −6

(continued)

Table 16.3 (continued)

	HTN-2	OSLO RDN	Prague-15	DENERHTN
Changes in 24-h SBP (mmHg) (RDN vs. control)	−11/−3	−10/−21	−8.6 vs. −8.1	−15.4 vs. −9.5
Changes in 24-h DBP (mmHg) (RDN vs. control)	−7/−1	−7/−11	−6 vs. −5	−9.7 vs. −6.6
Δ in changes in 24-h SBP between groups (mmHg) (RDN vs. control)	−8	NA	−0.5 (NS)	−5.9
Changes in daytime SBP (mmHg) (RDN vs. control)	NA	−10 vs. −19	−9 vs. 9	−15.8 vs. −9.9
Δ in changes in daytime SBP between groups (mmHg) (RDN vs. control)	NA	9	1.9	−5.9
RDN device	Symplicity	Symplicity	Symplicity	Symplicity
Assessment of medication adherence	Diary	Investigator witnessed intake of their antihypertensive morning medications	Plasma drug concentrations	Morisky score plus drug concentration

SSAHT standardized stepped-care antihypertensive regimen, *NA* not available

Prague-15 study, a prospective, randomized, open-label multicenter trial, evaluated the efficacy of catheter-based RDN (Symplicity, Medtronic) ($n=52$) versus intensified pharmacological treatment including spironolactone (if tolerated) ($n=54$) in patients with dRHTN [10]. This was confirmed by 24-h ambulatory BP monitoring after excluding secondary HTN and confirmation of adherence to therapy by measurement of plasma antihypertensive drug levels before enrollment. Regarding the primary end point of the study, a significant reduction in 24-h average systolic BP after 6 months (−8.6mmHg; $p<0.001$ in RDN versus −8.1 mmHg $p=0.001$ in the pharmacological group) was observed, which was comparable in both groups. Similarly, a significant reduction in systolic office BP (−12.4 mmHg; $p<0.001$ in RDN versus −14.3 mmHg; $p<0.001$ in the pharmacological group) was observed. Between-group differences in change were not significant. Prague-15 showed that RDN is not superior to intensified pharmacotherapy in dRHTN in reducing BP but it is important to note that the average number of antihypertensive drugs used was significantly higher (+0.3 drugs; $p<0.001$) and the serum creatinine was significantly increased in the pharmacological group at 6 months post RDN.

Table 16.4 HTN-3 randomized, blind, and sham-controlled RDN studies: effects on blood pressure

	HTN-3	Symplicity flex
	RDN vs. sham arm	RDN vs. sham arm
NCT	01418261	01656096
First author/year of publication	Bhatt [14]/2014	Desch [23]/2015
n	364 vs. 171	35 vs. 36
Age (years)	57.9 vs. 56.2	64.5 vs. 57.4
Baseline office BP (mmHg)	180/97 vs. 180/99	NA
Baseline 24 h BP (mmHg)	159/88 vs. 160/91	140/78 vs. 140/81
Baseline daytime BP (mmHg)	163/91 vs. 164/94	144/80 vs. 143/82
Baseline nighttime BP (mmHg)	152/82 vs. 151/84	130/68 vs. 132/73
Baseline 24-h heart rate (bpm)	71/72	NA
Baseline number of medications	5.1 vs. 5.2	4.4 vs. 4.3
Changes in office SBP at 6 months (mmHg)	−14 vs. −12	NA
Changes in 24-h SBP at 6 months (mmHg)	−6.7 vs. −4.8	−7 vs. −3.5 (intention to treat, p=ns) −8.3 vs. −3.5 (per protocol, p=0.042)
Changes in 24-h DBP at 6 months (mmHg)	−4.1 vs. −3.1	−2.8 vs. −2.1
Δ in changes in office systolic BP at 6 months between groups (mmHg)	−2.39 (ns)	NA
Δ in changes in ambulatory systolic BP at 6 months between groups (mmHg)	−1.96 (ns)	NA
Changes in 24-h heart rate (bpm)	−1.4 vs. 1.3	NA
RDN device	Symplicity	Symplicity

The small randomized OSLO study investigated the BP-lowering effect of RDN (n=9, performed with Symplicity catheter) versus clinically adjusted drug treatment (n=10), with the use of noninvasive integrated hemodynamic measurements of impedance cardiography with the HOTMAN System in true dRHTN after excluding patients with confounding poor drug adherence [12]. For the definition of dRHTN, ambulatory daytime SBP >135 mmHg after witnessed intake of antihypertensive drugs was required. The investigators stopped the study earlier because systolic and diastolic BP were significantly lower in the drug-adjusted group at 6 months and absolute changes in SBP were larger in the drug-adjusted group (p=0.008). Ambulatory BPs changed in parallel to office BPs. This study suggested that adjusted drug treatment has superior BP-lowering effects compared with RDN in patients with true dRHTN. However, the study results should be evaluated with caution because of methodological limitations and questionable clinical extrapolations (there are small number of studied patients, the decision to prematurely interrupt the study as "unethical" is not statistically justified, conclusions are based on an interim analysis of an underpowered study, the HOTMAN System has not been applied to the RDN arm and in the BEAUTY study the selection of antihypertensive drugs guided by the HOTMAN system did not resulted in greater BP reduction compared to the conventional selection of medications, etc).

The Renal Denervation for Hypertension (DENERHTN) trial was a prospective, open-label randomized controlled trial with blinded end point evaluation in 106 patients with dRHTN from 15 French tertiary care centers specialized in HTN management [13]. Eligible patients (aged 55 years old) received a standardized stepped-care antihypertensive treatment (SSAHT) of indapamide 1.5 mg, ramipril 10 mg (or irbesartan 300 mg), and amlodipine 10 mg daily for 4 weeks to confirm treatment resistance by ambulatory BP monitoring before randomization. Patients were then randomly assigned (1:1) to receive either RDN plus the abovementioned SSAHT regimen (RDN group) or the same SSAHT regimen alone (control group). The randomization sequence was generated by computer and stratified by centers. For SSAHT, after randomization, spironolactone 25 mg per day, bisoprolol 10 mg per day, prazosin 5 mg per day, and rilmenidine 1 mg per day were sequentially added from months two to five in both groups if home BP was more than or equal to 135/85 mmHg. The primary end point, i.e., the mean change in daytime ambulatory systolic BP at 6 months, was met: −15.8 mmHg in the RDN group and −9.9 mmHg in the control group with a baseline-adjusted difference of −5.9 mmHg (−11.3 to −0.5; $p=0.0329$). The number of antihypertensive drugs and drug adherence at 6 months were similar between the two groups. Accordingly, the carefully designed and conducted DENERHTN study concluded that in patients with well-defined dRHTN, RDN was effective in decreasing ambulatory BP at a 6-month follow-up period.

Symplicity HTN-Japan is a prospective, randomized, controlled trial comparing RDN with standard pharmacotherapy treatment of dRHTN. When Symplicity HTN-3 failed to meet the primary efficacy end point, the HTN-Japan enrollment was discontinued before completion and consequently was underpowered for the primary end point analysis. Accordingly, the available data at a 6-month follow-up period (for 22 patients in RDN group and 19 patients in the control group) showed that the between-group difference in SBP change was not significant [20].

16.5 Registries: Real-World Data

In addition to prospective observational and randomized RDN trials, the safety and efficacy of RDN has been assessed in real-world patients with dRHTN. In this setting, a first report from the Global Symplicity Registry, a prospective, open-label, and multicenter registry with 6-month outcome for 998 resistant hypertensive patients, was published in 2015 [21]. Baseline systolic office and ambulatory BP (163 and 151 mmHg, respectively) were reduced by 11.6 and 6.6 mmHg, respectively. This registry also confirmed that RDN-induced BP-lowering effect is directly related to the height of baseline BP. Accordingly, in the subcohort ($n=323$) with comparable BP entry criteria to the HTN-3 trial, office systolic BP was reduced by 20.3 and ambulatory systolic by 8.9 mmHg at 6 months post RDN.

In the UK experience, 253 patients with dRHTN (office BP, 185/102 mmHg) from 18 centers were treated with the use of five different RDN ablation systems (Symplicity flex, Simplicity spiral, Boston Vessix, EnligHTN, and OneShot) [22]. Office and ambulatory BP was significantly reduced by 22/9 and 12/7 mmHg, respectively, at an average follow-up of 11 months.

16.6 Randomized Sham-Controlled Studies

16.6.1 Symplicity HTN-3 Trial

The results of Symplicity HTN-3 trial tempered the enthusiasm of the scientific community and industry toward RDN. The Symplicity HTN-3 study was a prospective, randomized (2:1), masked (sham) procedure, single-blind study, which aimed to establish the safety and efficacy of RDN in 535 resistant hypertensive patients in the USA [14]. Inclusion criteria were similar to those of Symplicity HTN-1 and HTN-2, with the additional confirmation of 24-h ambulatory BP ≥ 135 mmHg. Before randomization, patients were receiving a stable antihypertensive regimen for at least 2 weeks involving maximum tolerated doses of at least three antihypertensive drugs, including a diuretic. The primary safety end point was met but the primary efficacy end point was not achieved. Office systolic BP at 6 months dropped by −14.1 in the RDN and −11.7 in the control (sham) group, respectively, with the difference of 2.39 mmHg not reaching statistical significance ($p=0.26$, with a superiority margin of 5 mmHg). The change in ambulatory BP at 6 months was −6.7 mmHg in the RDN and −4.7 mmHg in the sham ablation arm (difference of −1.96 mmHg) ($p=0.98$, with a 2 mmHg superiority margin). The observations regarding systolic BP were consistent when diastolic BP was examined.

A study from Germany by S. Desch examined the effectiveness of RDN in patients ($n=71$) with mildly elevated BP (daytime systolic BP 135–149 and diastolic BP 90–94 mmHg on 24-h ambulatory measurement). Patients were randomized in a 1:1 ratio to RDN with the Symplicity flex catheter (Medtronic) or an invasive sham procedure [23]. In patients with mild resistant hypertension, RDN failed to show a significant reduction in the primary end point of 24-h systolic BP at 6 months between groups in the intention to treat analysis, but in the per-protocol cohort, which is likely a better indicator of biological effectiveness of the intervention, 24-h systolic BP was significantly reduced. Due to the small sample and the discrepant results between the intention to treat and per-protocol population, these results should be perceived as explanatory and be interpreted with caution.

16.7 Controversial BP Reduction Post RDN: Possible Explanations

Symplicity HTN-3, except from the fact that was larger than the first two Symplicity studies (Symplicity 1 and 2), was a well-designed study with the use of sham procedure in the control group. However, the execution of the study has been questioned [24–26]. Some months later after the publication of Symplicity HTN-3, a subsequent comprehensive subanalysis by Kandzari et al. along with interesting new preclinical data regarding the location and distribution of renal fibers in the renal arterial wall highlighted a number of potential confounding factors that may explain, at least partially, the unexpected BP responses in both RDN and sham ablation groups as well as the huge variability in BP response post RDN. The list of these confounders includes incomplete denervation, poor antihypertensive medications stability and adherence, selection of non-appropriate population and selection of office BP as end point of RDN efficacy [27–32].

16.7.1 Incomplete Renal Denervation in Many Patients

Symplicity HTN-3 was a US trial with 88 sites and no fewer than 111 operators performing the procedure. The procedure per operator ratio is approximately 3.3, while 34 % of the interventionists carried out only one single procedure raising concerns about the "learning curve" effect [27, 31, 32]. Additionally, proctoring in the study sites was largely undertaken by nonclinical staff. In a recent post hoc analysis of the Symplicity 3 when procedural data were carefully evaluated, it was found that the BP response increased with increasing number of ablations delivered and the successful delivery of circumferential (four-quadrant) ablations. The mean number of ablation attempted (energy application) per artery was 4.7, whereas in Symplicity HTN-1, the corresponding number was 8.6, suggesting a "dose-response" dependency between the number of ablation attempts and the efficacy of RDN. Additionally, in Symplicity HTN-3 only a small proportion of patients ($n = 19$) had successful ablation across all four quadrants of the renal artery. Similarly, in HTN-3, it was shown that a successful four-quadrant ablation in both renal arteries was associated with the greatest BP drop (office systolic) of 24.3 mmHg, while with one-artery four-quadrant ablation, BP reduced to 16.1 mmHg and with no four-quadrant ablation, BP reduced to 14.2 mmHg.

In the years following the first studies on RDN, our view on the technique has significantly changed; RDN is now recognized as a complex, specialized therapy with a large list of influencing factors and uncertainties. Accordingly, our knowledge about the peri-arterial renal nerve distribution in chronically hypertensive patients is very limited and it is unclear to what extent preclinical results can be applied to vessels subjected to atherosclerosis. The optimal degree of pressure against the wall, the depth of ablation, and time/amount of energy delivered to provide the best procedural results are still being investigated. Recently, it has been shown that the highest average number of nerves was observed in the proximal and middle segments of the renal artery and the lowest in the distal segments [28, 29]. Even more important, the mean distance from the lumen to the nerve was the longest in the proximal and the lowest in the distal segments. These clinical and some preclinical observations suggest that asymmetric and most probably distal renal artery targeting is required to achieve effective ablation of renal sympathetic nerves. However in many clinical trials including HTN-3, ablation wasn't performed in this area, potentially reducing the efficacy of the procedure.

The lack of reliable markers of procedural success to establish on time whether denervation has been completely achieved in a specific patient remains the major unmet need [33, 34]. As a result, it remains uncertain whether the negative trials arise from suboptimal application of the technology or whether the technique in the way it was applied is not effective. A number of efficacy markers have been explored (i.e., acute changes in renal hemodynamics, changes in BP after high-frequency stimulation in the renal artery, etc.), but there is no consensus on their usefulness [34, 35].

16.7.2 Medication Stability and Adherence

Medication stability and patient adherence is critical at study baseline and during study [36]. Post hoc analysis of HTN-3 indicated that frequent drug changes and variable medication adherence may have interfered with the observed BP reduction post RDN [27]. In HTN-3, 38 % of patients have changes in their medications, while in the positive DENERHTN study, a standardized treatment protocol was followed. In HTN-3, the prespecified subgroup analysis for ethnicity deserves specific attention, and perhaps changes in the adherence rate may contribute in the discrepancy of RDN efficacy. Changes in office systolic BP in the African-American subgroup were not significant largely due to the large drop in BP in the sham group (−17.8 mmHg). In the non-African-American subgroup (in which more than 95 % were Caucasians), a significant difference in office systolic BP was observed (−15.2 in the denervation and −8.6 mmHg in the control (sham) group, $p=0.012$). Similarly, in the Global Symplicity Registry, the subset of non-African-American individuals with similar clinical characteristics to those included in the HTN-3 trial had a mean office systolic BP drop of 17.3 mmHg which was quite identical to the systolic BP reduction observed in the RDN group of HTN-3 [21]. Differences in the rate of adherence may explain, at least partially, these unexpected effects in HTN-3. For this reason, European experts on RDN suggest that in future RDN trials, it is crucial to standardize concomitant antihypertensive therapy (preferentially all treated with the combination of a renin-angiotensin blocker, calcium channel blocker, and diuretic) with a stable run-in period of at least 4–8 weeks and to monitor drug adherence as potential confounder of BP response (pill counting, electronic pill dispenser, toxicological drug analysis) [37]. However, it needs to be highlighted that the abovementioned confounders of BP response to RDN come from a post hoc analysis of the study. Therefore, the findings should be considered as exploratory and hypothesis generating and should be confirmed by appropriately designed prospective studies addressing these issues.

16.7.3 Appropriate Hypertensive Population for RDN: Identification of Responders Post RDN

All the RDN trials have clearly shown a pronounced heterogeneity in the BP response post RDN: BP is excessively reduced in some patients; some other patients experience a modest but still clinically significant BP reduction, whereas in some patients the BP is either minimally decreased or even increased [6–14,

21]. The heterogeneity of BP response to RDN is not surprising and should be considered in the general context of drug- and/or device-based antihypertensive therapy [37]. Accordingly, historical data with sympathetic splanchnicectomy showed that only 45 % of the surgically treated patients experienced a substantial BP reduction [1]. Besides that, HTN, and particularly dRHTN, is a multifactorial disease with several mechanisms involved in its pathogenesis [5, 6]. The long experience for pharmaceutical trials in HTN clearly shows that inhibition of any mechanism implicated in BP elevation is effective only in a certain percentage of patients (30–50 %). Based on the above, it is of paramount importance to identify predictors of BP response to RDN that will help identify the "right patient" for this interventional approach. Up to now, only largely elevated BP (systolic >180 mmHg) has been associated with greater reductions of BP, a fact that is evident with drug therapy as well [38]. This does not mean that all patients with largely elevated BP respond to RDN [21]. From a pathophysiological point of view, it seems rational to assume that RDN would be effective in patients with evident sympathetic overactivity, but there is a lack of clinically applicable measures of "increased sympathetic activity" that could be used to guide treatment decisions [39]. However, up to now there is no clear established link between SNS activity and response to RDN and clearly, there is a need for more research on this topic [40].

Preliminary data indicate that isolated systolic HTN, the predominant hypertensive subtype in elderly patients, is associated with limited response to RDN [41]. Accordingly, increased central pulse pressure indicative of aortic stiffness is related to worse BP response after RDN. It can be questioned whether older patients or patients with long-standing HTN may respond, compared to younger patients, given their commonly lower degree of SNS activation and their increased aortic stiffness. It has also been postulated that the most suitable population for RDN would be patients with earlier stages of HTN whereas the ultimate risk/benefit ratio of RDN remains to be elucidated [37, 41, 42].

16.7.4 Blood Pressure Measurements: Ambulatory-Office Blood Pressure Disparity

Data from trials using antihypertensive medications show that there was a disproportionally greater decrease in systolic office BP than in ambulatory BP which, for both office and ambulatory BP, seems to depend on the pretreatment BP levels [43–45]. Two meta-analyses comparing ambulatory and office BP reduction in patients with essential HTN revealed that the ambulatory response to drug treatment is about two-thirds of the office BP response [44]. Similarly, an in-depth overview of the published studies with RDN reveals a marked disparity between office and ambulatory BP reductions: the dramatic falls in office systolic and diastolic BP are not accompanied by similar reductions in ambulatory values. The absence of ambulatory BP measurements has been considered as a weakness of earlier RDN trials. Indeed, in the proof-of-concept study (Symplicity 1) and the randomized study (Symplicity 2), ambulatory systolic BP reduction was only 41 % and 38 % of the observed office BP pressure reduction, respectively. The white coat effect, which is very frequently encountered in dRHTN, might have contributed to this marked disparity [38, 43, 44]. It is well accepted that ambulatory BP is less susceptible to bias, placebo effect, regression to the mean, Hawthorn effect and day-to-day variability than office BP, can easily be analyzed blind to the allocation of treatment, and allows appropriate selection of patients for RDN. Patients with white coat HTN are not likely to show any effect on BP. Accordingly, 346 patients from ten centers from Germany and Australia who were enrolled following the extended Symplicity protocol were classified to true resistant HTN ($n=303$) (office and ambulatory systolic BP of 172 and 154 mmHg, respectively) and to pseudoresistant HTN ($n=43$) (office and ambulatory systolic BP of 161 and 121 mmHg, respectively) [46]. At 6 months post RDN, systolic ambulatory BP decreased by 10.2 mmHg in patients with true dRHTN, which is similar to the 24-h BP decline observed in Symplicity HTN-2, while there was no effect on ambulatory BP monitoring in pseudoresistant patients, whereas office BP was reduced to a similar extent. Similarly, participants in Symplicity HTN-3, whereas the white coat effect was excluded per protocol, did not demonstrate a significant difference between groups for both office and ABPM. In contrast, the French DENERHTN study, a prospective open-label randomized trial with blinded end point evaluation, used ambulatory BP as primary objective demonstrating a greater daytime BP response in the RDN group than in the control group.

16.7.5 Durability of BP Reduction: Long-Term Effects of RDN on BP

Experimental findings suggest regeneration mainly of renal efferent sympathetic fibers post RDN. Whether reinnervation actually takes place in humans, and if so whether the reinnervation is functional and not only anatomic, remains questionable [47]. However, data from clinical trials and registries indicate that changes in BP persist long term (available follow-up to 3 years) in patients with dRHTN after RDN [19].

In 88 out of 135 patients enrolled in the HTN-1, from a mean BP of 175/98 mmHg at baseline, office BP dropped by −32/−14 mmHg after 36 months, with a response rate of 93 % at 36 months [16]. The absence of any relapse or attenuation of the antihypertensive effect suggests that there is no evidence of functional reinnervation at 3 years.

In the entire population of the EnligHTN I ($n=46$), reduction in office BP at 24 months from baseline was −29/−13 mmHg, while the reduction in 24-h ambulatory

BP and in home BP at 24 months was −13/−7 mmHg and −11/−6 mmHg, respectively ($p<0.05$ for all cases) [17, 18].

According to HTN-3 protocol, subjects in the sham group meeting eligibility requirements could undergo RDN. Therefore, in denervation subjects, the 12-month office systolic BP change was greater than that observed at 6 months (−18.9 vs. −15.5 mmHg, $p=0.025$) but the 24 h systolic BP change was not significantly different at 12 months [48]. Thus, all of the above indicate that there is evidence that RDN results in a decline in office systolic BP and that this is maintained over a longer period of follow-up albeit in a smaller patient group.

16.8 RDN Efficacy on BP Reduction: Where Do We Stand?

In the latest guidelines of the European Society of Hypertension/European Society of Cardiology (ESH/ESC) for HTN management, the recommendation of treatment strategies in hypertensive patients with dRHTN suggested that in case of ineffectiveness of drug treatment, invasive procedures such as RDN may be considered as last resort [6]. However, after the publication of the Symplicity HTN-3 trial, the design, conduct, and interpretation of all RDN trials have been discussed extensively. On one hand, whatever the associated shortcoming of each trial may be, there is strong possibility that the observed BP reductions were due to the placebo effect, the Hawthorne effect, regression to the mean, drug changes and adherence, study population, and procedural methods or other biases. On the other hand, current evidence also seems insufficient to declare the technology a proven failure. Given that not one RDN study provided any serious safety concerns, all agree that a second chance is really needed to test the effectiveness of this new therapeutic approach. In this setting, a clinical consensus conference provided some considerations on future RDN clinical trials: selection of population, design of study, and study outcome (Box 16.1) [37]. Accordingly, the SPYRAL HTN Global Clinical Trial Program (using the Symplicity Spyral multielectrode renal denervation catheter) is designed to address limitations associated with predicate studies and provide insight into the impact of pharmacotherapy on RDN efficacy and already has enrolled patients in the USA and Europe [49]. The two initial trials of the program focus on the effect of RDN in hypertensive patients in the absence (SPYRAL HTN OFF-MED) and presence (SPYRAL HTN ON-MED) of antihypertensive medications. The SPYRAL HTN ON-MED study requires patients to be treated with a consistent mono or double or triple-therapy antihypertensive regimen, whereas the SPYRAL HTN OFF-MED study includes a 3–4-week drug washout period followed by a 3-month efficacy and safety end point in the absence of antihypertensive medications. The studies will randomize patients with combined systolic-diastolic HTN to RDN or sham procedure. Both studies allow RDN treatments in renal artery branches and accessories. Of similar design was the ongoing RE-INFORCE study

Box 16.1: Recommendation for Future Randomized Controlled Trials on Renal Denervation in Hypertensive Patients

Study Population

- Include patients with moderate rather than resistant hypertension reflecting the pathogenetic importance of sympathetic activity in earlier stages.
- Exclude patients with stiff large arteries (e.g., isolated systolic hypertension).

Study Design

- Perform washout period only in highly experienced centers (safety concerns).
- Standardize concomitant antihypertensive therapy (preferentially all treated with the combination of a RAS-blocker, calcium channel blocker, and diuretic in the run-in period).
- Monitor drug adherence as potential confounder of blood pressure response (e.g., pill counting, electronic pill dispensers, toxicological drug analysis).

Study Outcomes

- Use change in ambulatory blood pressure as the primary efficacy end point (strictly standardized), while change in office blood pressure should be considered as secondary parameter.
- Delineate clinically easy accessible predictors for blood pressure efficacy.

(using the Vessix RDN system) with the primary end point of ambulatory BP changes at 8 weeks post intervention. Table 16.5 summarizes the on going randomized RDN trials using different technology for ablating the renal fibers (radiofrequency, ultrasound, chemical etc).

Hopefully these ongoing and future appropriately designed trials will eventually resolve most of the uncertainties regarding the BP effects of RDN and help defining its place in clinical practice without denying an effective therapy in those patients who really need it and without putting those at risk from procedures that aren't beneficial. Until more evidence is available concerning the long-term BP efficacy and safety of RDN, it is recommended that these procedures remain in the hands of experienced operators while diagnosis and follow-up should be restricted to hypertension centers.

Table 16.5 On-going RDN clinical trials in hypertension

Trial	Sponsor	Key characteristics of the study	Ablation system	Study population	Primary efficacy end point of study
SPYRAL HTN–OFF MED	Medtronic	Multi center, randomized, blinded study with sham ablation arm (1:1) Main body and branch ablation No specific baseline medication requirement	SYMPLICITY SPYRAL System for delivery of radiofrequency energy	100 patients	Change in ambulatory systolic BP at 3 months
SPYRAL HTN–ON MED	Medtronic	Multi center, randomized, blinded study with sham ablation arm (1:1) Main body and branch ablation Fixed drug regimen: 1 vs 2 vs 3 medications, classes, max dose	SYMPLICITY SPYRAL System for delivery of radiofrequency energy	100 patients	Change in ambulatory systolic BP at 3 months
REINFORCE	BOSTON	2:1 Randomization	Vessix™ Renal Denervation System Balloon-based technology for delivery of radiofrequency energy	100 hypertensive patients	Changes in ambulatory 24 h systolic BP at 2 months
EnligHTNed	SJM	Randomized, sham-controlled, blinded Standardizing antihypertensive regimen Testing for adherence	EnligHTN™ Renal Denervation System for endovascular delivery of energy	525 subjects on triple antihyperyensive drugs (350 treatment, 175 control)	Reduction in ambulatory 24-hour systolic BP at 6 months compared to baseline
The RADIANCE-HTN Trial		FDA Approved study. Global multi-center, randomized, sham-controlled, blinded Solo cohort: patients off HTN medication Trio cohort: patients on a standardized, single pill, fixed dose triple HTN medication regimen	The PARADISE system for endovascular delivery of ultrasound	292 hypertensive Patients	Difference in daytime ambulatory systolic BP at 2 months post RDN
WAVE IV	KONA	Double blind, prospective, Randomized Sham Controlled Clinical Trial	Non-invasive renal denervation by *using externally delivered focused ultrasound*	132 randomized (1:1) subjects with uncontrolled HTN	Changes in office BP at 6 months follow up
The Peregrine Post -Market Study	Ablative Solutions Inc	Post-Market Study Single arm, open label	Alcohol-mediated renal denervation based on the peregrine system™	100 hypertensive patients	Change in 24-mean ABPM at 6 months

References

1. Smithwick RH, Thompson JE (1953) Splanchnicectomy for essential hypertension; results in 1,266 cases. JAMA 152(16):1501–1504
2. DiBona GF (2005) Physiology in perspective: the wisdom of the body. Neural control of the kidney. Am J Physiol Regul Integr Comp Physiol 289(3):R633–R641
3. Julius S, Majahalme S (2000) The changing face of sympathetic overactivity in hypertension. Ann Med 32(5):365–370
4. Krum H, Schlaich M, Whitbourn R, Sobotka PA, Sadowski J, Bartus K et al (2009) Catheter-based renal sympathetic denervation for resistant hypertension: a multicenter safety and proof-of-principle cohort study. Lancet 373:1275–1281
5. Schmieder RE, Redon J, Grassi G, Kjeldsen SE, Mancia G, Narkiewicz K et al (2013) Updated ESH position paper on interventional therapy of resistant hypertension. EuroIntervention 9(Suppl R):R58–R66
6. Mancia G, Fagard R, Narkiewicz K, Redón J, Zanchetti A, Böhm M, et al; Task Force Members (2013) 2013 ESH/ESC Guidelines for the management of arterial hypertension: the Task Force for the management of arterial hypertension of the European Society of Hypertension (ESH) and of the European Society of Cardiology (ESC). J Hypertens 31(7):1281–1357.
7. Worthley SG, Tsioufis CP, Worthley MI, Sinhal A, Chew DP, Meredith IT et al (2013) Safety and efficacy of a multi-electrode renal sympathetic denervation system in resistant hypertension: the EnligHTN I trial. Eur Heart J 34(28):2132–2140
8. Sievert H, Schofer J, Ormiston J, Hoppe UC, Meredith IT, Walters DL et al (2015) Renal denervation with a percutaneous bipolar radiofrequency balloon catheter in patients with resistant hypertension: 6-month results from the REDUCE-HTN clinical study. EuroIntervention 10(10):1213–1220
9. Esler MD, Krum H, Sobotka PA, Schlaich MP, Schmieder RE, Böhm M (2010) Renal sympathetic denervation in patients with treatment-resistant hypertension (The Symplicity HTN-2 Trial): a randomised controlled trial. Lancet 376(9756):1903–1909
10. Rosa J, Widimský P, Toušek P, Petrák O, Čurila K, Waldauf P et al (2015) Randomized comparison of renal denervation versus intensified pharmacotherapy including spironolactone in true-resistant hypertension: six-month results from the Prague-15 study. Hypertension 65:407–413
11. Verheye S, Ormiston J, Bergmann MW, Sievert H, Schwindt A, Werner N, Vogel B, Colombo A (2015) Twelve-month results of the rapid renal sympathetic denervation for resistant hypertension using the OneShotTM ablation system (RAPID) study. EuroIntervention 10(10):1221–1229
12. FadlElmula FE, Hoffmann P, Larstorp AC, Fossum E, Brekke M, Kjeldsen SE, Gjønnæss E, Hjørnholm U, Kjær VN, Rostrup M, Os I, Stenehjem A, Høieggen A (2014) Adjusted drug treatment is superior to renal sympathetic denervation in patients with true treatment-resistant hypertension. Hypertension 63(5):991–999
13. Azizi M, Sapoval M, Gosse P, Monge M, Bobrie G, Delsart P, et al; Renal Denervation for Hypertension (DENERHTN) investigators (2015) Optimum and stepped care standardised antihypertensive treatment with or without renal denervation for resistant hypertension (DENERHTN): a multicentre, open-label, randomised controlled trial. Lancet 385(9981):1957–1965
14. Bhatt DL, Kandzari DE, O'Neill WW, D'Agostino R, Flack JM, Katzen BT et al (2014) A controlled trial of renal denervation for resistant hypertension. N Engl J Med 370(15):1393–1401
15. Calaresu FR, Stella A, Zanchetti A (1976) Haemodynamic responses and renin release during stimulation of afferent renal nerves in the cat. J Physiol 255(3):687–700
16. Krum H, Schlaich MP, Sobotka PA, Böhm M, Mahfoud F, Rocha-Singh K, Katholi R, Esler MD (2014) Percutaneous renal denervation in patients with treatment-resistant hypertension: final 3-year report of the Symplicity HTN-1 study. Lancet 383(9917):622–629

17. Papademetriou V, Tsioufis CP, Sinhal A, Chew DP, Meredith IT, Malaiapan Y, Worthley MI, Worthley SG (2014) Catheter-based renal denervation for resistant hypertension: 12-month results of the EnligHTN I first-in-human study using a multielectrode ablation system. Hypertension 64(3):565–572
18. Tsioufis CP, Papademetriou V, Dimitriadis KS, Kasiakogias A, Tsiachris D, Worthley MI et al (2015) Catheter-based renal denervation for resistant hypertension: twenty-four month results of the EnligHTN I first-in-human study using a multi-electrode ablation system. Int J Cardiol 201:345–350
19. Esler MD, Bohm M, Sievert H, Rump CL, Schmieder RE, Krum H et al (2014) Catheter-based renal denervation for treatment of patients with treatment-resistant hypertension: 36 month results from the Symplicity HTN-2 randomized clinical trial. Eur Heart J 35(26):1752–1759
20. Kario K, Ogawa H, Okumura K, Okura T, Saito S, Ueno T, et al; SYMPLICITY HTN-Japan Investigators (2015) SYMPLICITY HTN-Japan – first randomized controlled trial of catheter-based renal denervation in Asian patients. Circ J 79:1222–1229
21. Böhm M, Mahfoud F, Ukena C, Hoppe UC, Narkiewicz K, Negoita M et al (2015) First report of the Global SYMPLICITY Registry on the effect of renal artery denervation in patients with uncontrolled hypertension. Hypertension 65(4):766–774
22. Sharp AS, Davies JE, Lobo MD, Bent CL, Mark PB, Burchell AE et al (2016) Renal artery sympathetic denervation: observations from the UK experience. Clin Res Cardiol. 105(6): 544–552 [Epub ahead of print]
23. Desch S, Okon T, Heinemann D, Kulle K, Röhnert K, Sonnabend M et al (2015) Randomized sham-controlled trial of renal sympathetic denervation in mild resistant hypertension. Hypertension 65(6):1202–1208
24. Papademetriou V, Rashidi AA, Tsioufis C, Doumas M (2014) Renal nerve ablation for resistant hypertension: how did we get here, present status, and future directions. Circulation 129(13):1440–1451
25. Papademetriou V, Tsioufis C, Doumas M (2014) Renal denervation and Symplicity HTN-3: "Dubium sapientiae initium" (doubt is the beginning of wisdom). Circ Res 115(2):211–214
26. Tsioufis C (2014) Hypertension: is the sham procedure 'toxic' for renal denervation? Nat Rev Nephrol 10(4):186–187
27. Kandzari DE, Bhatt DL, Brar S, Devireddy CM, Esler M, Fahy M et al (2015) Predictors of blood pressure response in the SYMPLICITY HTN-3 trial. Eur Heart J 36(4):219–227
28. Tzafriri AR, Mahfoud F, Keating JH, Markham PM, Spognardi A, Wong G et al (2014) Innervation patterns may limit response to endovascular renal denervation. J Am Coll Cardiol 64(11):1079–1087
29. Sakakura K, Ladich E, Cheng Q, Otsuka F, Yahagi K, Fowler DR et al (2014) Anatomic assessment of sympathetic peri-arterial renal nerves in man. J Am Coll Cardiol 64(7):635–643
30. Lüscher TF, Mahfoud F (2014) Renal nerve ablation after SYMPLICITY HTN-3: confused at the higher level? Eur Heart J 35(26):1706–1711
31. Mahfoud F, Bhatt DL (2013) Catheter-based renal denervation: the black box procedure. JACC Cardiovasc Interv 6(10):1092–1094
32. Mahfoud F, Lüscher TF (2015) Renal denervation: simply trapped by complexity? Eur Heart J 36(4):199–202
33. Tsioufis C, Mahfoud F, Mancia G, Redon J, Damascelli B, Zeller T et al (2014) What the interventionalist should know about renal denervation in hypertensive patients: a position paper by the ESH WG on the interventional treatment of hypertension. EuroIntervention 9(9):1027–1035
34. Tsioufis C, Papademetriou V, Dimitriadis K, Tsiachris D, Thomopoulos C, Park E et al (2013) Catheter-based renal sympathetic denervation exerts acute and chronic effects on renal hemodynamics in swine. Int J Cardiol 168(2):987–992
35. Tsiachris D, Tsioufis C, Dimitriadis K, Kordalis A, Thomopoulos C, Kasiakogias A, Papalois A, Papademetriou V, Tousoulis D, Stefanadis C (2014) Electrical stimulation of the renal arterial nerves does not unmask the blindness of renal denervation procedure in swine.Int J Cardiol. 176(3):1061–1063

36. Burnier M, Wuerzner G, Struijker-Boudier H, Urquhart J (2013) Measuring, analyzing, and managing drug adherence in resistant hypertension. Hypertension 62(2):218–225
37. Mahfoud F, Lüscher TF, Andersson B, Baumgartner I, Cifkova R, Dimario C et al (2013) Expert consensus document from the European Society of Cardiology on catheter-based renal denervation. Eur Heart J 34(28):2149–2157
38. Schmieder RE, Schmidt ST, Riemer T, Dechend R, Hagedorn I, Senges J et al (2014) Disproportional decrease in office blood pressure compared with 24-hour ambulatory blood pressure with antihypertensive treatment: dependency on pretreatment blood pressure levels. Hypertension 64(5):1067–1072
39. Grassi G, Seravalle G, Brambilla G, Trabattoni D, Cuspidi C, Corso R et al (2015) Blood pressure responses to renal denervation precede and are independent of the sympathetic and baroreflex effects. Hypertension 65(6):1209–1216
40. Hering D, Lambert EA, Marusic P, Walton AS, Krum H, Lambert GW et al (2013) Substantial reduction in single sympathetic nerve firing after renal denervation in patients with resistant hypertension. Hypertension 61(2):457–464
41. Ewen S, Ukena C, Linz D, Kindermann I, Cremers B, Laufs U et al (2015) Reduced effect of percutaneous renal denervation on blood pressure in patients with isolated systolic hypertension. Hypertension 65(1):193–199
42. Ott C, Mahfoud F, Schmid A, Ditting T, Sobotka PA, Veelken R et al (2013) Renal denervation in moderate treatment-resistant hypertension. J Am Coll Cardiol 62(20):1880–1886
43. Mancia G, Omboni S, Parati G, Ravogli A, Villani A, Zanchetti A (1995) Lack of placebo effect on ambulatory blood pressure. Am J Hypertens 8(3):311–315
44. Doumas M, Anyfanti P, Bakris G (2012) Should ambulatory blood pressure monitoring be mandatory for future studies in resistant hypertension: a perspective. J Hypertens 30(5):874–876
45. Redon J, Campos C, Narciso ML, Rodicio JL, Pascual JM, Ruilope LM (1998) Prognostic value of ambulatory blood pressure monitoring in refractory hypertension: a prospective study. Hypertension 31(2):712–718
46. Mahfoud F, Ukena C, Schmieder RE, Cremers B, Rump LC, Vonend O et al (2013) Ambulatory blood pressure changes after renal sympathetic denervation in patients with resistant hypertension. Circulation 128(2):132–140
47. Booth LC, Nishi EE, Yao ST, Ramchandra R, Lambert GW, Schlaich MP, May CN (2015) Reinnervation of renal afferent and efferent nerves at 5.5 and 11 months after catheter-based radiofrequency renal denervation in sheep. Hypertension 65(2):393–400
48. Bakris G, Townsend R, Liu M, Cohen S, D'Agostino R, Flack J, Kandzari D, Katzen B, Leon M, Mauri L, Negoita M, O'Neil W, Oparil S, Roscha-Singh K, Bhatt D (2015) Impact of renal denervation on 24 hour ambulatory blood pressure: results from SYMPLICITY HTN -3. J Am Coll Cardiol 65(13):1314–1321
49. Kandzari DE, Kario K, Mahfoud F, Cohen SA, Pilcher G, Pocock S, Townsend R, Weber MA, Böhm M (2016) The SPYRAL HTN Global Clinical Trial Program: rationale and design for studies of renal denervation in the absence (SPYRAL HTN OFF-MED) and presence (SPYRAL HTN ON-MED) of antihypertensive medications. Am Heart J 171(1):82–91
50. Symplicity HTN-1 Investigators. Catheter-based renal sympathetic denervation for resistant hypertension: durability of blood pressure reduction out to 24 months. Hypertension. 2011;57:911–7

Effects of Renal Denervation on Intermediate End Points

17

Kyriakos Dimitriadis, Dimitrios Tousoulis, and Costas Tsioufis

Abbreviations

BP	Blood pressure
dRHTN	Drug-resistant hypertension
LV	Left ventricle
RDN	Renal denervation
SNS	Sympathetic nervous system

17.1 Introduction

Enhanced sympathetic nervous system (SNS) activity constitutes an important pathway involved in the initiation and progression of the hypertensive disease [1, 2]. Sympathetic overactivity increases progressively and in parallel with hypertension stages, while accelerated cardiac damage reflected by left ventricular (LV) hypertrophy compared to normal geometry is accompanied by greater norepinephrine spillover [3]. The latter is typical of the hypertensive phenotype characterized by increased heart rate, cardiac output, and renovascular resistance. Similarly, the hallmark of renal disease is sympathetic overdrive, and microneurography studies revealed high muscle sympathetic nerve activity in patients with renal dysfunction [3, 4]. In these lines, SNS activation is related with the pathogenesis of arrhythmias, as well as it is involved in glucose metabolism regulation [3, 5]. Thus in this chapter,

K. Dimitriadis (✉) • D. Tousoulis • C. Tsioufis
1st Cardiology Clinic, National and Kapodistrian University of Athens, Hippokration Hospital, Athens, Greece
e-mail: dimitriadiskyr@yahoo.gr

C. Tsioufis et al. (eds.), *Interventional Therapies for Secondary and Essential Hypertension*, Updates in Hypertension and Cardiovascular Protection,
DOI 10.1007/978-3-319-34141-5_17

the effect of sympathetic nervous system modulation by means of renal denervation (RDN) on the intermediate end points related to the heart, kidney, arteries, arrhythmias, and glucose metabolism will be analyzed.

17.2 Effects of RDN on Kidney Damage

Even the beginning of end-stage renal disease is accompanied by significantly high levels of catecholamines indicating the importance of SNS activation in the initiation of the detrimental effects of adrenergic overdrive on renal tissue [1, 11]. Recently it was shown that in patients with a stable and moderate chronic renal failure (mean estimated glomerular filtration rate, 40.7 mL/min per 1.73 m^2), SNS activity is already elevated as compared to age-matched healthy controls, and the sympathetic overdrive exhibits an inverse relationship with renal function [6]. In a cross-sectional study of 496 subjects of the general population including hypertensives, urinary albumin excretion was strongly related with plasma norepinephrine, even after exclusion of patients with renal disease and accounting for age, body mass index, and ambulatory blood pressure (BP) [3]. SNS overdrive could mediate early glomerular permeability damage, as reflected by heightened albuminuria before or in parallel with clinical renal function decline, and this is genetically supported [7].

Animal studies provide promising data on the potential renoprotective effect of RDN. For example, in Dahl salt-sensitive rats, RSD causes decrease in albuminuria, less glomerulosclerosis, and overall less podocyte damage [3, 8]. In normal dogs and rats, surgical removal of basal renal sympathetic nerve did not alter renal blood flow, whereas studies in healthy rabbits revealed that RDN resulted in augmentation of renal flow [3, 9]. Electrocoagulation to achieve RDN in male Wistar rats caused increase in cortical flow, and similarly resistive index was significantly reduced by the RDN procedure in acute and chronic setting. In another study however, performed in Sprague Dawley rats, RDN did not influence either renal blood flow or renal vascular resistance [3, 9]. These discrepancies might be due to differences among animal species as well as the method of RDN. In a recent study, it was shown that catheter-based RDN by radiofrequency ablation exerts acute effects on renal hemodynamics in a healthy animal model that persist at 1 month after the procedure [9]. More specifically, RDN augmented average peak velocity and renal blood flow, whereas reduced resistive index and renal flow reserve acutely and after 1 month [9]. The absence of sympathetic tone due to radiofrequency ablation leads to a maximal vascular dilatory state that cannot be altered to a further degree by intrarenal administration of a powerful stimulus such as dopamine. Accordingly, RDN shifted the autoregulatory kidney mechanisms to a state of greater baseline renal blood flow with a lessened flow reserve range due to successful withdrawal of basal effective SNS outflow on renal microcirculation. Nevertheless, renal hemodynamic changes after radiofrequency RDN could be also used as an invasive but readily available tool to determine procedural success directly in the catheterization laboratory.

Coming to the human clinical setting of percutaneous transluminal RDN in the Symplicity HTN-1 trial, renal safety assessed by renal angiography and/or magnetic resonance angiogram revealed no instances of renal artery aneurysm, or stenosis, or other long-term adverse events [10]. Although participating patients were repeatedly exposed to contrast media during serial angiographies, renal function was not compromised. Paired baseline and 6-month follow-up estimated glomerular filtration rate (eGFR) data were available in 25 patients and were 79 ± 21 and 83 ± 25 mL/min/1.73 m^2. Notably, patients with low eGFR before RDN exhibited a trend for greater increase in eGFR [10].

In the first year of the extended Symplicity HTN-1 cohort, eGFR remained stable, and after 2 years, there were no cases of doubling of serum creatinine, developing class IV chronic kidney disease or requiring dialysis [11]. However, it is of note that in ten patients in whom there are post-procedure renal data at 24 months show an average reduction of eGFR = −16 ml/min/1.73 m^2. This drop of eGFR was attributed to the inclusion of anti-aldosterone therapy (spironolactone) in five hypertensives after the 1 year follow-up. In the other five patients without the newly added spironolactone, an inferior decrease of 7.8 ml/min/1.73 m^2 was shown [11]. This fall, evident after the first 6 months period, is larger compared to the one presented in studies with antihypertensive drugs like ramipril (−1.96 mL/min/1.73 m^2) and telmisartan (−3.05 mL/min/1.73 m^2) for the same follow-up period in the Ongoing Telmisartan Alone and in Combination With Ramipril Global Endpoint Trial in high-risk patients but not in the resistant hypertension setting [3]. This observation can be explained partially by the fact that these patients had initially excessively high BP levels that although BP was reduced by percutaneous RDN, most subjects were still hypertensives at 2 years of follow-up. Moreover, the extent of renal function decline within 12 months was favorably less than expected based on current evidence.

In Symplicity HTN-2, serum creatinine, eGFR, and cystatin C levels were unchanged from baseline in both groups at 6 months [12]. However, in the abovementioned Symplicity and EnligHTN I studies, patients with impaired eGFR < 45 ml/min/1.73 m^2 were excluded, and more insight on the renal impact of RSD in lower levels of baseline kidney function was not available [12–14]. In the randomized sham-controlled study Symplicity HTN-3, an increase of >50 % in glomerular filtration rate was observed in 1.4 % of the patients in the RDN group and 0.6 % in the sham-ablation arm with no statistical difference [15]. Focusing in the EnligHTN-1, population renal function as assessed by eGFR changed from 12 to 18 months but remained stable up to 24 months [14]. Some decline in eGFR is to be expected over time in this high-risk population with drug-resistant hypertension dRHTN and several comorbidities. In the absence of matched controls, however, it is difficult to assess whether it is procedure related. The change is small and unlikely to be due to effects of RDN.

Microalbuminuria is an established marker of diffuse vascular dysfunction and target organ damage. In 59 dRHTN patients with elevated albumin to creatinine ratio at baseline underwent catheter-based RDN using the Symplicity Flex™ catheter, a significant reduction in albuminuria occurred in all patients, irrespective of baseline presence of microalbuminuria [16]. Regression analysis revealed a modest positive relationship between the decrease of albuminuria and the fall of systolic BP independent of renal function that remained unchanged after RDN [16]. In another landmark study of Mahfoud et al., average albuminuria did not change significantly after RDN at 3 and 6 months [17]. However, the number of patients with normal albumin to excretion ratio increased by 5 % and 12 % at 3 and 6 month timepoint, respectively, whereas the number of patients with micro- and macroalbuminuria decreased by 10 % and 23 %, respectively. In the same study 3 and 6 months after the procedure, ultrasound renal resistive index decreased significantly after RDN, whereas there were no significant changes in renal resistive index in control patients during follow-up [17]. Interestingly, the decrease in renal resistance did not correlate with systolic BP reduction after 6 months, and systolic BP reduction showed no correlation to renal resistive index at baseline. In these lines, in EnligHTN-1 study microalbuminuria was reduced 24 months after RDN by 10 mg/g in the entire population.

In summary, although there is a current need for more evidence on the long-term effects of RDN on renal end points in diverse settings of the hypertensive disease, studies up to now have verified the neutral and/or beneficial effect of the procedure on kidney function regulation.

17.3 Effects of RDN on Cardiac Function and Structure

In experimental animal models, administration of norepinephrine causes augmentation of left ventricle (LV) mass, while chronic activation of SNS leads to hypertrophy via interaction with inflammatory pathways [3, 6, 18]. Furthermore, in humans, LV hypertrophy state identified by echocardiography or magnetic resonance imaging is accompanied by increased cardiac norepinephrine spillover and muscle sympathetic nerve traffic [3, 18]. Even in the absence of hypertrophied myocardium, SNS overdrive is also linked to unfavorable alterations of LV geometry [3].

Starting from the case-report study of a patient with resistant hypertension, there was evidence that RDN results in LV mass reduction from 184 to 169 g at 1 year after the procedure [3]. These findings were further supported and extended by a pioneer study including 46 patients with resistant hypertension enrolled in Symplicity HTN-2 trial [19]. LV mass index was reduced by 13 % after 1 month and 17 % after 6 months reflecting a drop of LV hypertrophy incidence from 63 % at baseline to 33 % after 6 months [19]. The beneficial effect of RDN on LV is correlated with the degree of hypertrophy before the procedure, and it is more evident in those with LV hypertrophy at baseline. Left atrium size was significantly reduced at follow-up and those with left atrium diameter above 44 mm were 55 % at baseline but after RSD decreased by 20 %. Patients without initial LV hypertrophy did not result in cardiac atrophy, and some patients did not exhibit regression of LV mass. The control group of resistant hypertensives did not achieve, despite optimal antihypertensive drug therapy, the above beneficial alterations in cardiac structure [19]. In the same study, the improvement in systolic function after RDN was reflected by the attenuated LV end-systolic volume accompanied by an increase in LV ejection fraction [19]. Mitral E-wave deceleration time shortened after RDN as well as isovolumic relaxation time. The ratio of mitral inflow velocity to annular relaxation velocity (lateral E/E') that reflects LV diastolic filling pressure was decreased early after RDN at 1 month and continued to drop to 6 months. From a more clinical point of view, patients with normal LV filling pressures presenting an E/E' ratio ≤8 were 38 % at baseline but increased to 58 % and 68 % at 1 and 6 months period respectively [19]. In these lines, the percentage of patients with E/E' ≥ 12 (increased LV filling pressures) was reduced from 29 to 4 % after RDN. The decrease in the E/E' was significant in those with baseline LV hypertrophy and those with higher E/E' [119]. Focusing on the confounding effect of BP reduction by RDN on the beneficial impact on LV structure and function, further analysis was made, showing that the higher the BP drop, the higher the reduction in LV mass and E/E'. However, patients exhibiting < 10 mmHg lowering after 6 months although characterized as "non-responders" had a significant reduction in LV mass index, suggesting an effect of RDN on these cardiac indices independently of RDN-induced BP control [3, 18, 19]. After RDN, in the EnligHTN-1 study, the mitral valve E'/A' ratio increased at 6 months, 12 months, and 24 months respectively, and the mitral lateral E/E' was reduced. There was a significant reduction of left atrial diameter and left atrial volume at 6 months after RDN, but the corresponding changes at 12 months and 24 months after RDN were not significant when compared with baseline [20, 21]. In the echocardiographic study of the Symplicity 2 patients, left atrial diameter at 6 months post RDN was reduced from 45.2 to 42.5 mm, while a recent meta-analysis confirmed at 6 months the reduction of left atrium studies by echocardiography but showed no changes when left atrium is assessed by cardiac magnetic resonance [18].

In a subgroup of the EnligHTN-1 population [20, 21], LV mass index was reduced at 6 months and continuously at 12 and 24 months respectively. Most importantly, after RDN, 9 (52.9 %), 10 (58.8 %), and 12 (70.6 %) patients showed improvements in the degree of LV hypertrophy at 6 months, 12 months, and 24 months, respectively, with nine patients improved by one level, two patients improved by two levels, and one patient improved by three levels from baseline at 24 months [21]. The number of patients with severely abnormal or moderately abnormal level of LV hypertrophy decreased from 9 (52.9 %) patients at baseline to 7 (41.2 %), 6 (35.3 %), and 5 (29.4 %) patients at 6 months, 12 months, and 24 months, respectively; the number with mildly abnormal level of LV hypertrophy decreased from 8 (47.1 %) patients at baseline to 5 (29.4 %) patients at 6 months, but increased back to 8 (47.1 %) patients at 12 months and then decreased again to 6 (35.5 %) patients at 24 months; and the number with LV mass/height$^{2.7}$ achieved the normal range increased from none at baseline to 5 (29.4 %), 3 (17.6 %), and 6 (35.3 %) patients at 6 months, 12 months, and 24 months, respectively. No statistically significant association was observed between the changes in office and ambulatory BP and the changes in LV mass index at any study timepoints [20, 21] (Fig. 17.1).

Apart from studies using echocardiography [19–21], cardiac magnetic resonance imaging [22, 23] has verified the beneficial effects of RDN on LV mass. In the study by Doltra A et al., LV mass index was reduced 6 months post RDN from

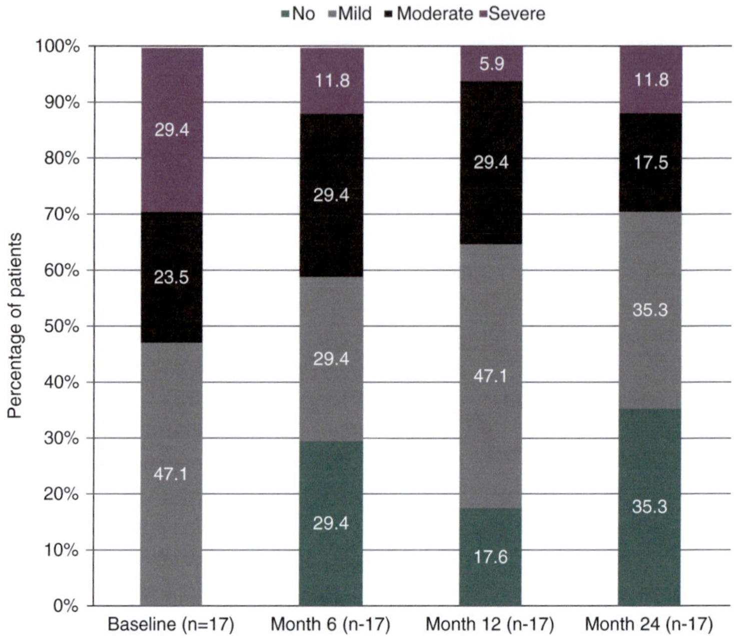

Fig. 17.1 Degree of LV hypertrophy at baseline and 6, 12, and 24 months post RDN in patients with dRHTN

41.83 ± 10.20 g/m$^{1.7}$ to 37.72 ± 7.44 g/m$^{1.7}$ ($p = 0.001$), similar to the reduction in a work by Mahfoud F et al., exhibiting a drop of LV mass index from 46.3 ± 13.6 g/m$^{1.7}$ to 43.0 ± 12.6 g/m$^{1.7}$ ($p < 0.001$) [22, 23]. Contrariwise, in another magnetic resonance imaging study, mean body surface area indexed LV mass decreased by 3 % in 44 patients with dRHTN showing no important impact of RDN on LV mass, despite reduction of ambulatory BP [24] (Table 17.1).

The above results could be attributed from a pathophysiological point of view, to the fact that RDN improves LV structure and function by affecting not only both beta- and alpha-receptor-mediated sympathetic nervous system hyperactivity but also by attenuating insulin concentration, myocardial fibrosis, as well as renin-angiotensin-system overdrive [3, 6, 18–24]. In this sense, cardiac alterations are not a result of BP reduction per se in patients after RDN but a synergistic effect of beneficial pathways of myocardial unloading and remodeling. Moreover, the extent of LV mass beneficial alterations is larger than that observed in previous pharmacological studies and at the same time of a greater degree compared to other settings of pressure-overload removal, such as in aortic stenosis [3]. The diverse impact of sympathetic modulation on LV, diastolic function, and left artium size as well as the variability in the degree of the beneficial effect through the course of time could be attributed to the complex interplay of mechanisms related with subclinical inflammation, heart remodeling, and hormonal axis along with changes of the hemodynamic burden induced by this intervention [3, 6, 18].

Table 17.1 Major studies of RDN effect on LV mass in patients with dRHTN

Study	Treatment	Patients	Time of follow-up	Change in BP after RDN	Method of LV mass estimation and baseline LV mass	LV mass changes in RDN group
Brandt et al. [19]	RDN Optimal medical therapy	46 18	6 months	↓27.8/8.8 mmHg (office)	Echocardiography [53.9 ± 15.6 g/$m^{2.7}$ (112.4 ± 33.9 g/m^2)]	↓ 9.2 g/$m^{2.7}$ (−17.5 g/m^2) (p<0.001)
Doltra et al. [22]	RDN Optimal medical therapy	23 5	6 months	↓17.2/5.2 mmHg (office)	Cardiac MRI [41.83 ± 10.20 g/$m^{1.7}$]	↓4.11 g/$m^{1.7}$ (p=0.001)
Mafhoud et al. [23]	RDN Optimal medical therapy	55 17	6 months	↓22/8 mmHg (office)	Cardiac MRI [46.3 ± 13.6 g/$m^{1.7}$]	↓3.3 g/$m^{1.7}$ (p<0.001)
Tsioufis et al. [20]	RDN Optimal medical therapy	18 10	6 months	↓42/16 mmHg (office)	Echocardiography [136.1 ± 20.1 g/m^2 (56.5 ± 8.7 g/$m^{2.7}$)]	↓13.3 g/m^2 (5.3/$m^{2.7}$) (p=0.004)
Verloop et al. [24]	RDN	54	12 months	↓7/5 mmHg (ambulatory)	Cardiac MRI [88 ± 20 g/m^2]	↓3 g/m^2 (p=NS)
Tsioufis et al. [21]	RDN	17	6, 12, and 24 months	↓41/17 mmHg, ↓30/11 mmHg and ↓39/16 mmHg (at 6, 12 and 24 months respectively)	Echocardiography [141.1 ± 16.8 g/m^2 (58.4 ± 7.8 g/$m^{2.7}$)]	↓13.6 g/m^2 (5.3 g/$m^{2.7}$) at 6 months ↓16.7 g/m^2 (6.5 g/$m^{2.7}$) at 12 and ↓22.8 g/m^2 (48.6 g/$m^{2.7}$) at 24 months (p<0.05)

LV left ventricle, *MRI* magnetic resonance imaging, *RDN* renal denervation, *dRHTN* drug-resistant hypertension

17.4 Effects of RDN on Arrhythmias

Alterations of the SNS-baroreflex axis constitute independent predictors of arrhythmogenic death even after accounting for reduced ejection fraction [6, 25]. The increase in SNS activation to the heart increases abnormal calcium cycling and decreases the myocardial contractility. Patients with arrhythmias detected in Holter monitoring (ventricular ectopy, atrial fibrillation (AF), sudden cardiac death) are characterized by higher muscle sympathetic nerve traffic further supporting the arrhythmogenic nature of SNS activation in the heart. It is well established that SNS activation and heightened plasma catecholamines are accompanied by increased heart rate and may exert direct pro-arrhythmic effects by facilitating reentry, triggered activity, automaticity or increasing excitability [25]. In animal models episodes of atrial fibrillation during short-term rapid atrial pacing or mediated through tracheal occlusion could be decreased by RDN. This beneficial impact of RDN on arrhythmic burden and heart rate could be attributed to the reduction of central sympathetic cardiac driving although the latter is not consistently exhibited in all studies. Improvement in BP control and regression of LV hypertrophy could also play a role in the decrease of cardiac arrhythmias.

In humans, Pokushalov et al. studied 27 moderately hypertensive patients with atrial fibrillation treated with pulmonary vein isolation alone and in combination with RDN and resulted in decreased atrial fibrillation relapse with RDN plus pulmonary vein isolation compared with the latter alone (69 % versus 29 %) [26]. In these lines, patients with paroxysmal atrial fibrillation or persistent atrial fibrillation and moderate dRHTN or severe dRHTN were randomized to pulmonary vein isolation or pulmonary vein isolation with RDN. At 12 months, 63 % were atrial fibrillation free in the RDN group compared to 41 % in the non-RDN group. The superior efficacy of adding RDN was most apparent in persistent atrial fibrillation and severe hypertension [6, 26]. Currently there are many ongoing randomized controlled studies examining the efficacy and safety of RDN as an add-on therapy to AF ablation.

Besides the important effect of RDN on heart rate and arrhythmic events, a significant improvement in both the time and frequency heart rate variability (HRV) parameters was evident in patients with dRHTN at 1 month and was even more pronounced at 6 months after the procedure [25]. The findings of this study regarding the impact of RDN on heart rate variability parameters are concordant with pharmacological reduction of sympathetic overactivity after long-term β-blocker therapy.

From a clinical point of view, RDN may provide a novel approach to attenuate heart rate and improve the arrhythmia profile and heart rate variability status in patients with dRHTN beyond BP reduction. Toward this end, 21 patients with persistent atrial fibrillation and hypertension underwent RDN and completed 7-day follow-up evaluations, including 24-h Holter monitoring. It was shown that RDN improved ventricular heart rate control in patients with persistent atrial fibrillation, slowing conduction in baseline heart rate-dependent manner [26].

Lastly, the potential of RDN to favorably modulate ventricular tachycardia in humans has been studied in small population. Based on these preliminary results in diverse clinical settings of ischemic, dilated, and hypertrophic cardiomyopathy, RDN proved its beneficial impact on ventricular ectopy [26]. Whether RDN has an antiarrhythmic effect beyond normalization of blood pressure and LV mass, amelioration remains to be determined.

17.5 RDN Effect on Arterial Properties

The impact of sympathetic modulation on large arteries has not been extensively explored. In a pioneer controlled study of 110 hypertensive patients, bilateral RDN caused a reduction of aortic augmentation index and carotid to femoral pulse wave velocity at 6 months after the procedure [6]. Consistently, ejection duration and aortic systolic pressure load were significantly diminished, indicating improvement of cardiac work load by RDN. In this work, no significant changes were obtained in the control arm for any of the abovementioned parameters. Assessing sympathetic nerve activity in addition to arterial stiffness alterations by RDN in dRHTN provides valuable clinical information as shown in the study by Hering D et al. [27] in which RDN significantly reduced BP, augmentation index, and muscle sympathetic nerve activity. Of note, changes in augmentation index with RDN were unrelated to systolic BP and diastolic BP (as well as muscle sympathetic nerve activity changes). There were no changes in BP, augmentation index, and sympathetic drive in the non-RDN group. However, in another report of 54 dRHTN patients, there is a lack of beneficial effect of RDN on pulse wave velocity that was increased, whereas augmentation index did not change 12 months post RDN [24]. Therefore, the changes on arterial properties by RDN should be further investigated in adequately powered controlled studies in order to elucidate the confounding effect of BP reduction and neuromodulation.

17.6 Effects of RDN on Glucose Metabolism

SNS overdrive is involved in glucose metabolism and decreasing insulin secretion, and vice versa insulin resistance causes further SNS overdrive [6, 28–30]. In various experimental models, which include obesity-induced hypertension, deoxycorticosterone acetate-induced hypertension, and aortic coarctation, the magnitude of hypertension has been reduced during the observation period post RDN. Central sympathetic output reduction causing an alteration in afferent sympathetic action, an inhibition of the renin-angiotensin-aldosterone-system, a decrease in vascular alpha adrenergic tone resulting in skeletal muscle vasodilation, and an improved glucose transport to the skeletal muscle are suggested mechanisms linking RDN with glucose regulation.

In animals made hyperinsulinemic by insulin infusion via osmotic minipumps implanted subcutaneously, surgically bilateral RDN prevented the development of hyperinsulinemia-induced hypertension, suggesting that RDN not only prevents hypertension but also reverses the pressor effects of insulin [6, 29].

Table 17.2 Major studies of RDN effect on glucose status

Study	Treatment	Patients	Time of follow-up	Change in BP after RDN	Glucose metabolism parameters changes
Mahfoud et al. [28]	RDN Optimal medical therapy	37 with dRHTN 13 with dRHTN	3 months	↓32/12 mmHg (office)	↓ Fasting glucose by 10 mg/dL ↓ Insulin levels by 11.5 mIU/mL ↓C-peptide levels by 2.3 ng/mL ↓ Homeostasis model assessment–insulin resistance (HOMA-IR by 3.6)
Witkowski et al. [30]	RDN	10 with dRHTN and metabolic syndrome	6 months	↓34/13 mmHg (office)	↓ Plasma glucose concentration 2-h after oral glucose tolerance test by 0.6 mmol/L ↓HbA1c by 0.5 %
Verloop Wi et al. [31]	RDN	29 patients with metabolic syndrome	12 months	↓6/5 mmHg (ambulatory)	No significant changes in fasting glucose and insulin sensitivity

RDN renal denervation, *dRHTN* drug-resistant hypertension

Based on this pathophysiological evidence, catheter-based RDN was tested on glycemic control. The landmark study in this field is the one by Mahfoud et al. [28], investigating the effect of RDN on glucose metabolism and insulin resistance in patients with dRHTN. Three months after RDN, besides mean BP reduction, fasting glucose was statistically significantly reduced from 118 to 108 mg/dL, insulin levels from 20.8 to 9.3 mIU/mL, C-peptide levels decreased from 5.3 to 3.0 ng/mL, and homeostasis model assessment–insulin resistance (HOMA-IR) improved from 6.0 to 2.4, while no BP reduction and metabolic marker changes were observed in the control group (Table 17.2).

The favorable effect of RDN on glucose metabolism is also shown in a report for two female patients with polycystic ovary syndrome in whom fasting plasma glucose declined and insulin sensitivity improved 3 months after RDN, and this was accompanied by reduction of SNS activity assessed by muscle sympathetic drive and norepinephrine spillover [29]. Another study carried out in ten obese dRHTN patients with obstructive sleep apnea syndrome in whom plasma glucose concentration of 2-h after oral glucose tolerance test significantly reduced from 7.0 to 6.4 mmol/L and HbA1c decreased from 6.1 to 5.6 % at 6 months after neuromodulation therapy [30].

Nevertheless, the denervation of the renal arteries in the metabolic syndrome (DREAMS-Study) investigating the effects of RDN on insulin sensitivity and BP in patients with metabolic syndrome, questioned the beneficial impact of RDN on insulin metabolism. More specifically, 29 patients fulfilling the criteria for metabolic syndrome and who used a maximum of one antihypertensive and one antidiabetic drug or one of both were treated by RDN. Median insulin sensitivity as assessed by the simple index assessing insulin sensitivity oral glucose tolerance test did not change at 6- and 12-month follow-up. Measurements of sympathetic activity showed no reduction in SNS activity [31] (Table 17.2). The results are limited by the non-randomized nature of the design, the lack of control group, and the fact that patients with type 2 diabetes were underrepresented in the total population. Currently there is a need for randomized controlled studies in hypertensive patients with metabolic syndrome and/or diabetes mellitus in order to better define the effect of RDN on the glucose status.

References

1. Mancia G, Grassi G, Giannattasio C, Seravalle G (1999) Sympathetic activation in the pathogenesis of hypertension and progression of organ damage. Hypertension 34:724–728
2. Tsioufis C, Kordalis A, Flessas D et al (2011) Pathophysiology of resistant hypertension: the role of sympathetic nervous system. Int J Hypertens 2011:642416
3. Tsioufis C, Dimitriadis K, Thomopoulos C, Doumas M, Papademetriou V, Stefanadis C (2014) Renal and cardiac effects of renal sympathetic denervation and carotid baroreceptor stimulation. Curr Vasc Pharmacol 12(1):55–62
4. Schlaich MP, Socratous F, Hennebry S et al (2009) Sympathetic activation in chronic renal failure. J Am Soc Nephrol 20:933–939
5. McArdle MJ, deGoma EM, Cohen DL, Townsend RR, Wilensky RL, Giri J (2016) Beyond blood pressure: percutaneous renal denervation for the management of sympathetic hyperactivity and associated disease states. J Am Heart Assoc 4(3). pii: e001415. doi:10.1161/JAHA.114.001415
6. Grassi G, Quarti Trevano F, Seravalle G et al (2011) Early sympathetic activation in the initial stages of chronic renal failure. Hypertension 57:846–851
7. Rao F, Wessel J, Wen G, Zhang L et al (2007) Renal albumin excretion. Twin studies identify influences of heredity, environment, and adrenergic pathway polymorphism. Hypertension 49:1015–1031
8. Vink EE, Blankestijn PJ (2012) Evidence and consequences of the central role of the kidneys in the pathophysiology of sympathetic hyperactivity. Front Phys 3:29, Epub 2012 Feb 20
9. Tsioufis C, Papademetriou V, Dimitriadis K, Tsiachris D, Thomopoulos C, Park E, Hata C, Papalois A, Stefanadis C (2013) Catheter-based renal sympathetic denervation exerts acute and chronic effects on renalhemodynamics in swine. Int J Cardiol 168(2):987–992
10. Krum H, Schlaich M, Whitbourn R et al (2009) Catheter-based renal sympathetic denervation for resistant hypertension: a multicentre safety and proof-of-principle cohort study. Lancet 373:1275–1281
11. Krum H, Barman N, Schlaich M et al (2011) Catheter-based renal sympathetic denervation for resistant hypertension: durability of blood pressure reduction out to 24 months. Hypertension 57:911–917
12. Esler MD, Krum H, Sobotka PA, Schlaich MP, Schmieder RE, Bohm M (2010) Renal sympathetic denervation in patients with treatment-resistant hypertension (The Symplicity HTN-2 Trial): a randomised controlled trial. Lancet 376:1903–1909
13. Worthley SG, Tsioufis CP, Worthley MI, Sinhal A, Chew DP, Meredith IT, Malaiapan Y, Papademetriou V (2013) Safety and efficacy of a multi-electrode renal sympathetic denervation system in resistant hypertension: the EnligHTN I trial. Eur Heart J 34(28):2132–2140

14. Tsioufis CP, Papademetriou V, Dimitriadis KS, Kasiakogias A, Tsiachris D, Worthley MI, Sinhal AR, Chew DP, Meredith IT, Malaiapan Y, Thomopoulos C, Kallikazaros I, Tousoulis D, Worthley SG (2015) Catheter-based renal denervation for resistant hypertension: twenty-four month results of theEnligHTN I first-in-human study using a multi-electrode ablation system. Int J Cardiol 201:345–350
15. Bhatt DL, Kandzari DE, O'Neill WW, D'Agostino R, Flack JM, Katzen BT, Leon MB, Liu M, Mauri L, Negoita M, Cohen SA, Oparil S, Rocha-Singh K, Townsend RR, Bakris GL; SYMPLICITY HTN-3Investigators (2014) A controlled trial of renal denervation for resistant hypertension. N Engl J Med 370(15):1393–1401
16. Ott C, Mahfoud F, Schmid A, Ditting T, Veelken R, Ewen S, Ukena C, Uder M, Böhm M, Schmieder RE (2014) Improvement of albuminuria after renal denervation. Int J Cardiol 173(2):311–315
17. Mahfoud F, Cremers B, Janker J, Link B, Vonend O, Ukena C, Linz D, Schmieder R, Rump LC, Kindermann I, Sobotka PA, Krum H, Scheller B, Schlaich M, Laufs U, Böhm M (2012) Renal hemodynamics and renal function after catheter-based renal sympathetic denervation in patients with resistant hypertension. Hypertension 60(2):419–424
18. Lu D, Wang K, Liu Q, Wang S, Zhang Q, Shan Q (2016) Reductions of left ventricular mass and atrial size following renal denervation: a meta-analysis. Clin Res Cardiol. [Epub ahead of print]
19. Brandt M, Mahfoud F, Reda S et al (2012) Renal sympathetic denervation reduces left ventricular hypertrophy and improves cardiac function in patients with resistant hypertension. J Am Coll Cardiol 59:901–909
20. Tsioufis C, Papademetriou V, Dimitriadis K, Tsiachris D, Thomopoulos C, Kasiakogias A, Kordalis A, Kefala A, Koutra E, Lau EO, Grassi G, Stefanadis C (2015) Effects of multielectrode renal denervation on cardiac and neurohumoral adaptations in resistant hypertension with cardiac hypertrophy: an EnligHTN I substudy. J Hypertens 33(2):346–353
21. Tsioufis C, Papademetriou V, Dimitriadis K, Kasiakogias A, Kordalis A, Andrikou E, Milkas A, Liatakis I, Oi-Yan Lau E, Tousoulis D (2016) Long-term effects of multielectrode renal denervation on cardiac adaptations in resistant hypertensive patients with left ventricular hypertrophy. J Hum Hypertens. doi:10.1038/jhh.2015.127. [Epub ahead of print]
22. Doltra A, Messroghli D, Stawowy P, Hassel JH, Gebker R, Leppänen O, Gräfe M et al (2014) Potential reduction of interstitial myocardial fibrosis with renal denervation. J Am Heart Assoc 3(6):e001353. doi:10.1161/JAHA.114.001353
23. Mahfoud F, Urban D, Teller D, Linz D, Stawowy P, Hassel JH et al (2014) Effect of renal denervation on left ventricular mass and function in patients with resistant hypertension: data from a multi-centre cardiovascular magnetic resonance imaging trial. Eur Heart J 35:2224–2231
24. Verloop WL, Vink EE, Spiering W, Blankestijn PJ, Doevendans PA, Bots ML, Vonken EJ, Voskuil M, Leiner T (2015) Effects of renal denervation on end organ damage in hypertensive patients. Eur J Prev Cardiol 22(5):558–567
25. Tsioufis C, Papademetriou V, Tsiachris D, Dimitriadis K, Kasiakogias A, Kordalis A, Antonakis V, Kefala A, Thomopoulos C, Kallikazaros I, Lau EO, Stefanadis C (2014) Drug-resistant hypertensive patients responding to multielectrode renal denervation exhibit improved heart rate dynamics and reduced arrhythmia burden. J Hum Hypertens 28(10):587–593
26. Kosiuk J, Hilbert S, Pokushalov E, Hindricks G, Steinberg JS, Bollmann A (2015) Renal denervation for treatment of cardiac arrhythmias: state of the art and future directions. J Cardiovasc Electrophysiol 26(2):233–238
27. Hering D, Lambert EA, Marusic P, Ika-Sari C, Walton AS, Krum H, Sobotka PA, Mahfoud F, Böhm M, Lambert GW, Esler MD, Schlaich MP (2013) Renal nerve ablation reduces augmentation index in patients with resistant hypertension. J Hypertens 31(9):1893–1900
28. Mahfoud F, Schlaich M, Kindermann I et al (2011) Catheter-based renal sympathetic denervation on glucose metabolism in patients with resistant hypertension: a pilot study. Circulation 123:1940–1946

29. Pan T, Guo JH, Teng GJ (2015) Renal denervation: a potential novel treatment for type 2 diabetes mellitus? Medicine (Baltimore) 94(44):e1932
30. Witkowski A, Prejbisz A, Florczak E, Kądziela J, Śliwiński P, Bieleń P, MichałowskaI I, Kabat M, Warchoł E, Januszewicz M, Narkiewicz K, Somers VK, Sobotka PA, Januszewicz A (2011) Effects of renal sympathetic denervation on blood pressure, sleep apnea course, and glycemic control in patients with resistant hypertension and sleep apnea. Hypertension 58(4):559–565
31. Verloop WL, Spiering W, Vink EE, Beeftink MM, Blankestijn PJ, Doevendans PA, Voskuil M (2015) Denervation of the renal arteries in metabolic syndrome: the DREAMS-study. Hypertension 65(4):751–757

Renal Denervation for Chronic Heart Failure

18

Michael Böhm, Sebastian Ewen, Ina Zivanovic, and Felix Mahfoud

Abbreviations

BP	Blood pressure
HF	Heart failure
HTN	Hypertension
SNS	Sympathetic nervous system

18.1 Activation of the Sympathetic Nervous System in Heart Failure

In chronic heart failure (HF), the activation of the sympathetic nervous system (SNS) [1] and the renin-angiotensin system [2] as well as pro-inflammatory activation [3] is associated with remodeling processes and maladaptive cardiac signal transduction [4]. Sympathetic activation plays a crucial role and is closely related to cardiovascular outcomes as judged from circulating norepinephrine (NE) concentrations [5, 6]. It is also likely to be involved in progression of the syndrome because norepinephrine concentrations are already increased in asymptomatic left ventricular dysfunction before clinical relevant heart failure symptoms develop [7].

M. Böhm, MD (✉) • S. Ewen • I. Zivanovic • F. Mahfoud
Universitätsklinikum des Saarlandes, Klinik für Innere Medizin III, Kardiologie, Angiologie und Internistische Intensivmedizin, Kirrberger Str. 1, Homburg/Saar, DE 66424, Germany
e-mail: michael.boehm@uks.eu

C. Tsioufis et al. (eds.), *Interventional Therapies for Secondary and Essential Hypertension*, Updates in Hypertension and Cardiovascular Protection,
DOI 10.1007/978-3-319-34141-5_18

Sympathetic activation is generated by the nucleus tractus solitarius in the midbrain and rostral ventrolateral medulla [8]. Efferent signaling to the heart adapts cardiac output to peripheral stress situations with an increase of chronotropy, inotropy, and dromotropy as well as increasing intraventricular conduction velocity (bathmotropy). After long-standing activation, cardiac phenotypes can change resulting in hypertrophy and fibrosis making the heart more prone to arrhythmia development, as well as pump function and relaxation disturbances. In HF, vasoconstriction and sodium retention are the results of α-adrenoceptor stimulation [9], whereas after long-standing neuroendocrine stimulation, endothelial dysfunction and oxidative stress are harbingers of structural changes of the vasculature [8] and end-organ damage, in particular impaired renal function [10, 11]. In the liver, SNS activation increases gluconeogenesis and glycogenolysis. Furthermore, SNS activation by α-adrenoceptor-mediated vasoconstriction shifts the blood flow away from insulin-sensitive organs and might make patients more prone to develop impaired glucose tolerance and diabetes mellitus type 2 [12, 13]. In the central nervous system, CO_2 sensitivity is enhanced contributing to dyspnea and in conditions like HF [14], in particular with congestion and volume overload [15]. Furthermore, sleep apnea is associated with sympathetic activation in hypertensives and patients with chronic HF [16, 17]. Blood pressure (BP) is upregulated by an increase of β1-adrenoceptor-mediated renin activation, sodium retention, and an impairment of renal blood flow [8]. All these conditions resemble those disturbances that are observed in chronic HF and in patients presenting with impaired myocardial function, associated with a high likelihood of developing comorbidities like diabetes mellitus type 2, renal impairment, and arrhythmias like atrial fibrillation or even sudden cardiac death [18]. The interaction of centrally generated sympathetic drive with peripheral organs is summarized in Fig. 18.1.

Among these mechanisms, the interplay between renal sympathetic activity and the central nervous system is crucial [19]. While activated efferents from the brain activate sodium retention and reduce renal blood flow, the renal afferents provide feedback to the brain with some of the signals being mediated by adenosine, oxidative stress, ischemia, and acidosis [11, 20, 21]. Afferent stimulation of the brain further increases sympathetic efferent activation leading to a vicious cycle in the interaction between the brain and kidneys to further enhance total body SNS activity [8, 11]. It has been shown that SNS activation occurring in different forms of hypertension (HTN) [22] is further enhanced in HF [1] and its comorbidities like metabolic syndrome [13] and renal failure [23]. Thus, a sympathetically cardiorenovascular continuum occurs during the progression from mild to severe organ damage and contributes to cardiac or renal-associated comorbidities.

18.2 Maladaptive Beta-Adrenergic Signal Transduction

Norepinephrine released from the sympathetic nerves in the heart produces excessive beta-adrenergic receptor stimulation [24]. As a consequence, beta receptors are downregulated [25], and post-receptor events like an increase of inhibitory G-proteins [26] produce an impaired effectiveness of cAMP-dependent positive inotropic agents like beta-adrenergic agonists and phosphodiesterase type 3 inhibitors [25, 26]. Beyond the receptor and post-receptor defects, there is a depletion of

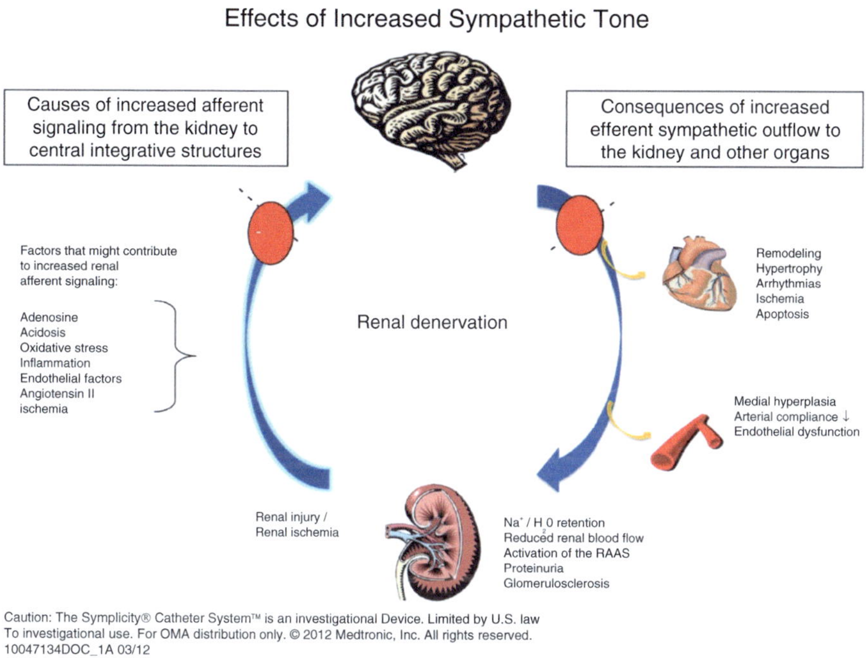

Fig. 18.1 Pathophysiological interaction between the brain, the kidney, and other peripheral organs like the heart, liver, and vasculature after sympathetic activity is enhanced. Generated in the sympathetic nervous system, efferent signals stimulate the heart and other organs producing maladaptive responses. In the kidney, sympathetic activation reduces renal blood flow, increases sodium retention, and activates renin-angiotensin system. Efferents further enhance sympathetic outflow providing a vicious cycle in the stepwise increase of the sympathetic activation in the interaction between the heart and the brain (Modified from Böhm et al. [11])

cardiac norepinephrine storing and a defect of uptake in the failing heart [27, 28] (Fig. 18.2). Serum norepinephrine concentrations are associated with mortality in chronic heart failure [5, 6]. In addition, not only cardiac but also renal norepinephrine spillover is increased and related to the severity of heart failure ([29], Fig. 18.3). Interestingly, also renal spillover is associated with poor outcomes ([30], Fig. 18.4). Abovementioned aspects gave the pathophysiologic background for the hypothesis that an intervention at the renal SNS could influence the outcome in chronic heart failure by reducing detrimental sympathetic activation.

18.3 Renal Denervation in Hypertension

The first clinical studies on lumbar splanchnicectomy involving sympathetic renal denervation (RDN) were done in severe HTN in the 1950s. Total paralumbar splanchnicectomy led to an increase of survival rates in patients with severe HTN and cardiovascular disease [31–33]. Severe adverse effects and high mortality were observed, and the method was left after the development of efficient and tolerable antihypertensive drugs.

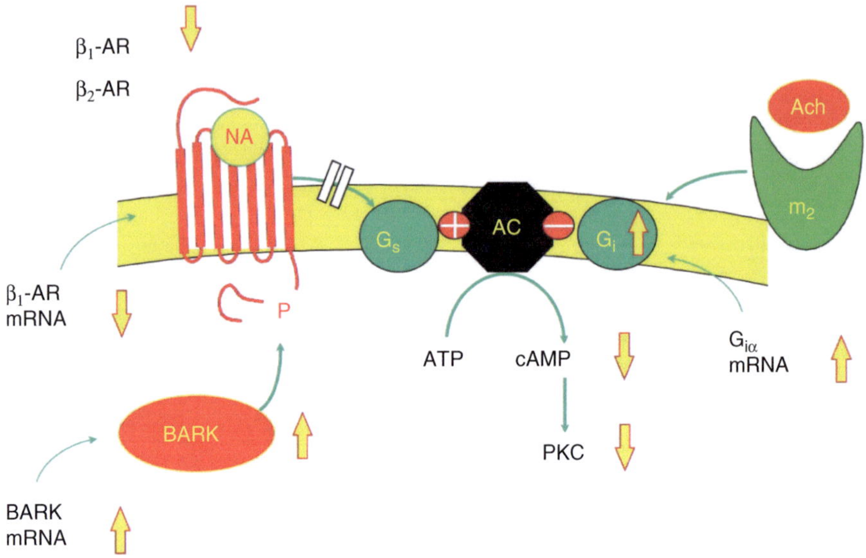

Fig. 18.2 Summary of beta-adrenergic signal transduction in heart failure [28]

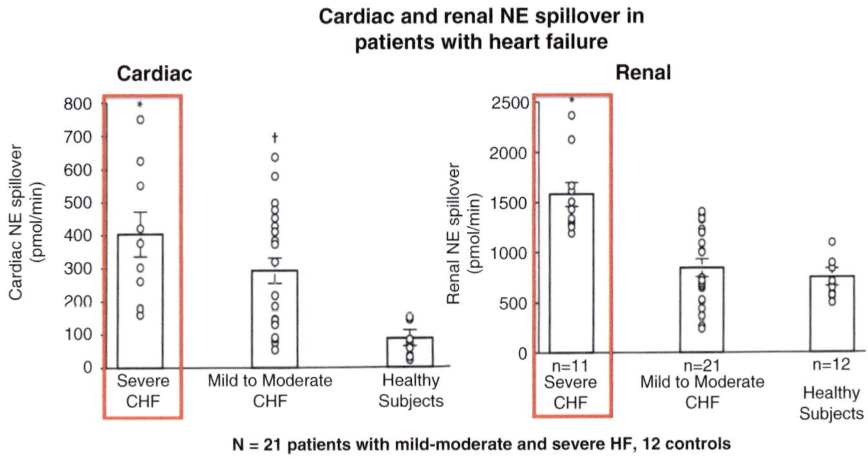

Fig. 18.3 Cardiac (*left*) and renal (*right*) norepinephrine (NE) spillover in patients with chronic heart failure. Spillover in the kidney and the heart, respectively, is more activated in severe and in mild to moderate heart failure and healthy subjects (Modified from Hasking et al. [29])

18.4 Interventional Renal Denervation

Renal sympathetic denervation was performed in patients with resistant HTN (patients being on three or more drugs, one has to be a diuretic, not achieving an optimal blood pressure control). The associated BP reduction was not accompanied by chronotropic incompetence [34-39], but was able to reduce peripheral artery

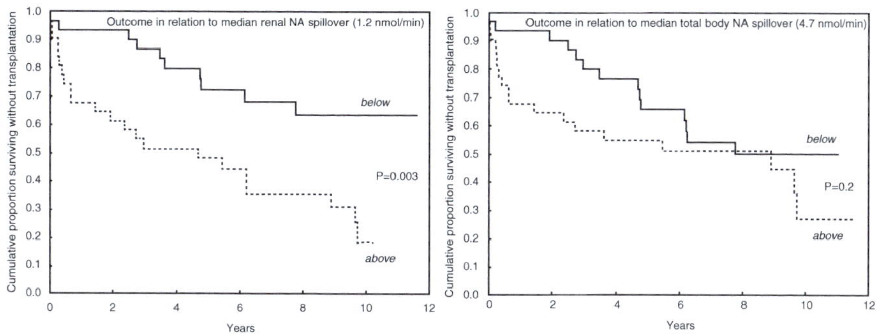

Fig. 18.4 Kaplan-Meier curves showing the portion of surviving without heart transplantation according to renal norepinephrine spillover (*left*), total body norepinephrine spillover (*right*) in individuals with chronic heart failure (Modified from Petersson et al. [30])

stiffness [40] and reduces myocardial hypertrophy, at least partly BP independent [41]. These studies in hypertensives provided evidence that reducing sympathetic activity is able to reduce cardiovascular function due to reducing myocardial hypertrophy [41], thus setting the stage to perform trials in heart failure.

18.5 Pilot Studies in Heart Failure

Heart failure is often affected by low BP hampering the possibilities to apply evidence-proven drugs often associated with further BP reductions to improve the outcomes. For this reason, a first pilot study (REACH, NCT 01639378) has studied HF in patients with reduced ejection fraction and a BP above 120 mmHg systolic [42]. Blood pressure before and after RDN remained stable in these patients at 6 months follow-up. Interestingly, after RDN there was an increase of 6 min walk test despite no change in BP. The reason might be that RDN might redistribute the blood flow after reduction of sympathetic activation and counteract the sympathetically mediated reduction of the venous reservoir and sodium-water retention, thereby reducing congestion [43].

18.6 Accompanying Diseases in Heart Failure

18.6.1 Atrial Fibrillation and Sleep Apnea

Atrial fibrillation is due to functional changes of the atria, which follows the progressive remodeling of the ventricles in hypertrophy with preserved or impaired left ventricular fraction. There is a high prevalence and incidence of atrial fibrillation in HF which produces a symptomatic burden in these patients and also increases the risk of stroke [18]. Furthermore, HF is associated with sleep apnea, which in turn is associated with atrial fibrillation. In an experimental study, intermittent negative

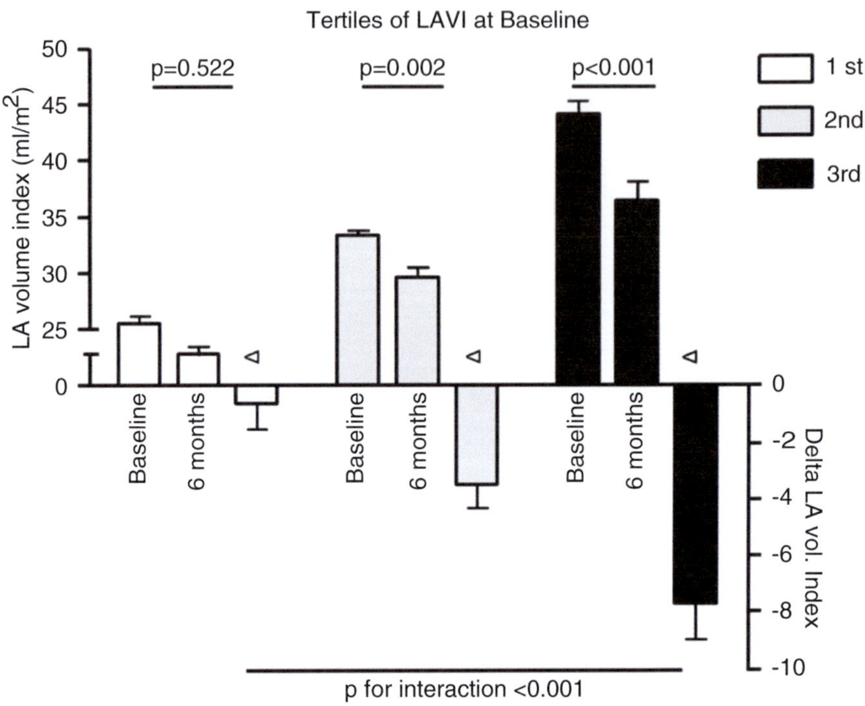

Fig. 18.5 Left atrial remodeling according to tertiles of left ventricular and left atrial volume index at baseline (Modified according to Schirmer et al. [49])

tracheal pressure was associated with an enhanced inducibility of atrial fibrillation, which was accompanied by a shortening of the atrial effective refractory period [44]. Renal denervation abolished the electrophysiological effect and reduced atrial fibrillation by 70% [45]. The atrial fibrillation cycle length was not affected, but there was a better rate control reflected by an increase of the cycle length of the ventricle during atrial fibrillation. Trials are ongoing to study the effect of RDN on atrial remodeling and the recurrence rate after pulmonary vein isolation [46]. Interestingly, RDN was associated with a reduction of atrial size as judged by echocardiography [47] and magnetic resonance imaging [48]. Remodeling of the atria was observed to be independent of BP, but related to fewer atrial ectopies (Fig. 18.5) [49]. In a sheep model of atrial remodeling, RDN inhibited the renal sympathetic nerve sprouting in the atria [50].

18.6.2 Ventricular Arrhythmias

In a model with acute myocardial ischemia and reperfusion in pigs, RDN reduced ventricular ectopies and ventricular fibrillation [51]. This effect was not accompanied by action-potential changes and was not occurring during reperfusion

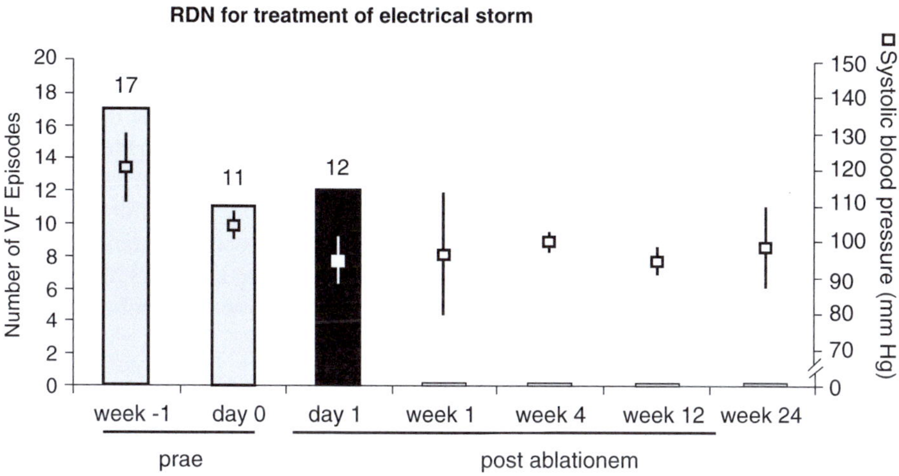

Fig. 18.6 Effect of renal denervation in a patient with dilated cardiomyopathy presenting with an electrical storm. Depicted are the numbers of ventricular fibrillation episodes (*left*) and the systolic blood pressure values (*right*). It becomes clear that after 1 week of renal denervation no further charges of the intracardiac cardioverter defibrillator (ICD) were detected. The blood pressure was particularly low in this patient, but remained stable over time (Modified according to Ukena et al. [52])

showing that abolition of ventricular fibrillation during ischemia might be directly due to an effect of sympathetic withdrawal by RDN. There is a preliminary report on two patients with cardiomyopathy suffering an electrical storm. In these patients RDN on the background of full antiarrhythmic therapy and optimized heart failure treatments abolished discharges from an implanted cardiac defibrillator [52] (Fig. 18.6). More data and larger case series have been recently presented [53].

18.6.3 Renal Dysfunction

In patients with resistant HTN, the method was safe in terms of deterioration of renal function in the Symplicity-HTN trials. However, in these trials only patients with a glomerular filtration rate (GFR) >45 ml/min were enrolled. In preliminary studies it was shown that BP reduction was similar in patients with impaired renal function [36] or terminal renal failure [54]. Even at lower levels of GFR, there was no signal of deterioration of renal function, at least when RDN was performed by investigators experienced with the technique and careful use of contrast medium [36, 54]. Indeed, RDN was able to reduce microalbuminuria, most likely by an improvement of intrarenal hemodynamics [55]. In sleep apnea induced in pigs, RDN was able to abolish the drop in renal perfusion and attenuated the rise in renin activation after obstructive episodes [56]. Data on the long-term renal effects in conditions other than HTN are presently lacking.

18.6.4 Diabetes

Patients with symptomatic HF suffer from insulin resistance and diabetes in 50 % of the cases. Insulin resistance is depending on SNS activation and is most likely due to a shift of blood flow away from insulin-sensitive organs [11–14]. In patients with resistant HTN, RDN has been shown to improve an impaired fasting glucose level. Furthermore, there was a reduction of fasting insulin and fasting C-peptide concentrations. Insulin sensitivity was improved in patients with glucose intolerance and resistant HTN as judged from the HOMA index [57]. However, it appears likely that RDN could provide an upstream therapy for the development of metabolic disease in situations where SNS activation is enhanced.

18.7 Perspective

Heart failure is associated with activation of the SNS which presumably results in a progression of the syndrome and thereby in poor outcome. Renal denervation should be studied in conditions with enhanced SNS activity. In HF, the first studies are ongoing assessing whether RDN can improve myocardial function and signs and symptoms of HF in patients with both preserved and reduced ejection fraction. It is necessary to study clinical outcomes in larger prospective trials involving sham procedures because symptomatic improvements are affected by placebo and Hawthorne effects in interventional trials. Furthermore, novel interventional approaches [58], devices, and trial designs [59] according to recent consensus conferences [60] must be taken into consideration. Renal denervation is a promising approach to improve outcome in patients with different cardiovascular disease including chronic HF.

Conflict of Interests MB received scientific support and speaker's honoraria from Bayer, Boehringer Ingelheim, Medtronic, and Servier. MB is supported by the Deutsche Forschungsgemeinschaft and FM by the Hochdruckliga and the German Cardiac Society.

References

1. Floras JS (2009) Sympathetic nervous system activation in human heart failure: clinical implications of an updated model. J Am Coll Cardiol 54:375–385
2. Holmer S, Rinne B, Eckardt KU, Le Hir M, Schricker K, Kaissling B, Riegger G, Kurtz A (1994) Role of renal nerves for the expression of renin in adult rat kidney. Am J Physiol 266:F738–F745
3. Hofmann U, Frantz S (2013) How can we cure a heart "in flame"? A translational view on inflammation in heart failure. Basic Res Cardiol 108:356
4. Heineke J, Molkentin JD (2006) Regulation of cardiac hypertrophy by intracellular signalling pathways. Nat Rev Mol Cell Biol 7(8):589–600
5. Cohn JN, Levine TB, Olivari MT, Garberg V, Lura D, Francis GS, Simon AB, Rector T (1984) Plasma norepinephrine as a guide to prognosis in patients with chronic congestive heart failure. N Engl J Med 311:819–823

6. Rector TS, Olivari MT, Levine TB, Francis GS, Cohn JN (1987) Predicting survival for an individual with congestive heart failure using the plasma norepinephrine concentration. Am Heart J 114:148–152
7. Francis GS, Benedict C, Johnstone DE, Kirlin PC, Nicklas J, Liang CS, Kubo SH, Rudin-Toretsky E, Yusuf S (1990) Comparison of neuroendocrine activation in patients with left ventricular dysfunction with and without congestive heart failure. A substudy of the Studies of Left Ventricular Dysfunction (SOLVD). Circulation 82:1724–1729
8. Esler M (2010) The 2009 Carl Ludwig Lecture: Pathophysiology of the human sympathetic nervous system in cardiovascular diseases: the transition from mechanisms to medical management. J Appl Physiol 108:227–237
9. DiBona GF, Sawin LL (1991) Role of renal nerves in sodium retention of cirrhosis and congestive heart failure. Am J Physiol 260:R298–R305
10. Campese VM (1997) Neurogenic factors and hypertension in chronic renal failure. J Nephrol 10:184–187
11. Böhm M, Linz D, Ukena C, Esler M, Mahfoud F (2014) Renal denervation for the treatment of cardiovascular high risk-hypertension or beyond? Circ Res 115:400–409
12. Huggett RJ, Scott EM, Gilbey SG, Stoker JB, Mackintosh AF, Mary DA (2003) Impact of type 2 diabetes mellitus on sympathetic neural mechanisms in hypertension. Circulation 108: 3097–3101
13. Mancia G, Bousquet P, Elghozi JL, Esler M, Grassi G, Julius S, Reid J, Van Zwieten PA (2007) The sympathetic nervous system and the metabolic syndrome. J Hypertens 25:909–920
14. Sobotka PA, Krum H, Böhm M, Francis DP, Schlaich MP (2012) The role of renal denervation in the treatment of heart failure. Curr Cardiol Rep 14:285–292
15. Dunlap ME, Sobotka PA (2013) Fluid re-distribution rather than accumulation causes most cases of decompensated heart failure. J Am Coll Cardiol 62:165–166
16. Peppard PE, Young T, Palta M, Skatrud J (2000) Prospective study of the association between sleep-disordered breathing and hypertension. N Engl J Med 342:1378–1384
17. Logan AG, Perlikowski SM, Mente A, Tisler A, Tkacova R, Niroumand M, Leung RS, Bradley TD (2001) High prevalence of unrecognized sleep apnoea in drug-resistant hypertension. J Hypertens 19:2271–2277
18. McMurray JJ, Adamopoulos S, Anker SD, Auricchio A, Böhm M, Dickstein K, Falk V, Filippatos G, Fonseca C, Gomez-Sanchez MA, Jaarsma T, Køber L, Lip GY, Maggioni AP, Parkhomenko A, Pieske BM, Popescu BA, Rønnevik PK, Rutten FH, Schwitter J, Seferovic P, Stepinska J, Trindade PT, Voors AA, Zannad F, Zeiher A, ESC Committee for Practice Guidelines (2012) ESC Guidelines for the diagnosis and treatment of acute and chronic heart failure 2012: The Task Force for the Diagnosis and Treatment of Acute and Chronic Heart Failure 2012 of the European Society of Cardiology. Developed in collaboration with the Heart Failure Association (HFA) of the ESC. Eur Heart J 33:1787–1847
19. Ljungqvist A, Wågermark J (1970) The adrenergic innervation of intrarenal glomerular and extra-glomerular circulatory routes. Nephron 7:218–229
20. Stella A, Zanchetti A (1991) Functional role of renal afferents. Physiol Rev 71:659–682
21. Katholi RE, Whitlow PL, Hageman GR, Woods WT (1984) Intrarenal adenosine produces hypertension by activating the sympathetic nervous system via the renal nerves in the dog. J Hypertens 2:349–359
22. Esler M, Lambert G, Jennings G (1989) Regional norepinephrine turnover in human hypertension. Clin Exp Hypertens A Suppl 1:75–89
23. Hausberg M, Kosch M, Harmelink P, Barenbrock M, Hohage H, Kisters K, Dietl KH, Rahn KH (2002) Sympathetic nerve activity in end-stage renal disease. Circulation 106:1974–1979
24. Swedberg K, Viquerat C, Rouleau JL, Roizen M, Atherton B, Parmley WW, Chatterjee K (1984) Comparison of myocardial catecholamine balance in chronic congestive heart failure and in angina pectoris without failure. Am J Cardiol 54:783–786
25. Böhm M, Beuckelmann D, Brown L, Feiler G, Lorenz B, Näbauer M, Kemkes B, Erdmann E (1988) Reduction of beta-adrenoceptor density and evaluation of positive inotropic responses in isolated, diseased human myocardium. Eur Heart J 9:844–852

26. Böhm M, Gierschik P, Jakobs KH, Pieske B, Schnabel P, Ungerer M, Erdmann E (1990) Increase of Gi alpha in human hearts with dilated but not ischemic cardiomyopathy. Circulation 82:1249–1265
27. Goldstein DS, Brush JE Jr, Eisenhofer G, Stull R, Esler M (1988) In vivo measurement of neuronal uptake of norepinephrine in the human heart. Circulation 78:41–48
28. Böhm M, La Rosée K, Schwinger RH, Erdmann E (1995) Evidence for reduction of norepinephrine uptake sites in the failing human heart. J Am Coll Cardiol 25:146–153
29. Hasking GJ, Esler MD, Jennings GL, Burton D, Johns JA, Korner PI (1986) Norepinephrine spillover to plasma in patients with congestive heart failure: evidence of increased overall and cardiorenal sympathetic nervous activity. Circulation 73:615–621
30. Petersson M, Friberg P, Eisenhofer G, Lambert G, Rundqvist B (2005) Long-term outcome in relation to renal sympathetic activity in patients with chronic heart failure. Eur Heart J 26:906–913
31. Page IH (1934) The effect on renal efficiency of lowering arterial blood pressure in cases of essential hypertension and nephritis. J Clin Invest 13:909–915
32. Page IH, Heuer GJ (1935) The effect of renal denervation on the level of arterial blood pressure and renal function in essential hypertension. J Clin Invest 14:27–30
33. Smithwick RH, Thompson JE (1953) Splanchnicectomy for essential hypertension; results in 1,266 cases. J Am Med Assoc 152:1501–1504
34. Krum H, Schlaich M, Whitbourn R, Sobotka PA, Sadowski J, Bartus K, Kapelak B, Walton A, Sievert H, Thambar S, Abraham WT, Esler M (2009) Catheter-based renal sympathetic denervation for resistant hypertension: a multicentre safety and proof-of-principle cohort study. Lancet 373:1275–1281
35. Symplicity HTN-1 Investigators (2011) Catheter-based renal sympathetic denervation for resistant hypertension: durability of blood pressure reduction out to 24 months. Hypertension 57:911–917
36. Hering D, Mahfoud F, Walton AS, Krum H, Lambert GW, Lambert EA, Sobotka PA, Böhm M, Cremers B, Esler MD, Schlaich MP (2012) Renal denervation in moderate to severe CKD. J Am Soc Nephrol 23:1250–1257
37. Symplicity HTN-2 Investigators, Esler MD, Krum H, Sobotka PA, Schlaich MP, Schmieder RE, Böhm M (2010) Renal sympathetic denervation in patients with treatment-resistant hypertension (The Symplicity HTN-2 Trial): a randomised controlled trial. Lancet 376:1903–1909
38. Esler MD, Krum H, Schlaich M, Schmieder RE, Böhm M, Sobotka PA, Symplicity HTN-2 Investigators (2012) Renal sympathetic denervation for treatment of drug-resistant hypertension: one-year results from the Symplicity HTN-2 randomized, controlled trial. Circulation 126:2976–2982
39. Ukena C, Mahfoud F, Kindermann I, Barth C, Lenski M, Kindermann M, Brandt MC, Hoppe UC, Krum H, Esler M, Sobotka PA, Böhm M (2011) Cardiorespiratory response to exercise after renal sympathetic denervation in patients with resistant hypertension. J Am Coll Cardiol 58:1176–1182
40. Brandt MC, Reda S, Mahfoud F, Lenski M, Böhm M, Hoppe UC (2012) Effects of renal sympathetic denervation on arterial stiffness and central hemodynamics in patients with resistant hypertension. J Am Coll Cardiol 60:1956–1965
41. Brandt MC, Mahfoud F, Reda S, Schirmer SH, Erdmann E, Böhm M, Hoppe UC (2012) Renal sympathetic denervation reduces left ventricular hypertrophy and improves cardiac function in patients with resistant hypertension. J Am Coll Cardiol 59:901–909
42. Davies JE, Manisty CH, Petraco R, Barron AJ, Unsworth B, Mayet J, Hamady M, Hughes AD, Sever PS, Sobotka PA, Francis DP (2013) First-in-man safety evaluation of renal denervation for chronic systolic heart failure: primary outcome from REACH-Pilot study. Int J Cardiol 162:189–192
43. Fallick C, Sobotka PA, Dunlap ME (2011) Sympathetically mediated changes in capacitance: redistribution of the venous reservoir as a cause of decompensation. Circ Heart Fail 4: 669–675

44. Linz D, Schotten U, Neuberger HR, Böhm M, Wirth K (2011) Negative tracheal pressure during obstructive respiratory events promotes atrial fibrillation by vagal activation. Heart Rhythm 8:1436–1443
45. Linz D, Mahfoud F, Schotten U, Ukena C, Neuberger HR, Wirth K, Böhm M (2012) Renal sympathetic denervation suppresses postapneic blood pressure rises and atrial fibrillation in a model for sleep apnea. Hypertension 60:172–178
46. Ahmed H, Miller MA, Dukkipati SR, Cammack S, Koruth JS, Gangireddy S, Ellsworth BA, D'Avila A, Domanski M, Gelijns AC, Moskowitz A, Reddy VY (2013) Adjunctive renal sympathetic denervation to modify hypertension as upstream therapy in the treatment of atrial fibrillation (H-FIB) study: clinical background and study design. J Cardiovasc Electrophysiol 24:503–509
47. Schirmer SH, Sayed MM, Reil JC, Ukena C, Linz D, Kindermann M, Laufs U, Mahfoud F, Böhm M (2014) Improvements in left ventricular hypertrophy and diastolic function following renal denervation: effects beyond blood pressure and heart rate reduction. J Am Coll Cardiol 63:1916–1923
48. Mahfoud F, Urban D, Teller D, Linz D, Stawowy P, Hassel JH, Fries P, Dreysse S, Wellnhofer E, Schneider G, Buecker A, Schneeweis C, Doltra A, Schlaich MP, Esler MD, Fleck E, Böhm M, Kelle S (2014) Effect of renal denervation on left ventricular mass and function in patients with resistant hypertension: data from a multi-centre cardiovascular magnetic resonance imaging trial. Eur Heart J 35:2224–2231
49. Schirmer SH, Sayed MM, Reil JC, Lavall D, Ukena C, Linz D, Mahfoud F, Böhm M (2015) Atrial remodeling following catheter-based renal denervation occurs in blood pressure- and heart rate-independent manner. JACC Cardiovasc Interv 8:972–980
50. Linz D, van Hunnik A, Hohl M, Mahfoud F, Wolf M, Neuberger HR, Casadei B, Reilly SN, Verheule S, Böhm M, Schotten U (2015) Catheter-based renal denervation reduces atrial nerve sprouting and complexity of atrial fibrillation in goats. Circ Arrhythm Electrophysiol 8: 466–474
51. Linz D, Wirth K, Ukena C, Mahfoud F, Pöss J, Linz B, Böhm M, Neuberger HR (2013) Renal denervation suppresses ventricular arrhythmias during acute ventricular ischemia in pigs. Heart Rhythm 10:1525–1530
52. Ukena C, Bauer A, Mahfoud F, Schreieck J, Neuberger HR, Eick C, Sobotka PA, Gawaz M, Böhm M (2012) Renal sympathetic denervation for treatment of electrical storm: first-in-man experience. Clin Res Cardiol 101:63–67
53. Ukena C, Mahfoud F, Ewen S, Bollmann A, Hindricks G, Hoffmann BA, Linz D, Musat D, Pavlicek V, Scholz E, Thomas D, Wilems S, Böhm M, Steinberg JS Renal denervation for treatment of ventricular arrhythmias: data from an international multicenter registry. Clin Res Cardiol, in press
54. Schlaich MP, Bart B, Hering D, Walton A, Marusic P, Mahfoud F, Böhm M, Lambert EA, Krum H, Sobotka PA, Schmieder RE, Ika-Sari C, Eikelis N, Straznicky N, Lambert GW, Esler MD (2013) Feasibility of catheter-based renal nerve ablation and effects on sympathetic nerve activity and blood pressure in patients with end-stage renal disease. Int J Cardiol 168: 2214–2220
55. Mahfoud F, Cremers B, Janker J, Link B, Vonend O, Ukena C, Linz D, Schmieder R, Rump LC, Kindermann I, Sobotka PA, Krum H, Scheller B, Schlaich M, Laufs U, Böhm M (2012) Renal hemodynamics and renal function after catheter-based renal sympathetic denervation in patients with resistant hypertension. Hypertension 60:419–424
56. Linz D, Hohl M, Nickel A, Mahfoud F, Wagner M, Ewen S, Schotten U, Maack C, Wirth K, Böhm M (2013) Effect of renal denervation on neurohumoral activation triggering atrial fibrillation in obstructive sleep apnea. Hypertension 62:767–774
57. Mahfoud F, Schlaich M, Kindermann I, Ukena C, Cremers B, Brandt MC, Hoppe UC, Vonend O, Rump LC, Sobotka PA, Krum H, Esler M, Böhm M (2011) Effect of renal sympathetic denervation on glucose metabolism in patients with resistant hypertension: a pilot study. Circulation 123:1940–1946

58. Tzafriri AR, Mahfoud F, Keating JH, Markham PM, Spognardi A, Wong G, Fuimaono K, Böhm M, Edelman ER (2014) Innervation patterns may limit response to endovascular renal denervation. J Am Coll Cardiol 64:1079–1087
59. Mahfoud F, Böhm M, Azizi M, Pathak A, Durand Zaleski I, Ewen S, Tsioufis K, Andersson B, Blankestijn PJ, Burnier M, Chatellier G, Gafoor S, Grassi G, Joner M, Kjeldsen SE, Lüscher TF, Lobo MD, Lotan C, Parati G, Redon J, Ruilope L, Sudano I, Ukena C, van Leeuwen E, Volpe M, Windecker S, Witkowski A, Wijns W, Zeller T, Schmieder RE (2015) Proceedings from the European clinical consensus conference for renal denervation: considerations on future clinical trial design. Eur Heart J 36:2219–2227
60. Kandzari DE, Kario K, Mahfoud F, Cohen SA, Pilcher G, Pocock S, Townsend R, Weber MA, The BM, SPYRAL HTN (2016) The SPYRAL HTN Global Clinical Trial Program: Rationale and design for studies of renal denervation in the absence (SPYRAL HTN OFF-MED) and presence (SPYRAL HTN ON-MED) of antihypertensive medications. Am Heart J 171: 82–91

Effects of Renal Denervation on Chronic Kidney Disease

19

Ana Vrdoljak, Vedran Premužić, and Bojan Jelaković

Abbreviations

ACR	Albumin-to-creatinine ratio
BP	Blood pressure
CKD	Chronic kidney disease
CV	Cardiovascular
dRHTN	Drug-resistant hypertension
eGFR	Estimated glomerular filtration rate
ESRD	End-stage renal disease
GFR	Glomerular filtration rate
HTN	Hypertension
MDRD	Modifications of diet in renal disease
MSNA	Muscle sympathetic nerve activity
RAAS	Renin-angiotensin-aldosterone system
RDN	Renal denervation

19.1 Introduction

Chronic kidney disease (CKD) is a worldwide problem, and its prevalence is continuing to increase considerably contributing to the global burden of cardiovascular (CV) morbidity and mortality.

A. Vrdoljak • V. Premužić • B. Jelaković (✉)
Department of Nephrology, Hypertension, Dialysis and Transplantation,
School of Medicine, University of Zagreb, University Hospital Centre Zagreb,
Kištpatićeva 12, Zagreb, Croatia
e-mail: jelakovicbojan@gmail.com

C. Tsioufis et al. (eds.), *Interventional Therapies for Secondary and Essential Hypertension*, Updates in Hypertension and Cardiovascular Protection,
DOI 10.1007/978-3-319-34141-5_19

In CKD patients, the risk of CV morbidity is higher then the risk of developing end stage renal disease (ESRD) and need for renal replacement therapy. Hypertension (HTN) is highly prevalent (65–95 %) in patients with CKD [1], the majority of patients are uncontrolled, and many of them could be classified as resistant hypertensive patients. Data from *Re*asons for *G*eographic *a*nd *R*acial *D*ifferences in *S*troke (REGARDS) cohort revealed an increasing prevalence and risk of true drug-resistant hypertension (dRHTN) among patients with lower glomerular filtration rate (GFR) and higher albuminuria and albumin-to-creatinine ratio (ACR) [2]. On the other hand, the prevalence of CKD, defined as estimated glomerular filtration rate (eGFR) < 60 ml/min among dRHTN, is remarkably high, being 40.1 and 37.8 % in the reduction of atherothrombosis for continued health (REACH) registry and national health and nutrition examination survey (NHANES) 2008, respectively [3]. In CKD hypervolaemia, inappropriately activated renin-angiotensin-aldosterone system (RAAS) and oxidative stress have important role in the pathogenesis of HTN. However, there is growing evidence that sympathetic overactivity contributes to the pathogenesis of HTN in CKD, and it was even questioned whether this is one of the most important determinants of increased CV risk in this particularly high-risk population. Furthermore, much of the increased sympathetic tone observed in essential HTN and heart failure is directed towards the kidney, forcing renin release, increasing GFR, tubular sodium reabsorption and pressure natriuresis. This has led to the concept of 'neurogenic hypertension' and the development of nerve ablation therapies to lower blood pressure (BP) [4]. Although renal sympathetic nerve activity is not measurable in humans, muscle sympathetic nerve activity (MSNA) and norepinephrine spillover are common findings particularly in younger patients with essential HTN. Growing evidence is proclaiming kidney to be both a target and a contributor in 'neurogenic hypertension' and in all other sympathetically driven diseases (diabetes mellitus, polycystic ovary syndrome and obesity). Kidney injury itself via increased afferent renal activity significantly contributes to increased sympathetic activity, making CKD patients potentially very appropriate candidates for sympathectomy and RDN.

19.2 Sympathetic Overactivity, Hypertension and CKD

Already in 1983, Ishii et al. [5] reported on elevated concentrations of plasma catecholamines in patients with CKD, and Converse [6] documented increased MSNA in ESRD patients undergoing dialysis. Various mechanisms contribute to increased sympathetic activity in CKD: impaired nitric oxide bioavailability (due to inflammation, oxidative stress, uraemia and accumulation of asymmetric dimethylarginine) [7, 8], increased concentration of angiotensin II which has sympathicoexcitatory effects [9, 10], reduced renalase availability [11], etc. However, there is growing evidence that kidney disease per se importantly contributes to sympathetic overactivity. Grassi et al. [12] documented increased adrenergic activation in the early stages of CKD, and the magnitude of sympathetic activity was related to the severity of CKD. Penne et al. [13] reported that severity of CKD correlates positively with MSNA. In animal models, it was found that minimal renal damage which did not alter GFR induced sustained HTN which was prevented by renal sympathectomy [14]. It was also observed that after intervention, BP could not be increased with infusion of adenosine. In humans with autosomal dominant polycystic kidney disease, MSNA was increased even in those with normal GFR [15]. In kidney-transplanted patients, normalization of renal function was not associated with reduction in MSNA, and this was achieved only after bilateral nephrectomy of native kidneys [16]. As already mentioned, MSNA is increased in dialysis patients, whereas after bilateral nephrectomy, it becomes similar to healthy subjects [17]. Unilateral nephrectomy for living kidney donation, which results in decreased renal mass but in the absence of renal parenchymal disease, did not affect MSNA measured several months after donation [18]. These data strongly indicate that the diseased kidneys, independent of renal function and CKD stage, contribute to sympathetic overdrive.

Kidneys are connected with the central nervous system with both efferent and afferent nerve fibres. The efferent fibres innervate predominately the renal vasculature, proximal tubules and juxtaglomerular cells. The main neurotransmitter of efferent fibres is norepinephrine, and the stimulation of efferent fibres leads to increased tubular sodium reabsorption (α-adrenoreceptors), reduced renal blood flow and glomerular filtration (at higher level) and increased renin release (β-adrenoreceptors on juxtaglomerular cells) [19]. All mechanisms significantly contribute to the development of systemic HTN. Importantly, juxtaglomerular and tubular cells are more sensitive to changes in sympathetic activity than other renal structures; thus tubular sodium and water reabsorption and renin release are present in cases with mild sympathetic activation even without vasoconstriction or reduction in GFR [20]. In addition to efferent activity, there is evidence that increased afferent activity can cause hypertension [21, 22]. Contrary to healthy kidneys where afferent activity is mostly inhibitory, in injured kidney, it is excitatory. The development of 'neurogenic hypertension' is a consequence, at least in some part in impaired renorenal reflex, as shown in animal studies [23]. The mechanisms of the hyperadrenergic state are manifold and include reflex and neurohumoral pathways [24–26]. Mechanism of afferent activation in kidney injury is not completely elucidated, and various processes and substances may be involved (ischaemia, RAAS activity, adenosine, chemoreflex activation, decreased nitric oxide and renalase availability) [27–29]. Recently, Muariello et al. [30] reported on the morphological basis underlying sympathetic hyperactivity in ESRD patients identifying an anatomical substrate. Patients undergoing dialysis showed a significant increase in nerve density in the internal area of the peri-adventitial tissue of renal arteries compared with the controls. Furthermore, hypertensive patients with signs of severe arteriolar damage had a greater number of nerve endings in the most internal adventitia, and this number was significantly higher compared with patients without hypertensive arteriolar damage. Finding of increased activity in sympathetic endings present only in the internal area of the adventitia, closest to the vessel wall, might have practical implication influencing the amount of energy required to achieve catheter-based RDN. This is in accordance with the results of Kiuchi et al. who achieved success in CKD patients probably because the number of applications of radiofrequency energy within the renal arteries (an average of nine in each artery) was higher than in other studies and routine work [31].

All mentioned data on increased sympathetic outflow associated with kidney impairment and other listed reasons indicate that RDN would be particularly useful in CKD patients starting from early renal impairment to ESRD.

19.3 RDN Across CKD Stages

Sympathetic overactivity occurs early in the course of CKD and parallels deterioration of kidney function. For several reasons mentioned in the previous paragraph, all CKD patients with dRHTN without anatomical or other contraindication are appropriate candidates for RDN.

In the first human study conducted on 15 patients with CKD stages 3 and 4, BP was reduced significantly during the 12-month follow-up period [32]. Significant restoration of a dipping pattern was observed which could be attributed to the achieved lower sympathetic activity after RDN. Recently, Kiuchi et al. [33] reported on the effect of RDN on 24 patients with dRHTN in CKD stages 2–4. At 180 days after the procedure, ambulatory BP significantly decreased to 132/80 mmHg which was associated with the improvement in kidney function. There were no major complications. The same group of authors followed 27 CKD patients for 12 months and concluded that improvement in renal function is related to BP control [34]. Ott et al. [35] in an observational study in patients with CKD stages 3 and 4 observed significant decrease of office and ambulatory BP after RDN. They failed to find correlation of eGFR with the change of ambulatory BP values and proposed that RDN may attenuate renal function decline independently of the effect on BP. Importantly, acute (24 h) reduction in BP after RDN was observed, and this effect sustained during the follow-up period [36]. RDN was reported to be effective in a patient with autosomal dominant polycystic kidney disease. After intervention BP significantly decreased, but it was also associated with rapid resolution of pain which was maintained at 12 month follow-up [37].

In ESRD, Schlaich et al. tested the feasibility of RDN in nine patients undergoing haemodialysis [38]. After RDN BP decreased significantly, change to normal dipping pattern was observed, and reduced number of antihypertensive drugs was needed to the end of 12-month follow-up. Those changes parallel reduced renal noradrenaline spillover and caused reduction in MSNA.

Besides this small study, only case reports were published on safety and significant BP decrease after RDN in patients undergoing dialysis [39–41].

High sympathetic activity is frequently present in patient after renal transplantation which is perpetuated by the preservation of renal afferent fibres from native kidneys. Schneider et al. [42] reported the effect of RDN in kidney-transplanted patients. Patients with resistant post-transplant HTN were randomized to receive RDN or medical therapy alone. The ablation catheter was introduced in each native renal artery, and six ablations were performed in both renal arteries. At the end of follow-up, office BP was significantly lower in RDN group. There were no differences in ambulatory BP values, but in the RDN group, more patients converted from non-dippers to dippers. There were no difference in renal outcome, and no adverse events were reported. This study demonstrated feasibility and safety of RDN in kidney-transplanted patients. However, more results are needed before RDN could be suggested as effective method for post-transplant resistant HTN.

19.4 Effects of RDN on Renal Function

There is particular concern of RDN impact on renal function in all patients undergoing this intervention and particularly in CKD patients.

Animal studies have shown beneficial effects of lowering sympathetic drive on renal function and proteinuria [29, 43]. In patients with advanced CKD (GFR <30 ml/min/1.73 m^2), it was reported that moxonidine, the sympatholytic agent, slowed down progression of kidney impairment and decreased proteinuria in diabetic nephropathy independently of blood pressure [44, 45].

However, concerns have been raised because of the limited follow-up data on whether RDN might negatively influence renal function [46]. As eGFR lower than 45 ml/min/1.73 m^2 was arbitrarily chosen as a contraindication for RDN, there is even less evidence about the effect of RDN in moderate-to-severe CKD.

A significant reduction in renal resistive index and office BP was reported in a group of 88 patients with dRHTN and preserved renal function at 6 months after the RDN. eGFR (cystatin C) was unchanged, and the proportion of patients with normal urinary albumin excretion increased by 12 %, while proportion of patients with microalbuminuria and macroalbuminuria decreased by 10 and 23 %, respectively [47]. In 19 patients with normal renal function, renal perfusion and renal vascular resistance were noninvasively assessed by magnetic resonance imaging with arterial spin labelling [48]. After 3 months, renal perfusion was not statistically different while renal vascular resistance dropped. There were no changes in renal function at any time point. Thus, despite reduced systemic BP, renal perfusion and function did not change after RDN. Authors concluded that autoregulation of renal perfusion did not appear to be adversely affected and confirmed the absence of hyperfiltration after RDN in all patients, including those with diabetes. In another study, renal function was evaluated for up to 3 years prior and 1 year after RDN in 27 patients with CKD stages 3 and 4 [35]. Before RDN, eGFR (modifications of diet in renal disease (MDRD) equation) declined by -4.8 ± 3.8 ml/min/1.73 m^2 per year, and after RDN, eGFR improved by 1.5 ± 10 ml/min/1.73 m^2 at 12 months ($P<0.009$). According to the authors, these results indicate that treatment of HTN with RDN decreases BP and slows or even halts the decline of renal function in CKD patients at stages 3 and 4. Keeping in mind that patients with eGFR<45 ml/min/1.73 m^2 were excluded from Symplicity HTN-2, long-term follow-up data from this study showed no change in eGFR from the baseline at 3 years among patients who underwent RDN at enrolment (eGFR 76.7 ± 18.8 ml/min/1.73 m^2 versus 77.1 ± 18 ml/min/1.73 m^2). Finally, Kiuchi et al. reported on 30 patients with dRHTN and CKD stages 2–4 who underwent RDN [31]. At the end of 12-month follow-up, ambulatory blood pressure decreased significantly, eGFR (CKD-EPI equation) increased from 61.9±23.9 mL/min/1.73 m^2 to 88.0±39.8 mL/min/1.73 m^2 ($P<.0001$), and urine ACR decreased from 99.8 mg/g (IQR 38.0–192.1) to 11.0 mg/g (IQR 4.1–28.1; $P<.0001$ mg/g). Importantly, at the end of the follow-up period, 70% of patients were no longer classified as having CKD (eGFR >60 ml/min/1.73 m^2 and ACR<30 mg/g). These data support a potential renoprotective effect of RDN, either as a result of BP lowering alone or in conjunction with decreased global and/or renal sympathetic activity.

The majority of clinical studies indicate that RDN is not detrimental for kidney function; it is at least neutral and, according to some results, could be even beneficial. Murray Esler [49] raised several important questions related to the observed beneficial effects of RDN on renal function: Is this attributable to beneficial prerenal influences on GFR from the reduction in antihypertensive dosing? Or could RDN change vascular glomerular dynamics in such a way as to improve GFR and to lessen microalbuminuria? Could there really be improvement in renal parenchymal disease? If this is the case, he concluded that this will be the victory for the method. However, long-lasting prospective studies on renal function after RDN are warranted before final conclusion is reached. Several large trials with thousands of enrolled patients are currently underway (ClinicalTrials.gov; NCT numbers: 01418560, 01442883, 01534299). Blankestijn et al. are conducting the clinical trial SYMPATHY which will examine whether RDN added to standard care reduces ambulatory BP, and this will be analysed in specific GFR strata (20–60 ml/min/1.73 m^2 and>60 ml/min/1.73 m^2) [50].

19.5 Limitations, Concerns and Possible Solutions

Few concerns and a couple of issues regarding potential risks and questions on safety have arisen and deserve further consideration.

- First, renal anatomy and changes in haemodynamics. In patients with advanced CKD, and particularly in patients with ESRD, renal artery diameters are usually small, which in addition to low renal blood flow could induce overheating of tissue resulting in pain during the procedure and tissue damage. Consecutively, RDN may not be technically feasible in some ESRD patients. However, this is not the case in early CKD stages as shown by Kiuchi et al. [31].
- Second, the potential risk of renal artery stenosis. Catheter-based radiofrequency ablation induces intimal injury increasing the risk for renal artery stenosis. Data from the majority of follow-up studies are reassuring, while no signs of renal artery stenosis were found.
- Third, the risk of contrast-induced nephropathy. In all CKD patients, the risk of contrast-induced nephropathy is higher than in other patients undergoing this procedure as well as any other imaging procedure with radiocontrast media.

However, RDN is an elective procedure, thereby allowing adequate prehydration to minimize the risk of contrast nephropathy. Hydration before, during and after the procedure could protect CKD patients from this complication. It seems reasonable to propose adequate hydration with iv sodium bicarbonate (3 mL/kg) and 0.9 % saline for 1 h, as prophylaxis for attenuation of iodinated contrast media-associated nephrotoxicity, and at the end of procedure another infusion of sodium bicarbonate (1 ml/kg/h) for 6 h [31]. The other possibility to minimize administered radiocontrast volume is to use, where available, carbon dioxide angiography which reduces the risk of renal damage.

- Fourth, potential sympathetic reinnervation. However, sustained and long-lasting blood pressure reduction observed in various trials is a strong argument against reinnervation. Nevertheless, even longer period of follow-up is needed. Importantly, the cell bodies of afferent renal sympathetic nerves are located in the anterior horn of the spinal cord. Therefore, afferent regeneration would be much more difficult than efferent regeneration (which cell bodies lay in the ganglia around the renal artery).
- Fifth, one must be aware of increased susceptibility to the development of pseudoaneurysm at the femoral vascular access [38].

Keeping in mind the 'primum nil nocere' axiom and knowing that CKD patients have higher risk for all listed complications than other resistant hypertensive patients, they should be carefully selected, prepared and strictly monitored during long-term follow-up.

Conclusion

Increased sympathetic overflow is a characteristic of CKD; thus those patients should be considered prime candidates for RDN. However, there is scarce evidence on the effects of RDN in CKD because renal impairment was among the exclusion criteria in several landmark studies. Nevertheless, available data confirmed the presumption that this procedure is effective and safe in all CKD stages. However, because of higher risk of complications and less experience, CKD patients should be closely monitored during the procedure and during a longer period after intervention. It is important to notice that in CKD patients, RDN decreases BP, diminishes cardiovascular risk but also reduces progression of CKD which additionally lowers global risk. It is especially important to realize which patients are likely to benefit, i.e. proper patient selection based on the knowledge of the pathophysiology and anatomy is crucial. Unfortunately, there are no clinical characteristics that can predict response to RDN other than basal level of the office systolic BP and probably lower eGFR.

Finally, CKD patients with dRHTN should be considered for RDN. In this group of patients, this procedure is effective and keeping in mind several limitations could be safe as in all other patients.

References

1. Mahmoodi BK et al (2012) Associations of kidney disease measures with mortality and end-stage renal disease in individuals with or without hypertension: a meta-analysis. Lancet 380:1649–1661
2. Tanner RM et al (2013) Prevalence of apparent treatment-resistant hypertension among individuals with CKD. Clin J Am Soc Nephrol 8:1583–1590
3. Vemulapalli S et al (2014) Apparent treatment-resistant hypertension and chronic kidney disease: another cardiovascular- renal syndrome? Adv Chronic Kidney Dis 21(6):489–499
4. Larsen RN et al (2014) Regulation of the sympathetic nervous system by the kidney. Curr Opin Nephrol Hypertens 23(1):61–68
5. Ishii M et al (1983) Elevated plasma catecholamines in hypertensives with primary glomerular diseases. Hypertension 5:545–551
6. Converse RL Jr et al (1992) Sympathetic overactivity in patients with chronic renal failure. N Engl J Med 327(27):1912–1918
7. Zoccali C et al (2002) CREED investigators: left ventricular hypertrophy, cardiac remodeling and asymmetric dimethylarginine (ADMA) in hemodialysis patients. Kidney Int 62:339–345
8. Shi B et al (2010) Circulating levels of asymmetric dimethylarginine are an independent risk factor for left ventricular hypertrophy and predict cardiovascular events in pre-dialysis patients with chronic kidney disease. Eur J Intern Med 21:444–448
9. Ligtenberg G et al (1999) Reduction of sympathetic hyperactivity by enalapril in patients with chronic renal failure. N Engl J Med 340:1321–1328
10. Schiffrin EL et al (2007) Chronic kidney disease: effects on the cardiovascular system. Circulation 116(1):85–97
11. Li G et al (2008) Catecholamines regulate the activity, secretion, and synthesis of renalase. Circulation 117(10):1277–1282
12. Grassi G et al (2011) Early sympathetic activation in the initial clinical stages of chronic renal failure. Hypertension 57:846–851
13. Penne EL et al (2009) Sympathetic hyperactivity and clinical outcome in chronic kidney disease patients during standard treatment. J Nephrol 22:208–215
14. Ye S et al (1997) Renal afferent impulses, the posterior hypothalamus, and hypertension in rats with chronic renal failure. Kidney Int 51:722–727
15. Klein IH et al (2001) Sympathetic activity is increased in polycystic kidney disease and is associated with hypertension. J Am Soc Nephrol 12:2427–2433
16. Hausberg M et al (2002) Sympathetic nerve activity in end-stage renal disease. Circulation 106(15):1974–1979
17. Blankestijn PJ et al (2014) Pro: sympathetic renal denervation in hypertension and in chronic kidney disease. Nephrol Dial Transplant 29:1120–1123
18. Klein IH et al (2003) Sympathetic nerve activity is inappropriately increased in chronic renal disease. J Am Soc Nephrol 14:3239–3244
19. DiBona GF (2005) Physiology in prospective: the wisdom of the body. Neural control of the kidney. Am J Physiol Regul Integr Comp Physiol 289(3):R 633–R 641
20. Kopp UC (2011) Neural control of renal function. Chapter 5, Neural control of renin secretion rate. Morgan & Claypool Life Sciences, San Rafael
21. Kottke FJ et al (1945) The production of arterial hypertension by chronic renal artery-nerve stimulation. Am J Physiol 145:38–47
22. Calaresu FR et al (1976) Haemodynamic responses and renin release during stimulation of afferent renal nerves in the cat. J Physiol 255:687–700
23. Kopp U et al (2011) Impaired interaction between efferent and afferent nerve activity in SHR involves activation of alpha2-adrenoceptors. Hypertension 57:640–647
24. McGrath BP et al (1978) Catecholamines in peripheral venous plasma in patients on chronic haemodialysis. Clin Sci Mol Med 55:89–96

25. Grassi G (2010) Sympathetic neural activity in hypertension and related diseases. Am J Hypertens 23:1052–1060
26. Grassi G (2009) Assessment of sympathetic cardiovascular drive in human hypertension: achievements and perspectives. Hypertension 54:690–697
27. Neumann J et al (2004) Sympathetic hyperactivity in chronic kidney disease: pathogenesis, clinical relevance, and treatment. Kidney Int 65:1568–1576
28. Schlaich MP et al (2009) Sympathetic activation in chronic renal failure. J Am Soc Nephrol 20:933–939
29. Joles JA, Koomans HA (2004) Causes and consequences of increased sympathetic activity in renal disease. Hypertension 43:699–706
30. Mauriello A, Rovella V, Anemona L, Servadei F, Giannini E (2015) Increased sympathetic renal innervation in hemodialysis patients is the anatomical substrate of sympathetic hyperactivity in end-stage renal disease. J Am Heart Assoc 26;4(12). pii e002426. doi:10.1161/JAHA.115.002426
31. Kiuchi MG et al (2016) Long-term effects of renal sympathetic denervation on hypertensive patients With mild to moderate chronic kidney disease. J Clin Hypertens 18:190–196. doi:10.1111/jch.12724
32. Hering D et al (2012) Renal denervation in moderate to severe CKD. J Am Soc Nephrol 23:1250–1257
33. Kiuchi MG et al (2013) Effects of renal denervation with a standard irrigated cardiac ablation catheter on blood pressure and renal function in patients with chronic kidney disease and resistant hypertension. Eur Heart J 34:2114–2212
34. Kiuchi MG et al (2014) Renal sympathetic denervation in patients with hypertension and chronic kidney disease: does improvement in renal function follow blood pressure control? J Clin Hypertens (Greenwich) 16:794–800
35. Ott C et al (2015) Renal denervation preserves renal function in patients with chronic kidney disease and resistant hypertension. J Hypertens 33(6):1261–1266
36. Kiuchi MG et al (2015) Acute effect of renal sympathetic denervation on blood pressure in refractory hypertensive patients with chronic kidney disease. Int J Cardiol 190:29–31
37. Shetty SV et al (2013) Percutaneous transluminal renal denervation: a potential treatment option for polycystic kidney disease-related pain? Int J Cardiol 162:e58–e59
38. Schlaich MP et al (2013) Feasibility of catheter-based renal nerve ablation and effects on sympathetic nerve activity and blood pressure in patients with end-stage renal disease. Int J Cardiol 168(3):2214–2220
39. Prochnau D et al (2012) Catheter-based radiofrequency ablation therapy of the renal sympathetic-nerve system for drug resistant hypertension in a patient with end-stage renal disease. Int J Cardiol 154:e29–e30
40. Di DN et al (2012) Renal sympathetic nerve ablation for the treatment of difficult-to-control or refractory hypertension in a haemodialysis patient. Nephrol Dial Transplant 27:1689–1690
41. Ott C et al (2012) Renal denervation in a hypertensive patient with end-stage renal disease and small arteries: a direction for future research. J Clin Hypertens (Greenwich) 14:799–801
42. Schneider S et al (2015) Impact of sympathetic renal denervation: a randomized study in patients after renal transplantation (ISAR-denerve). Nephrol Dial Transplant 30(11):1928–1936
43. de Beus E et al (2014) Sympathetic activation secondary to chronic kidney disease: therapeutic target for renal denervation? J Hypertens 32:1751–1761
44. Vonend O et al (2003) Moxonidine treatment of hypertensive patients with advanced renal failure. J Hypertens 21:1709–1717
45. Strojek K et al (2001) Lowering of microalbuminuria in diabetic patients by a sympathicoplegic agent: novel approach to prevent progression of diabetic nephropathy? J Am Soc Nephrol 12(3):602–605

46. Petidis K et al (2011) Renal sympathetic denervation: renal function concerns. Hypertension 58:e19. doi:10.1161/HYPERTENSIONAHA.111.178145
47. Mahfoud F et al (2012) Renal hemodynamics and renal function after catheter-based renal sympathetic denervation in patients with resistant hypertension. Hypertension 60:419–424
48. Ott C et al (2013) Vascular and renal hemodynamic changes after renal denervation. Clin J Am Soc Nephrol 8(7):1195–1201
49. Esler M (2016) Renal denervation for the hypertension of chronic kidney disease: a special case? J Clin Hypertens 18:187–189. doi:10.1111/jch.12730
50. Zoccali C, Mallamaci F (2014) Moderator's view: renal denervation: the jury is still out and the verdict will be more complex than initially envisaged. Nephrol Dial Transplant 29(6):1124–1126

Effects of Renal Denervation on Sympathetic Nervous System Activity

20

Gino Seravalle, Gianmaria Brambilla, and Guido Grassi

Abbreviations

BP	Blood pressure
HTN	Hypertension
NTS	Nucleus tractus solitarius
RDN	Renal denervation
SNS	Sympathetic nervous system

20.1 The Sympathetic Nervous System

The sympathetic nervous system (SNS) has a fundamental role in maintaining the physiological homeostasis of the cardiovascular system. It is also involved in the genesis and progression of several cardiovascular and non-cardiovascular pathophysiological conditions other than hypertension (HTN).

After the initial studies on physiological-based mechanisms, the later pathophysiological evaluations and the clinical implication of the studies during the past century have brought renewed interest for the SNS. This vision is greatly changed

G. Seravalle
Cardiologia, Ospedale San Luca, IRCCS Istituto Auxologico Italiano, Milan, Italy

G. Brambilla • G. Grassi (✉)
Clinica Medica, Dipartimento di Scienze della Salute, Università Milano-Bicocca, Via Pergolesi 33-20052, Monza, Italy
e-mail: guido.grassi@unimib.it

C. Tsioufis et al. (eds.), *Interventional Therapies for Secondary and Essential Hypertension*, Updates in Hypertension and Cardiovascular Protection,
DOI 10.1007/978-3-319-34141-5_20

during the last 30 years due to the development of the modern neurobiology and the progressive improvement of methods to investigate the noradrenergic system.

This chapter will briefly overview the anatomical aspect of the SNS both at central and peripheral levels, the distribution in the kidney and in particular at the renal artery level, and the effects of non-pharmacological interventions (radio-frequency ablation of renal nerves) acting on the sympathetic drive on several pathophysiological conditions characterized by a sympathetic hyperactivity.

20.2 Anatomical Aspects: From Central to Peripheral Level

Starting from the studies of Dittmar and colleagues, the role of the vasomotor center in the nucleus tractus solitarius (NTS) and the different areas and loci in the medulla oblongata has been established [1, 2]. Cardiovascular sensory afferent fibers terminate in the dorsal part of the medulla oblongata, in the nucleus tractus solitarius. Their terminations are, in part, organized topographically based on the function of the receptor. NTS neurons also project to higher brain regions, and at each neural level, inputs arising from the periphery can integrate with others ascending and descending the neuraxis into more complex patterns of autonomic, behavioral, and endocrine responses [3, 4] (Fig. 20.1).

The SNS is organized at a spinal and peripheral level such that cell bodies within the thoracolumbar segments of the spinal cord provide preganglionic efferent

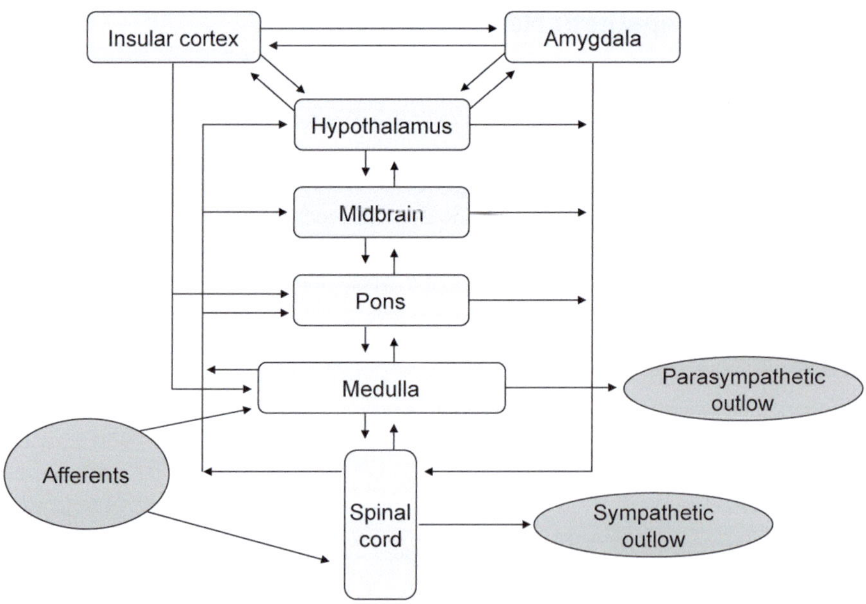

Fig. 20.1 Schematic diagram of the possible interconnections between regions of the central nervous system involved in the central nervous integration of cardiovascular control

innervation to sympathetic neurons that reside in ganglia dispersed in paravertebral, prevertebral, and previsceral or terminal ganglia. The outflow from the spinal cord to the peripheral ganglia is segmentally organized with some overlap (Fig. 20.2). The distribution of postsynaptic fibers also follows a regional pattern. Multiple supraspinal descending pathways provide a dense innervation of major autonomic cell groups in the spinal cord, but clearly specific topographic responses exist. Each preganglionic neuron innervates from 4 to 20 postganglionic sites, and each spinal outflow level may reach multiple peripheral ganglia. At each thoracic level, there are an estimated 5000 preganglionic neurons that have a powerful base to influence greater than 100,000 postganglionic neurons. The autonomic neuroeffector junction is generally a poorly defined synaptic structure. The unmyelinated postganglionic fibers become beaded with varicosities as they approach their targets. The number of varicosities varies from 10,000/mm^3 to over 2 million per mm^3 depending on the target

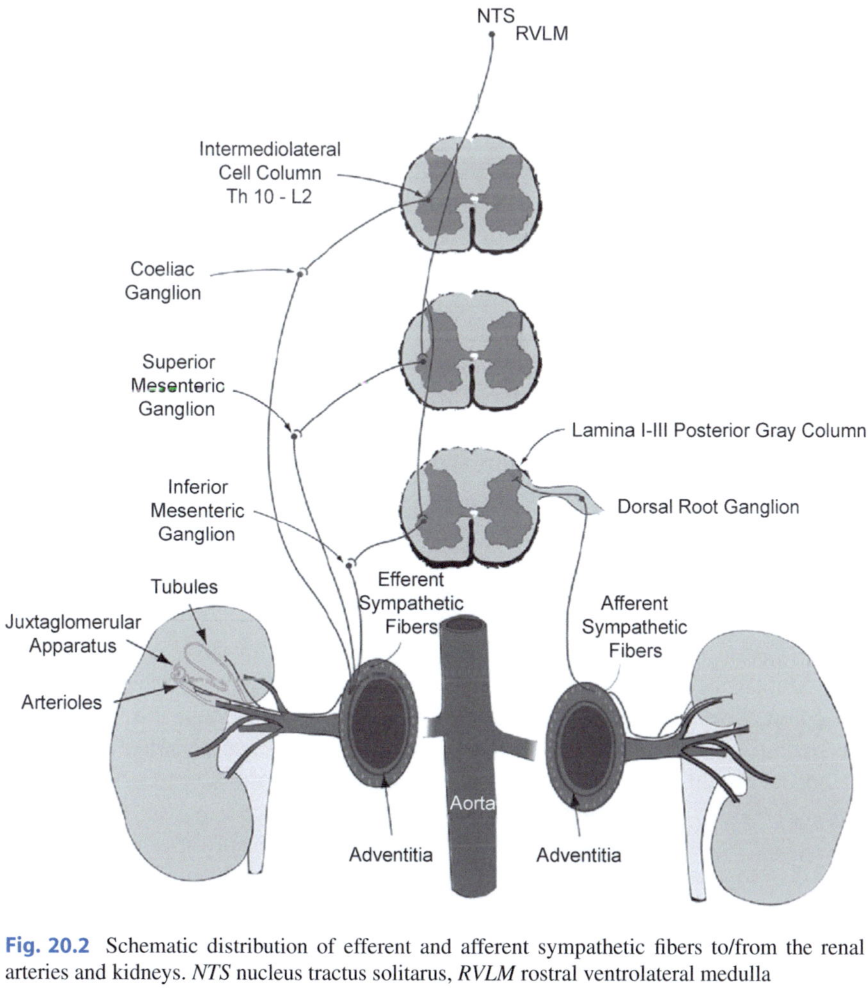

Fig. 20.2 Schematic distribution of efferent and afferent sympathetic fibers to/from the renal arteries and kidneys. *NTS* nucleus tractus solitarus, *RVLM* rostral ventrolateral medulla

being innervated. The varicosities are packed with mitochondria and vesicles containing various transmitters and are at different distances from their target organs. The principal neuronal phenotype in peripheral sympathetic ganglia is the noradrenergic neuron which is generally multipolar in character with synapses mainly located on dendrites. 80–95 % of ganglion cells contain catecholamines, while the remaining contain a mixture of transmitters or are postganglionic cholinergic cells [5, 6].

20.3 Methods to Evaluate the Sympathetic Nervous System

As previously described, there are multiple levels of the SNS with quantitative and qualitative differences: (1) central regions, (2) ganglionic transmission, (3) junctional modulation of neurotransmitters, (4) clearance and reuptake of neurotransmitter, (5) adrenergic receptors, and (6) the responsiveness of the effector. Due to this complexity, a single method is not able to obtain an overall assessment of the SNS [7, 8].

20.3.1 Heart Rate

Assessment of heart rate is based on the evidence that heart rate is regulated by the positive chronotropic effects of catecholamines and negative vagal parasympathetic inhibitory influence on the sinus node [9]. There are, however, several limitations to heart rate as specific markers of sympathetic activity due to the vagal cholinergic influences. There are also quantitative and qualitative differences between sympathetic activity to the heart and other districts like the kidney or skeletal muscle. It is possible to observe conditions characterized by an increase in norepinephrine spillover rate or muscle sympathetic nerve activity in which heart rate is in the normal range [10]. This suggests that heart rate may not reflect sympathetic overdrive to other important regional circulations and cannot be taken as a marker of cardiac sympathetic adrenergic activity.

20.3.2 Power Spectral Analysis

Power spectral analysis of heart rate has gained popularity for the assessment of cardiac sympathetic and parasympathetic cholinergic influences on the sinus node since it is noninvasive, relatively easy to perform, and inexpensive. Despite this, the method has significant limitations as a quantitative and specific indicator of cardiac SNS activity, and its insight does not extend beyond sympathetic control of heart rate [11].

20.3.3 Plasma Catecholamines

The advantages of this approach are the relatively easy performance and wide applicability. However, the sensitivity and reproducibility of the measurements are far from optimal [7, 8]. The sensitivity of the method is more challenging as a result of several factors. First, circulating norepinephrine levels are only a minor fraction of the amount secreted from sympathetic nerve terminals. As a result, plasma norepinephrine values may not reflect sympathetic neural drive and secretion of the neurotransmitter [12, 13]. There is also a conceptual limitation to the measurement of plasma norepinephrine as an indicator of sympathetic activity. In this case, the SNS is considered as a unit while, as mentioned before, there are multiple levels and components, and it is possible to observe profound regional differences in sympathetic nerve activity. It has also been shown that the reproducibility of the norepinephrine approach can be improved by increasing the number of blood samples. Three norepinephrine samples are required to achieve such a goal and to make reproducibility closer to the one of microneurography [14].

20.3.4 Norepinephrine Radiolabeled Technique

The norepinephrine isotope dilution method involving infusion of small doses of radiolabeled norepinephrine represents an approach that overcomes several limitations related to plasma norepinephrine measurement [7, 8]. During constant-rate infusion of radiolabeled norepinephrine, the regional rate of spillover of norepinephrine to plasma can be determined by isotope dilution according to the formula:

$$\text{Regional norepinephrine spillover} = \times\left[\left(C_{\mathrm{V}} - C_{\mathrm{A}}\right) + C_{\mathrm{A}} \times E\right] \times \mathrm{PF}$$

where C_V and C_A are the plasma concentrations of norepinephrine in regional venous and arterial plasma, E is the fractional extraction of tritiated norepinephrine at steady state in passage through the organ, and PF is the organ plasma flow [15]. This method allows precise quantification of the net release of the adrenergic neurotransmitter undergoing clearance from the bloodstream. Given the regional differences in sympathetic regulation, an advantage of the norepinephrine spillover method is its ability to quantify sympathetic drive selectively to several regional districts, like the kidney and heart. No other method currently available provides direct quantitative measurement of sympathetic adrenergic drive at these levels. An example of this advantage is the evidence that in normotensive obese humans, there are marked increases in renal norepinephrine spillover but decreases in cardiac nor epinephrine spillover, despite the frequent increase in heart rate values [16]. Limits of this technique are the use of radiolabeled norepinephrine in humans and the catheterization of renal vessels and the coronary sinus for assessment of renal and cardiac norepinephrine spillovers, respectively.

20.3.5 Efferent Postganglionic Nerve Traffic Recording

The intraneural recording of efferent postganglionic sympathetic nerve activity to the skeletal muscle and skin has contributed greatly to study the sympathetic cardiovascular drive in humans [17]. The microneurographic technique is minimally invasive, requiring the percutaneous insertion and positioning of tungsten recording electrode in superficial nerves (peroneal or radial nerve) [7, 8]. The advantages of this technique include (a) a direct measurement of the central nervous system sympathetic neural outflow either to skeletal muscle circulation or to the skin, (b) a continuous recording of sympathetic nerve traffic allowing a dynamic assessment of sympathetic drive in a given experimental session, (c) the ease of performing repeated recordings over time, and (d) the high reproducibility of the activity between recordings in two different nerves and over time [7]. This technique presents also several limitations. First, postganglionic sympathetic nerve traffic may not always reflect the release of the neurotransmitter at the neuroeffector junction. Second, microneurographic recordings do not provide direct information on sympathetic activity to visceral tissues such as the kidney and heart. In healthy humans, there are good relationships between the microneurographic data collected in the peripheral nerve and the ones characterizing the cardiac or the renal neural network, but this may not pertain in pathological states [7, 8]. The single-unit recording [18] coupled with catheterization and norepinephrine isotope dilution has recently shown that a relationship exists between single-unit firing patterns and cardiac and whole-body norepinephrine spillover to plasma [19]. Using microneurographic recording, evidences for a marked sympathetic overdrive have been obtained in several pathophysiological conditions [20–38].

All these pathophysiological conditions represent the target for pharmacological and non-pharmacological approaches able to reduce the hyperadrenergic state.

20.4 Renal Innervations

Nerves carrying fibers to or from the kidney are derived from the celiac plexus that consists of the aortic-renal ganglion, the celiac ganglion, and the major splanchnic nerves. The renal sympathetic nerves originate from the intermediolateral column of the spinal cord from T9 to T13. Several nuclei in the brainstem project to intermediolateral column, including the medullary raphe nuclei, the rostral ventrolateral medulla, and the paraventricular hypothalamic nucleus. Baroreceptor regulation of sympathetic outflow is regulated through the rostral ventrolateral medulla by neurons that control sympathetic outflow to various organs [39, 40].

Efferent nerves enter the kidney along renal artery and vein. The afferent renal nerves travel from the kidney toward the dorsal root ganglia along the spinal cord and have a role in the water and salt homeostasis. The efferent renal nerves are postganglionic, and the majority contain norepinephrine varicosities at their nerve terminals. They are distributed to all segments of the intrarenal vasculature in the renal cortex and outer medulla, including the interlobar, arcuate, and interlobular arteries and the afferent and efferent glomerular arterioles [41]. All parts of the nephron are innervated by sympathetic nerves [42].

Efferent renal nerve fibers are known to influence renal hemodynamics by modifying arteriolar vascular tone, renin release by a direct action on juxtaglomerular cells, and the excretion of sodium and water by changing tubular reabsorption of sodium and water at the different tubular levels [43, 44]. In animals, efferent renal sympathetic nerve activity is recorded by an amplified signal from an electrode placed around the central portion of a cut renal nerve bundle or placed around intact nerve (conscious animals). In basal conditions, these recordings most likely represent efferent activity [45]. In animals, the electrical stimulation of afferent renal nerve fibers can either increase or decrease systemic arterial pressure. The hypertensive response to electrical stimulation of renal afferents is the result of widespread activation of the sympathetic nervous system, leading to an increase in peripheral vascular resistance. Activation of afferent renal nerve fibers by an intraneural artery infusion of adenosine elicits increases in arterial pressure, heart rate, and cardiac output without changing total peripheral resistance, indicating reflex activation of the sympathetic nervous system, predominantly restricted to the heart [46]. There is evidence that tonically active contralateral renorenal reflexes, which are inhibitory in nature, mainly control the secretion of renin and the tubular reabsorption of sodium and water [47]. The potential of therapeutic denervation to attenuate hypertension and the progression of renal disease has been obtained in experimental studies. Dorsal rhizotomy prevents the rise of BP in 5/6 nephrectomy rat model of chronic renal failure and HTN [48], suggesting that afferent impulses from the kidney may be responsible for the increase in BP levels. The HTN induced by unilateral renal injury in rats is accompanied by increase in norepinephrine secretion from the posterior hypothalamus and increase in renal sympathetic efferent and afferent nerve activity of both kidneys [49]. Studies of the effects of increases in efferent renal SNS activity on renal function have most commonly applied electrical square-wave signals at different intensities and frequencies via electrodes placed around the peripheral portion of one renal nerve bundle. Numerous studies have shown that this technique results in frequency-dependent changes in renin secretion, urinary sodium excretion, and renal blood flow, resembling those elicited by reflex renal nerve stimulation and thus suggesting that this techniques mimics physiological changes in efferent renal sympathetic nerve activity [50, 51]. Surgical bilateral native renal removal, but not renal transplantation, is able to reverse sympathetic activation of end-stage renal disease and HTN [35, 52].

Given the importance of the renal afferent nerves in generating high sympathetic nervous activity in renal hypertension and end-stage renal disease and the relation between plasma concentration of norepinephrine and prediction of incidence of cardiovascular events and survival [53], there might be a special place for catheter-based RDN in the treatment of hypertension of renal disease. To this aim, two uncontrolled small studies reported positive results in renal hypertension and in end-stage renal disease [54, 55].

The technical problems that should be overcome are first the avoidance of radiocontrast nephropathy during the necessary angiographic procedure by the use of carbon dioxide imaging and second the need for the denervation procedure to be often performed on small-diameter renal arteries with low blood flow which increases the risk of damaging the artery.

20.5 Microanatomic Evaluation: From Animals to Humans

As percutaneous technologies have emerged, the swine model became the most frequently used because of its similarity to the renovascular anatomy and size in humans [56, 57].

Recent data in pigs have shown that nerve density is higher in proximal segments of the renal arteries, although with increasing distance from the aorta, nerve and ganglia are localized closer to the lumen. At a distance of about 3 mm from the aorta, nerves are localized at radial depths of 2–8 mm, whereas at a distance of 6 mm, nerves are localized at radial depths of 1–5 mm. These significant differences imply that 75 % of nerves were located within 9.3, 6.3, and 3.4 mm of the lumen of the aorta and 3 and 6 mm into the renal artery. Ganglion distributions display a similar trend with 75 % located within 10.8 mm from the lumen at the aorta. Circumferential distributions show differences with distance from the aorta, as shown by quadrant-level composite maps. At the aorta, nerves and ganglia are more abundant in the superior-posterior and particularly the superior-anterior quadrants, but most were localized at >5 mm from the lumen (Fig. 20.3). At 3 mm from the aorta, nerves were more abundant in the anterior and superior-posterior quadrants and were localized at >5 mm from the lumen. At 6 mm from the aorta, ganglia (but not nerves) are more abundant in the superior quadrants at >5 mm from the lumen [58]. Although generally similar to humans, caution should be warranted in translating animal findings to humans due to the differences in length, tortuosity, compliance, and calcification in human renal arteries.

Recent microanatomic studies have reported the evidence of renal sympathetic nerve distribution in humans [59]. Renal arteries were harvested from human autopsies, sectioned into three parts, and prepared for microscopy with hematoxylin and eosin staining to visualize the renal nerves. Nerve numbers have been obtained by manual count. The investigators have found a circumferential distribution of the nerves around the renal artery. In particular, the number of nerves appears to increase along the length of the artery due to the arborization pattern of the nerves [60, 61]. This is in contrast with the hypothesis that the renal sympathetic nerves increase in number near the ostium of the artery.

A micrometer measurement of radial distances from the lumen-intima interface allowed to group each nerve into 0.5 mm deep rings. It has been found that 90.5 % of all renal sympathetic nerves reside within 2 mm of the renal artery lumen (Fig. 20.4). The use of special stains has been employed in an effort to distinguish the efferent and afferent nerves. Functionally, these nerves differ in more ways than simply the direction of nerve traffic. For example, the efferent nerves use norepinephrine as its neurotransmitter (sympathetic fibers), and the afferent nerves (sensory fibers) use substance P or calcitonin gene-related peptide [62, 63].

This information represents an important tool for all subjects dedicated to the endovascular catheter-based approach using radiofrequency ablation and, in particular, to those using the single catheter method as an aid in the development of precise and more efficient procedures and technologies for renal ablation [64].

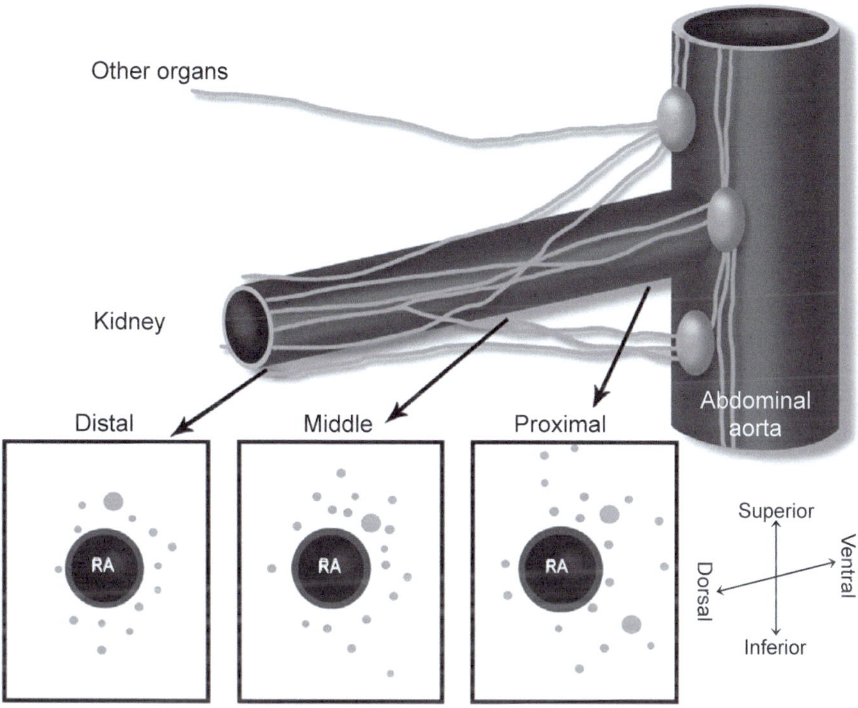

Fig. 20.3 The illustration shows the proposed diagram of renal artery and circumferential peri-arterial nerve location

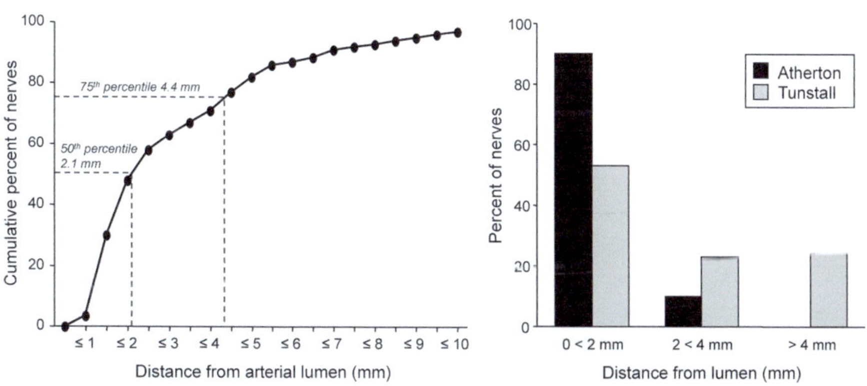

Fig. 20.4 Cumulative incidence of perirenal nerve distance from the renal arterial lumen (*left panel*) and distribution of renal nerve depth (*right panel*) (Modified by Refs. [59–61], with permission)

20.6 Sympathetic Deactivation: Physiological and Clinical Effects

With this background in mind, it is clear that sympathectomy could represent an effective approach to control high BP levels. Starting from 1930, sympathectomy, splanchnicectomy, and celiac ganglionectomy were used but poorly tolerated due to their significant side effects including orthostatic hypotension, palpitations, anhidrosis, and incidence of fatal events [65–67]. The surgical approach was abandoned despite the evidence for a consistent BP reduction. Recently, a renewed interest, accompanied by a more conservative approach, has been performed at the level of thoracic vertebra [68], but again, although with satisfactory results, the adverse systemic effects discouraged many from performing this. Then the attention has been shifted toward drug therapies to control severe HTN reserving sympathectomy for drug resistant HTN (dRHTN) not responsive to medications.

During the last years, evidences from physiological studies on the role of renal sympathetic efferent nerves and the development of a radiofrequency catheter-based procedure for selective RDN in humans induced a great and renewed enthusiasm. Although a big amount of data has been published on the effects of this procedure on BP values in resistant hypertensive subjects and in subjects with HTN-related pathological conditions, two main questions deserve to be better understood: the timing between sympathetic deactivation and clinical responses and how to test for achieved sympathetic deactivation.

20.6.1 Timing Effects of Sympathetic Deactivation

Studies on dRHTN have clearly shown in these patients a marked sympathetic activation and a baroreflex impairment [69] that could be reversed by RDN, but some studies provided conflicting results [70–73]. One study failed to detect any effect of the procedure on sympathetic nerve traffic [71], while others reported a significant reduction in sympathetic nerve traffic but of modest degree compared with the concomitant marked reduction in BP values [72, 73]. These studies have two common limitations: first, sympathetic activity has been assessed only once or twice after renal nerve ablation, thus failing to provide serial information over an extended follow-up period, and, second, these studies didn't measure the earliest post-RDN phases, thus lacking to determine whether the hypothesized sympathetic effects preceded were concomitant to or followed the BP ones. A recent study evaluated these aspects in true resistant hypertensives [74] by serial measurements of office and ambulatory BP and sympathetic nerve traffic according to a study design which included sessions performed before and after 2 weeks and 1,3, and 6 months after bilateral RDN. In this study, it is possible to observe that RDN had BP-lowering effect starting one month from the procedure but not at the early evaluation performed 15 days after the procedure. The decrease in BP was less pronounced for 24 h and finger than for office BP. Renal deactivation did not significantly affect heart rate. Regarding the effects on sympathetic nerve traffic, this parameter was unchanged 15 and 30 days after the procedure, whereas a significant reduction was

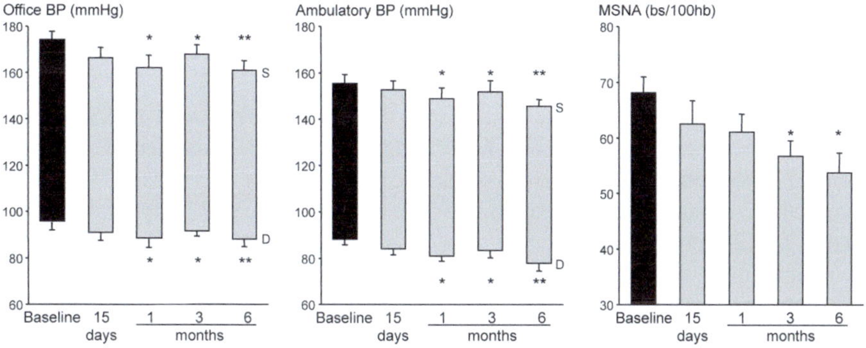

Fig. 20.5 Office (*left*) and ambulatory (*middle*) systolic (*S*) and diastolic (*D*) blood pressure values and muscle sympathetic nerve activity (*right panel*; MSNA) expressed as burst incidence corrected for heart rate values before (baseline), 15 days, 1 month, 3 months, and 6 months after bilateral renal denervation. Data are expressed as mean ± SEM. Asterisks (*$p<0.05$, **$p<0.01$) refer to the statistical significance between values recorded after the renal denervation procedure and those recorded before the intervention

observed after 3 and 6 months (Fig. 20.5). A specular behavior was also observed for baroreflex-muscle sympathetic nerve activity values. At the 6-month follow-up, the sympathetic nerve traffic reduction had a similar magnitude in patients displaying a BP reduction greater or lower the median value. Similarly, the BP reduction detected six months after renal deactivation was similar in patients displaying a sympathetic reduction greater or lower than the median value. The two major informations provided by the study are the following: (a) no quantitative relationship has been detected between BP and the sympathetic responses to the renal nerve ablation at any time during the 6-month follow-up, and (b) patients having a marked BP reduction in response to RDN can display a reduction in adrenergic tone superimposable to that observed in patients with a BP lesser pronounced. Thus, RDN can lower sympathetic activity even when BP is not or not yet reduced. Furthermore, when the denervation procedure markedly lowers BP, this can occur also in the absence of any similarly marked alterations of sympathetic drive and vice versa. These temporal, quantitative, and qualitative discrepancies suggest that the BP-lowering effects of renal deactivation are not necessarily dependent to, and thus not necessarily triggered by, a decrease in central sympathetic outflow. The observed improvement in baroreflex-sympathetic sensitivity is also unlikely to play a major role because, like the sympathetic nerve traffic, it shows a temporal discrepancy and no quantitative relationship with the BP effects. Thinking about other mechanisms, it is possible to suggest that (a) sympathetic nerve traffic does not reflect overall sympathetic deactivation, which is not in line with its close relation with general markers of sympathetic activity, such as plasma norepinephrine or norepinephrine spillover [75, 76], (b) BP reduction was accounted for by a better adherence of the patients to the prescribed drugs [77], (c) RDN might affect in a different way single fiber versus multifiber sympathetic nerve traffic recordings, taking into account that the single fiber approach has been shown to provide a more sensitive assessment of sympathetic nerve traffic when compared with the multifiber nerve recording [72],

(d) renal nerve ablation modifies the cardiovascular influence of neural pathways other than the sympathetic ones [78], or (e) factors such as reduction of blood volume and cardiac output by denervation diuresis are involved [79, 80].

Another interesting aspect coming from this study is that heart rate does not show any significant change in the short-term period after RDN in contrast with the marked concomitant sympathetic nerve traffic modifications. It is possible to speculate that the dissociation between the behavior of heart rate and peripheral sympathetic nerve activity reflects the fact that RDN, despite having peripheral sympathoinhibitory effects, does not affect cardiac sympathetic outflow. This data is confirmed in recent large-scale studies with a prolonged follow-up showing a significant increase of heart rate after RDN [81, 82].

20.6.2 Testing for Achieved Sympathetic Deactivation

The renal nerve ablation procedure necessitates that the effectiveness of denervation should be confirmed in studies of surgical RDN in experimental hypertension, documenting 90–95 % reduction in the kidney content of norepinephrine. RDN has been confirmed in the Symplicity HTN-1 trial by means of measuring norepinephrine spillover as a validated test for denervation. Measurement of regional norepinephrine spillover is well established as a valid test for sympathetic denervation, having been applied for two decades in the diagnosis of pure autonomic failure [83].

The degree of RDN achieved in the Symplicity HTN-1 trial was less than expected (on average 47 %) but was accompanied by an adequate antihypertensive response. It should be noted, however, that denervation is often incomplete and nonuniform between patients. It may be less than 25 %, which is inadequate for a full therapeutic effect. Although the denervation catheter technique might look easy, compared with other interventional procedures, achieving denervation is difficult. As previously described, some asymmetries in terms of nerve distribution around the artery are reported, favoring the ventral surface, but a significant number of nerves occupy each quadrant of the renal artery wall. These anatomic considerations suggest that the optimal renal nerve target injury zone may be the most distal of the renal artery where the nerves are closer to the catheter tip [59]. It remains unknown whether all renal nerve fibers must be ablated for successful BP lowering or if there is some critical threshold effect. Furthermore, it is unclear whether it is more important to interrupt efferent or afferent nerve traffic. Given that, these nerves travel together; they are injured simultaneously with the current renal ablation techniques.

20.7 Perspectives

All the studies, in which RDN procedures were delivered, were not accompanied by major complications both in the short- and long-term follow-up periods. It has been also shown that about 40 % of the denervated patients at the 18-month follow-up had achieved full BP control allowing them to substantially reduce in daily dosage of antihypertensive drugs. The evidence obtained by microanatomic studies has

Table 20.1 Different techniques of renal denervation

Approach	Technique	Device	Population
Invasive	RF ablation	Balloon:	
		OneShot	Human
		Vessix	Human
		Non-balloon:	
		Symplicity	Human
		Spiral	Human
		EnligHTN	Human
	Ultrasound	Paradise	Human
		Tivus	Human
	Others	Beta-Cath radiation	Human
Noninvasive	Ultrasound	Verve	Human
	Chemical	Cisplatin	Animal
		Vincristine	Animal
		Guanethidine	Animal
		Neurotoxin	Animal

clearly suggested that the nonselective partial RDN of both efferent and afferent nerve fibers (Table 20.1, 83) is likely to play a causative role for the effective treatment of resistant hypertension in the major trials like Symplicity HTN-1 [83] and Symplicity HTN-2 and EnligHTN [84]. While new devices will be disposable in the future, more attention should be obtained during the procedures with the application of thermal energy on the ventral region of proximal and middle arterial segments in which peri-arterial sympathetic nerve fibers are concentrated. The technological improvement both in the devices and in the ablative approach, accompanied by a demonstrated safety profile, will allow to apply this technique to several pathophysiological conditions characterized by a sympathetic overdrive and high cardiovascular risk other than subjects with difficult BP control.

References

1. Alexanders RS (1946) Tonic and reflex functions of medullary sympathetic cardiovascular centers. J Neurophysiol 9:205–17
2. Loewy AD (1990) Central autonomic pathways. In: Loewy AD, Spyer KM (eds) Central regulation of autonomic functions. Oxford University Press, Oxford, pp 88–103
3. Jordan D, Spyer KM (1986) Brainstem integration of cardiovascular and pulmonary afferent activity. Prog Brain Res 67:295–314
4. Coleridge HM, Coleridge JCG, Jordan D (1991) Integration of ventilator and cardiovascular control system. In: Crystal RG, West JB (eds) The lung: scientific foundations. Raven, New York, pp 1405–18
5. Janig W, Habler HJ (2000) Specificity in the organization of the autonomic nervous system: a basis for precise neural regulation of homeostatic and protective body functions. Prog Brain Res 122:351–67
6. Janig W (2006) The integrative action of the autonomic nervous system neurobiology of homeostasis. Cambridge University Press, Cambridge
7. Grassi G, Esler M (1999) How to assess sympathetic activity in humans. J Hypertens 17:719–34

8. Seravalle G, Dimitriadis K, Dell'oro R, Grassi G (2013) How to assess sympathetic nervous system activity in clinical practice. Curr Clin Pharmacol 8:182–8
9. Shen MJ, Zipes DP (2014) Role of the autonomic nervous system in modulating cardiac arrhythmias. Circ Res 114:1004–21
10. Grassi G, Vailati S, Bertinieri G, Seravalle G, Stella ML, Dell'Oro R, Mancia G (1998) Heart rate as a marker of sympathetic activity. J Hypertens 16:1635–9
11. Eckberg DL (1997) Sympathovagal balance: a critical appraisal. Circulation 96:3224–32
12. Esler M, Jennings G, Korner P, Blombery P, Zacharias N, Leonard P (1984) Measurement of total and organ-specific norepinephrine kinetics in humans. Am J Physiol 247:E21–8
13. Esler M, Jennings G, Korner P, Willett I, Dudley F, Hasking G, Anderson W, Lambert G (1988) Assessment of human sympathetic nervous system activity from measurements of norepinephrine turnover. Hypertension 11:3–20
14. Grassi G, Seravalle G, Dell'Oro R, Arenare F, Facchetti R, Mancia G (2009) Reproducibility patterns of plasma norepinephrine and muscle sympathetic nerve traffic in human obesity. Nutr Metab Cardiovasc Dis 19:469–75
15. Eisenhofer G, Esler MD, Goldstein DS, Kopin IJ (1991) Neuronal uptake, metabolism, and release of tritium-labeled norepinephrine during assessment of its plasma kinetics. Am J Physiol Endocrinol Metab 261:E505–15
16. Vaz M, Jennings G, Turner A, Cox H, Lambert G, Esler M (1997) Regional sympathetic nervous activity and oxygen consumption in obese normotensive human subjects. Circulation 96:3423–9
17. Hagbarth KE, Vallbo AB (1968) Pulse and respiratory grouping of sympathetic impulses in human muscle nerves. Acta Physiol Scand 74:96–108
18. Macefield VG, Wallin BG, Vallbo AB (1994) The discharge behavior of single vasoconstrictor motoneurones in human muscle nerves. J Physiol 481:799–809
19. Lambert EA, Schlaich MP, Dawood T, Sari C, Chopra R, Barton D, Kaye DM, Elam M, Esler M, Lambert GW (2011) Single-unit muscle sympathetic nervous activity and its relation to cardiac noradrenaline spillover. J Physiol 589:2597–605
20. Yamada Y, Miyajima E, Tochikubo O, Matsukawa AT, Ishii M (1989) Age-related changes in muscle sympathetic nerve activity in essential hypertension. Hypertension 13:870–7
21. Anderson EA, Sinkey CA, Lawton WJ, Mark AL (1989) Elevated sympathetic nerve activity in borderline hypertensive humans: evidence from direct intraneural recordings. Hypertension 14:177–83
22. Seravalle G, Lonati L, Buzzi S, Cairo M, Quarti Trevano F, Dell'oro R, Facchetti R, Mancia G, Grassi G (2015) Sympathetic nerve traffic and baroreflex function in optimal, normal and high-normal blood pressure states. J Hypertens 33:1411–7
23. Floras JS, Hara K (1993) Sympathoneural and hemodynamic characteristics of young subjects with mild essential hypertension. J Hypertens 11:647–55
24. Palatini P, Dorigatti F, Zaetta V, Mormino P, Mazzer A, Bortolazzi A, D'Este D, Pegoraro F, Milani L, Mos L, HARVEST Study Group (2006) Heart rate as a predictor of development of sustained hypertension in subjects screened for stage 1 hypertension: the HARVEST study. J Hypertens 24:1873–80
25. Grassi G, Seravalle G, Cattaneo BM, Bolla GB, Lanfranchi A, Colombo M, Giannattasio C, Brunani A, Cavagnini F, Mancia G (1995) Sympathetic activation in obese normotensive subjects. Hypertension 25:560–3
26. Kassab S, Kato T, Wilkins FC, Chen R, Hall JE, Kaiser J, Granger JP (1995) Renal denervation attenuates the sodium retention and hypertension associated with obesity. Hypertension 25:893–7
27. Anderson EA, Balon TW, Hoffman RP, Sinkey CA, Mark AL (1992) Insulin increases sympathetic activity but not blood pressure in borderline hypertensive humans. Hypertension 19:621–7
28. Julius S, Gundrandsson T, Jamerson K, Andersson O (1992) The interconnection between sympathetic, microcirculation and insulin resistance in hypertension. Blood Press 1:9–19

29. Grassi G, Dell'Oro R, Quarti Trevano F, Scopelliti F, Seravalle G, Paleari F, Gamba PL, Mancia G (2005) Noradrenergic and reflex abnormalities in patients with metabolic syndrome. Diabetologia 48:1359–65
30. Narkiewicz K, van de Borne PJ, Cooley RL, Dyken ME, Somers VK (1998) Sympathetic activity in obese subjects with and without obstructive sleep apnea. Circulation 98:772–6
31. Grassi G, Seravalle G, Quarti Trevano F, Mineo C, Lonati L, Facchetti R, Mancia G (2010) Reinforcement of the adrenergic overdrive in the metabolic syndrome complicated by obstructive sleep apnea. J Hypertens 28:1313–20
32. Huggett RJ, Scott EM, Gilbey SG, Stoker JB, Macintosh AF, Mary DA (2003) Impact of type 2 diabetes mellitus on sympathetic neural mechanisms in hypertension. Circulation 108:3097–101
33. Gordon RD, Backmann AW, Jackson RV, Saar N (1982) Increased sympathetic activity in renovascular hypertension in man. Clin Exp Pharmacol Physiol 9:277–81
34. Grassi G, Quarti Trevano F, Seravalle G, Arenare F, Volpe M, Furiani S, Dell'Oro R, Mancia G (2011) Early sympathetic activation in the initial stages of chronic renal failure. Hypertension 57:846–51
35. Hausberg M, Kosch M, Harmelink P, Barenbrock M, Hohage H, Kisters K, Dietl KH, Rahn KH (2002) Sympathetic nerve activity in end-stage renal disease. Circulation 106:1974–9
36. Leimbach WN Jr, Wallin BG, Victor RG, Aylward PE, Sundlof G, Mark AL (1986) Direct evidence from intraneural recordings for increased central sympathetic outflow in patients with heart failure. Circulation 73:913–9
37. Hasking GJ, Esler MD, Jennings GL, Burton D, Johns JA, Korner PI (1986) Norepinephrine spillover to plasma in patients with congestive heart failure evidence of increased overall and cardiorenal sympathetic nervous activity. Circulation 73:615–21
38. Grassi G, Seravalle G, Cattaneo BM, Lanfranchi A, Vailati S, Giannattasio C, Del Bo A, Sala C, Bolla GB, Pozzi M, Mancia G (1995) Sympathetic activation and loss of reflex sympathetic control in mild congestive heart failure. Circulation 92:3206–11
39. Smith HW (1951) The kidney: structure and function. Oxford Univ Press, New York
40. Smith HW (1937) The physiology of the kidney. Oxford Univ Press, New York
41. Muller J, Barajas L (1972) Electron microscopic and histochemical evidence for a tubular innervations in the renal cortex of the monkey. J Ultrastruct Res 41:533–49
42. Barajas L, Liu L, Powers K (1992) Anatomy of the renal innervations: intrarenal aspects and ganglia of origin. Can J Physiol Pharmacol 70:735–49
43. Bell-Reuss E, Trevino DL, Gottschalk CW (1976) Effects of renal sympathetic nerve stimulation on proximal water and sodium reabsorption. J Clin Invest 57:1104–7
44. Zanchetti A (1977) Neural regulation of renin release: experimental evidence and clinical implications in arterial hypertension. Circulation 56:691–8
45. LaGrange RG, Sloop CH, Schmid HE (1973) Selective stimulation of renal nerves in the anesthetized dog. Circ Res 33:704–12
46. Stella A (1992) The kidney as a sensor: functional evidence. J Hypertens 10:a113–s119
47. Zanchetti A, Stella A, Golin R, Genovesi S (1984) Neural control of the kidney – are there reno-renal reflexes? Clin Exp Hypertens 6:275–86
48. Campese VM (1997) Neurogenic factors and hypertension in chronic renal failure. J Nephrol 10:184–7
49. Ye S, Zhong H, Yanamadala V, Campese VM (2002) Renal injury caused by intraneural injection of phenol increases afferent and efferent renal sympathetic nerve activity. Am J Hypertens 15:717–24
50. Stella A, Zanchetti A (1991) Functional role of renal afferents. Physiol Rev 71:659–82
51. DiBona GF (2000) Neural control of the kidney: functionally specific renal sympathetic nerve fibers. Am J Physiol Regulatory Integrative Comp Physiol 279:R1517–24
52. Converse RL, Jacobsen TN, Toto RD, Jost CM, Cosentino F, Fouad-Tarazi F, Victor RG (1992) Sympathetic overactivity in patients with chronic renal failure. N Engl J Med 327:1912–8

53. Zoccali C, Mallamaci F, Parlongo S, Cutrupi S, Benedetto FA, Tripepi G, Bonanno G, Rapisarda F, Fatuzzo P, Seminara G, Cataliotti A, Stancanelli B, Malatino LS (2002) Plasma norepinephrine predicts survival and incident cardiovascular events in patients with end-stage renal disease. Circulation 105:1354–9
54. Hering D, Mahfoud F, Walton AS, Krum H, Lambert GW, Lambert EA, Sobotka PA, Bohm M, Cremers B, Esler M, Schlaich MP (2012) Renal denervation in moderate to severe CKD. J Am Soc Nephrol 23:1250–57
55. Schlaich MP, Bart B, Hering D, Walton A, Marusic P, Mahfoud F, Böhm M, Lambert EA, Krum H, Sobotka PA, Schmieder RE, Ika-Sari C, Eikelis N, Straznicky N, Lambert GW, Esler MD (2013) Feasibility of catheter-based renal nerve ablation and effects of sympathetic nerve activity and blood pressure in patients with end-stage renal disease. Int J Cardiol 168:2214–20
56. Rippy MK, Zarins D, Barman NC, Wu A, Duncan KL, Zarins CK (2011) Catheter-based renal sympathetic denervation: chronic preclinical evidence for renal artery safety. Clin Res Cardiol 100:1095–101
57. Tellez A, Rousselle S, Palmieri T, Rate WR IV, Wicks J, Degrange A, Hyon CM, Gongora CA, Hart R, Grundy W, Kaluza GL, Granada JF (2013) Renal artery nerve distribution and density in the porcine model: biologic implications for the development of radiofrequency ablation therapies. Transl Res 162:381–9
58. Tzafriri AR, Mahfoud F, Keating JH, Markham PM, Spognardi A, Wong G, Fujimaono K, Bohm M, Edelman ER (2014) Innervation patterns may limit response to endovascular renal denervation. J Am Coll Cardiol 64:1079–87
59. Atherton DS, Deep NL, Mendelsohn FO (2012) Microanatomy of the renal sympathetic nervous system: a human postmortem histologic study. Clin Anat 25:628–33
60. Sakakura K, Ladich E, Edelman ER, Markham P, Stanley JRL, Keating J, Kolodgie FD, Virmani R, Joner M (2014) Methodological standardization for the pre-clinical evaluation of renal sympathetic denervation. J Am Coll Cardiol Intv 7:1184–93
61. Tunstall RR, Winsor-Hines D, Butt M, Huibregtse B (2012) A preclinical comparative histological evaluation of the renal artery and nerves in the human cadaver and swine model. J Am Coll Cardiol 60(17):TCT 216. doi:10.1016/j.jacc.2012.08.238
62. Hua XY, Thodorsson-Norheim E, Lundberg JM, Kinn AC, Hockfelt T, Cuello AC (1987) Co-localization of tachykinins and calcitonin gene-related peptide in capsaicin-sensitive afferents in relation to motility effects on the human ureter in vitro. Neuroscience 23:693–703
63. Knight DS, Cicero S, Beal JA (1991) Calcitonin gene-related peptide-immunoreactive nerves in the rat kidney. Am J Anat 190:31–40
64. Mafeld S, Vasdev N, Haslam P (2012) Renal denervation for treatment resistant hypertension. Ther Adv Cardiovasc Dis 6:245–58
65. Grimson KS, Wilson H, Phemister DB (1937) The early and remote effects of total and partial paravertebral sympathectomy on blood pressure: an experimental study. Ann Surg 106:801–25
66. Grimson KS (1941) Total thoracic and partial to total lumbar sympathectomy and celiac ganglionectomy in the treatment of hypertension. Ann Surg 114:753–75
67. Smithwick RH, Thompson JE (1953) Splanchnicectomy for essential hypertension: results in 1266 cases. J Am Med Assoc 152:1501–4
68. Pfaff WW, Cade JR, De Quesada A, Jurkiewicz MJ (1968) Reevaluation of thoracic sympathectomy for the management of malignant hypertension. Surg Forum 19:172–4
69. Grassi G, Seravalle G, Brambilla G, Pini C, Alimento M, Facchetti R, Spaziani D, Cuspidi C, Mancia G (2014) Marked sympathetic activation and baroreflex dysfunction in true resistant hypertension. Int J Cardiol 177:1020–5
70. Schlaich MP, Sobotka PA, Krum H, Lambert E, Esler M (2009) Renal sympathetic nerve ablation for uncontrolled hypertension. N Engl J Med 361:932–4
71. Brickmann J, Heusser K, Schmidt BM, Menne J, Klein G, Bauersachs J, Haller H, Sweep FC, Diedrich A, Jordan J, Tank J (2012) Catheter-based renal nerve ablation and centrally

generated sympathetic activity in difficult-to-control hypertensive patients: prospective case series. Hypertension 60:1485–90
72. Hering D, Lambert EA, Marusic P, Walton AS, Krum H, Lambert GW, Esler MD, Schlaich MP (2013) Substantial reduction in single sympathetic nerve firing after renal denervation in patients with resistant hypertension. Hypertension 61:457–64
73. Hering D, Marusic P, Walton AS, Lambert EA, Krum H, Narkiewicz K, Lambert GW, Esler MD, Schlaich MP (2014) Sustained sympathetic and blood pressure reduction 1 year after renal denervation in patients with resistant hypertension. Hypertension 64:118–24
74. Grassi G, Seravalle G, Brambilla G, Trabattoni D, Cuspidi C, Corso R, Pieruzzi F, Genovesi S, Stella A, Facchetti R, Spaziani D, Bartorelli A, Mancia G (2015) Blood pressure responses to renal denervation precede and are independent of the sympathetic and baroreflex effects. Hypertension 65:1209–16
75. Mancia G, Grassi G (2014) The autonomic nervous system and hypertension. Circ Res 114:1804–14
76. Wallin BG, Thompson JM, Jennings GL, Esler MD (1996) Renal noradrenaline spillover correlates with muscle sympathetic activity in humans. J Physiol 49:881–7
77. Kjeldsen SE, Os I, Mahfoud F (2013) Treatment resistant hypertension and renal sympathetic denervation: drug adherence and the consolidation of blood pressure lowering effects. Eurointervention 9(suppl R):R7–9
78. DiBona GF, Esler M (2010) Translational medicine: the antihypertensive effect of renal denervation. Am J Physiol Regul Integr Comp Physiol 298:R245–53
79. Kubota J, Nishimura H, Ueyama M, Kawamura K (1993) Effects of renal denervation on pressure-natriuresis in spontaneously hypertensive rats. Jpn Circ J 57:1097–105
80. Wang Y, Denton KM, Golledge J (2013) Control of salt and volume retention cannot be ruled out as a mechanism underlying the blood pressure-lowering effect of renal denervation. Hypertens Res 36:1006–7
81. Ukena C, Mahfoud F, Spies A, Kindermann I, Linz D, Cremers B, Laufs U, Neuberger HR, Bohm M (2013) Effects of renal sympathetic denervation on heart rate and atrioventricular conduction in patients with resistant hypertension. Int J Cardiol 167:2846–51
82. Esler MD, Bohm M, Sievert H, Rump CL, Schmieder RE, Krum H, Mahfoud F, Schlaich MP (2014) Catheter-based renal denervation for treatment of patients with treatment-resistant hypertension: 36 month results from the SYMPLICITY HTN-2 randomized clinical trial. Eur Heart J 35:1752–9
83. Krum H, Schlaich M, Whitbourn R, Sobotka PA, Sadowski J, Bartus K, Kapelak B, Walton A, Sievert H, Thambar S, Abraham WT, Esler M (2009) Catheter-based renal sympathetic denervation for resistant hypertension: a multicentre safety and proof-of-principle cohort study. Lancet 373:1275–81
84. Worthley SG, Tsioufis CP, Worthley MI, Sinhal A, Chew DP, Meredith IT, Malalapan Y, Papademetriou V (2013) Safety and efficacy of a multi-electrode renal sympathetic denervation system in resistant hypertension: the EnligHTN-1 Trial. Eur Heart J 34:2132–40

Alternative Methods for Renal Denervation

21

Christian Ott and Roland E. Schmieder

Abbreviations

ABP	Ambulatory blood pressure
BP	Blood pressure
CTA	Computed tomography angiography
dRHTN	Drug-resistant hypertension
FSE	Fast spin echo
HIFU	High-intensity focused ultrasound
MRgHIFUS	Magnetic resonance-guided high-focused ultrasound
MRI	Magnetic resonance imaging
OCT	Optimal coherence tomography
RDN	Renal denervation

21.1 Introduction

To date, the main approaches and hence data about renal denervation (RDN) in drug resistant hypertension (dRHTN) are based on endovascular catheter-based delivery of "energy" for disrupting sympathetic (efferent) and sensory (afferent) nerve fibers running along the renal arteries. After the first success [1, 2], uncertainty or even disillusions have grown, since the apparently rigorously conducted randomized and sham-controlled Symplicity HTN-3 trial has failed to prove its primary efficacy end point [3]. However, post hoc analysis revealed

C. Ott, MD (✉) • R.E. Schmieder, MD
Department of Nephrology and Hypertension, University Hospital,
Friedrich-Alexander University Erlangen-Nürnberg, Ulmenweg 18, Erlangen 91054, Germany
e-mail: christian.ott@uk-erlangen.de; roland.schmieder@uk-erlangen.de

C. Tsioufis et al. (eds.), *Interventional Therapies for Secondary and Essential Hypertension*, Updates in Hypertension and Cardiovascular Protection,
DOI 10.1007/978-3-319-34141-5_21

Table 20.1 Clinical indications/scenarios for alternative methods of renal denervation

Anatomic abnormalities (e.g., narrow or short main trunk) or hemodynamically relevant stenosis of renal artery
History of prior renal artery intervention (e.g., balloon angioplasty or stenting)
Severe chronic kidney disease which is more prone to contrast nephropathy
Intolerance to antiplatelet agents or bleeding disorders
Unresponsiveness to endovascular approaches

methodological concerns [4], and additional preclinical data (e.g., autopsy study) showed that nerve fibers vary widely regarding distribution and depth from the lumen along the renal artery [5]. According to these data, currently used catheter-based radiofrequency systems may be unable to apply an adequate energy deposition from the intraluminal side to all nerves, thereby leaving a substantial number of nerve fibers unharmed. Moreover, several clinical conditions are known that limit the use of "traditional" endovascular catheter-based RDN (Table 20.1).

In the recent years, there was large effort for alternative approaches of RDN. Several technologies may overcome discussed limitations (e.g., insufficient energy deposition far away from the lumen side) by targeting the nerves from the extraluminal side. This chapter emphasizes these new alternative, non-endovascular methods of RDN. Since these approaches are at different stages of development and yet undergoing clinical evaluation, available data are limited.

21.2 Focused Ultrasound for RDN

Several approaches based on delivery of externally focused ultrasound have been developed or adapted from other interventional fields. The nature of this technique offers the opportunity of completely noninvasive RDN, thus overcoming several concerns of endovascular RDN (e.g., radiation exposure, contrast agent application). Moreover, it overcomes the anatomical limitation of a distinct minimum length of renal arteries, since external ablation can be achieved along a relatively short segment.

In general, a therapeutically focused ultrasound method is based on high-frequency sound waves (i.e., rapid mechanical oscillations) emitted by several piezoelectric transducers that are focused on a small tissue area and is a noninvasive method. In contrast to diagnostic imaging purposes of the ultrasound technique that uses low-intensity ultrasound with negligible tissue heating, the administered high-frequency ultrasound waves pass through the tissue and generate frictional heating of soft tissue in the proposed depth (hence resulting in a thermal ablation of, in this case, renal nerves along the renal artery) by directing several high-power ultrasound beams on a small tissue area. In principle, this technique enables the discrete damage of soft tissue within small boundary of less than ten cells wide [6].

21.2.1 Surround Sound System™

The Surround Sound System™ (Kona Medical Inc., Bellevue, Washington, USA) is a single mobile patient platform unit (Fig. 21.1), which consists of three major components: the generator, a treatment module with an imaging probe, and a water conditioner. The generator serves as the overall system controller, energizes and directs the treatment module, powers and processes signals from the targeting subsystem, and drives the applicator-positioning mechanisms.

Once the renal artery is localized with the imaging probe (a diagnostic 3-MHz ultrasound array with a focal range of 8–13 cm), the imaging probe is fixed to assure a secure imaging array. The treatment module contains a phased array therapeutic ultrasound transducer consisting of 220 individually phased elements to deliver high-energy ultrasound waves with water atop the transducer for cooling purposes and is positioned against the subject's skin for acoustic coupling. Necessarily, the imaging and the treatment module are interconnected, meaning that automatic tracking allows correction for slow motions of the kidney due to breathing in real time during the treatment (Fig. 21.2a). In case of excessive motions (e.g., whole snoring), which are beyond the tracking boundaries, administration of treatment ultrasound energy is automatically paused, but is completed after stable targeting and tracking has been achieved again.

The treatment itself contains nowadays delivery of focused therapeutic ultrasound energy in a specific annular pattern of 14 ellipsoid-shaped foci positioned within a 12-mm-diameter circle around the renal artery (Fig. 21.2b). Each individual ellipsoid-shaped focus has an average diameter of 2.3 mm on its short axis and about 15 mm along the long axis, i.e., the beam direction. The targeted tissue encompasses about 50% of the total focused ultrasound energy and according to

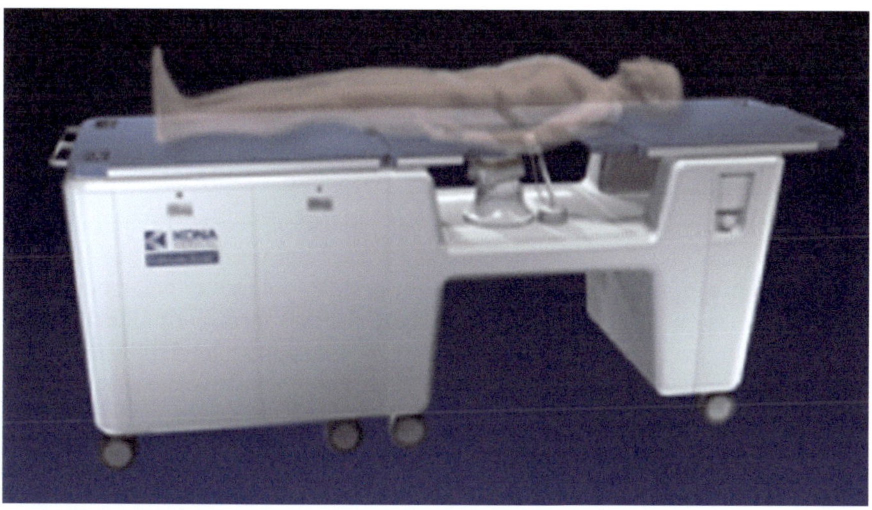

Fig. 21.1 Illustration of Surround Sound System™ (Kona Medical)

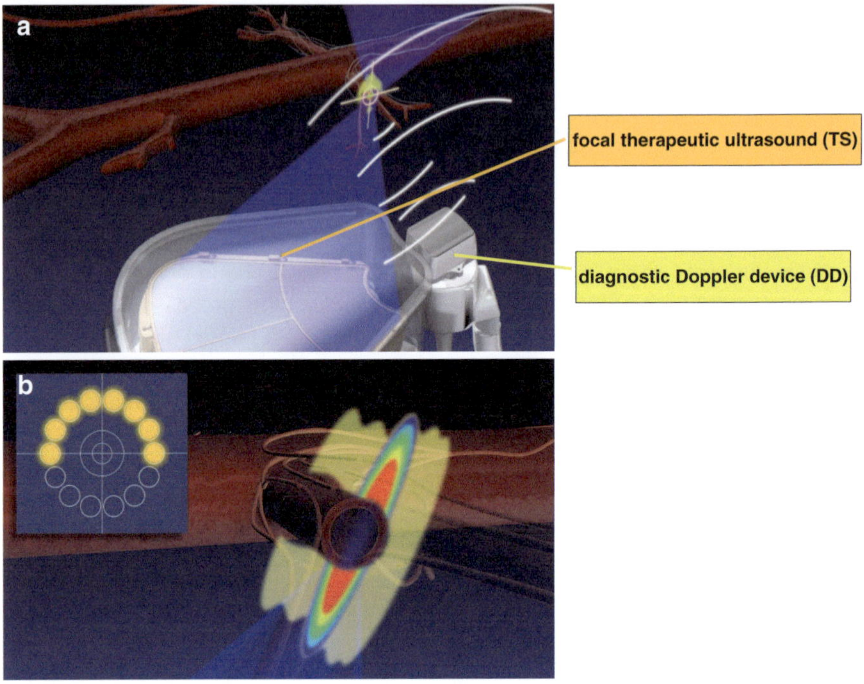

Fig. 21.2 (**a**) Illustration of externally delivered focused ultrasound to the renal artery and surrounding nerves. (**b**) Illustration of ablative field formation with 14 ellipsoid-shaped foci within a 12-mm-diameter circle relative to the renal artery

preexperiments is heated up to 50–75 °C. In contrast, although within the ultrasound field, the high-blood flow preserves a negligible rising of the temperature of the renal artery including its endothelium. The total treatment time is less than 3 min per side and each of the 14 energy delivery episodes lasts 7 s. The energy delivery is done in a robotic way and not dependent on the skills and experiences of the interventionalists.

21.2.1.1 Development/Evaluation Program

Based on the extensively conducted studies of simulation, bench working, and animal experiences, the energy delivery algorithm has been verified, and the development program comprised three consecutive prospective, multicenter, non-randomized smaller studies (WAVE I–III) using externally focused therapeutic ultrasound in subjects with uncontrolled hypertension (office systolic blood pressure [BP] >160 mmHg, although treated with at least three antihypertensive medications).

The WAVE I feasibility study, comprising 24 patients, assessed acute and chronic safety and efficacy. Subjects underwent RDN with externally focused ultrasound, effecting 18 focused lesions in about 13 min per side. However, for targeting and tracking reason, a 5-F intravascular catheter was inserted in the renal artery. This approach allowed understanding and assured correct delivery of focused ultrasound energy from an external position to the renal arteries and enabled subsequently the implementation of duplex-ultrasound image-guided targeting that takes renal artery movements due to normal breathing into account. An optimized treatment protocol was used in the WAVE II trial, causing 14 focused ellipsoid tissue lesions (in less than 3 min) per side [7]. A total of 18 subjects were enrolled in this study. Again an invasive catheter was inserted to direct and control energy delivery. In the WAVE III (NCT01926951) study, the first five patients underwent RDN by using also inserted catheter for targeting and the image-guided targeting of energy delivery to validate the performance and accuracy of a fully noninvasive duplex-ultrasound image-guided approach (Fig. 21.2). Thereafter, the other 22 patients with resistant hypertension included in WAVE III had a completely noninvasive duplex-ultrasound image-guided approach.

21.2.1.2 Efficacy

In total, the WAVE I–III studies comprise 69 patients with "severe" dRHTN, with at least 6 months of follow-up [8]. Office BP was 180 ± 19/98 ± 14 mmHg at baseline despite treatment with an average of 4.6 antihypertensive medications and was remarkably reduced by–24.6 ± 28/–9.0 ± 15 mmHg after 6 months, which remained stable (–23.8 ± 24/–10.3 ± 13 mmHg) after 12 months (N = 66) (Fig. 21.3). In addition, response rate (defined as decrement of office systolic BP ≥10 mmHg) was observed in 75 % of the patients after 6 months and 77 % after 12 months, respectively.

Specific attention is given to the subset of 22 patients (WAVE III study) who had a fully noninvasive externally delivered focused ultrasound approach. At 6-month follow-up, office BP was reduced by–19.8 ± 18/–6.2 ± 15 mmHg and at 12-month

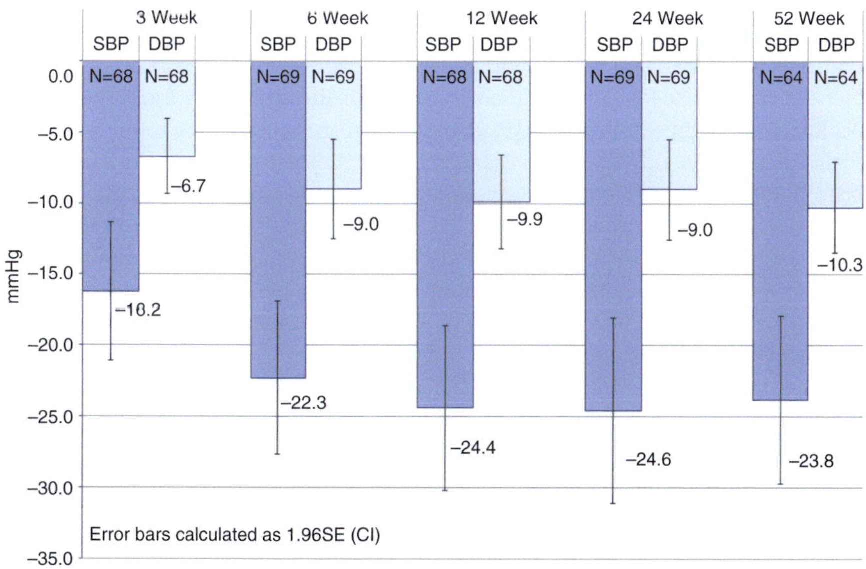

Fig. 21.3 WAVE I–III studies aggregate average office BP response (N = 69)

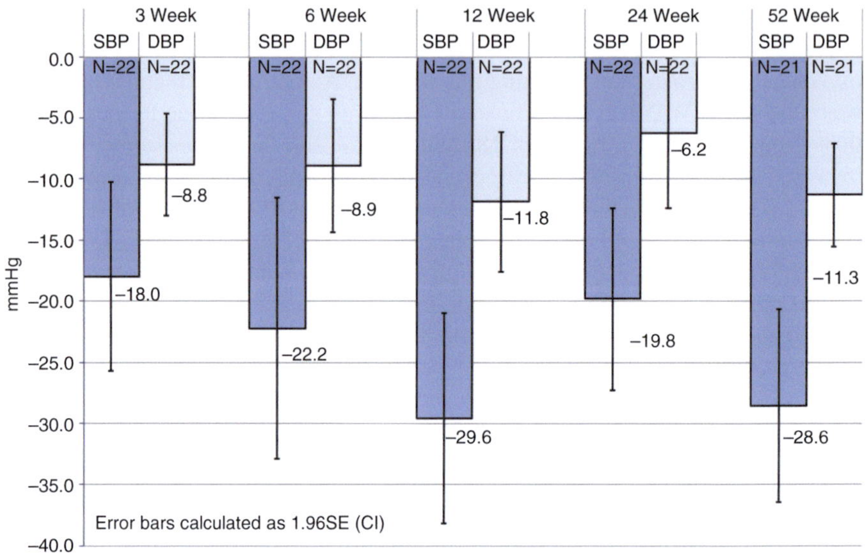

Fig. 21.4 WAVE III study average office BP response for patients with fully noninvasive RDN ($N=22$)

follow-up by–28.6 ± 19/–11.3 ± 10 mmHg, respectively (Fig. 21.4). Overall, BP reduction at 12-month follow-up in these noninvasively treated patients was comparable to the BP reduction observed in the whole study population (WAVE I–III).

21.2.1.3 Safety

Regarding safety emphasis has been given to local vascular injury, since thermal injury of the vessel wall may potentially lead to extensive media fibrosis, with the consequence of late renal artery stenosis, aneurysmatic dilation, or thromboembolic occlusions of segmental arteries [9, 10]. Indeed, case reports with development of renal artery stenosis after invasive endovascular radiofrequency-based RDN have been published [11–13]. Recent observations on post-procedural imaging of the renal vasculature with optical coherence tomography (OCT) raised concerns of vascular lesions induced by invasive endovascular RDN. Diffuse renal artery constriction and local tissue damage at the ablation site with edema and thrombus formation in varying extent have been described. Importantly, angiographic examinations were unable to detect these alterations [10, 14–16].

In face of these potential complications of invasive interventions of RDN, it is noteworthy to mention that in the WAVE I study, OCT of the renal artery was performed at baseline and immediately following RDN. In contrast to the described findings of invasive endovascular RDN, OCT examinations in five subjects revealed no evidence of thrombus formation, endothelial damage, or dissection of the renal artery after an externally delivered focused ultrasound for RDN (Fig. 21.5). In addition, control magnetic resonance imaging (MRI) scans at 3 weeks and 24 weeks posttreatment supported safety aspect by revealing no evidence of spasm, stenosis,

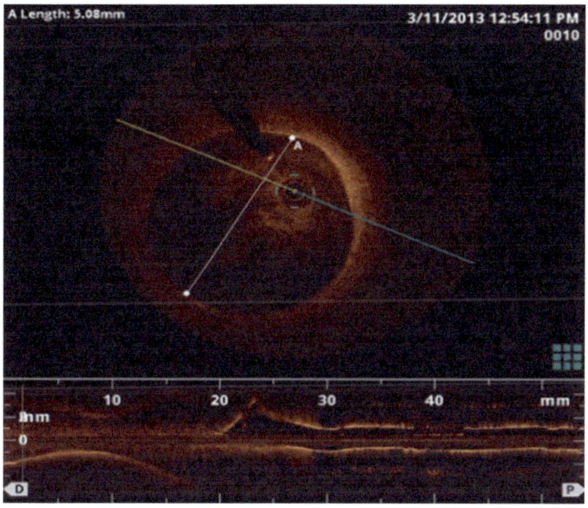

Fig. 21.5 Representative image of optical coherence tomography (WAVE I study), disclosing (immediately) vascular lesions induced by externally delivered focused ultrasound for RDN

thrombosis, dissection, aneurysm, pseudoaneurysm, fistula, or any other vascular abnormalities of the renal artery as well as alterations of the kidney and other abdominal surrounding organs [8].

The most common adverse event reported across the three studies was posttreatment back pain, which was reported in 32/69 subjects. However, these cases have to be classified as clinically insignificant, since no motor and sensory deficits were found, and back pain spontaneously resolved in the majority of patients within 3 days. Moreover, modifications of the energy delivery doses and pattern in WAVE I–III have resulted in a decreasing incidence of this complaint by the subjects.

21.2.1.4 Future

The WAVE IV trial (NCT02029885), a prospective randomized sham-controlled study using Kona Medical's Surround Sound® Renal Denervation System, has started enrollment. In total 132 patients with severe dRHTN (office systolic BP ≥160 mmHg and average systolic ambulatory blood pressure (ABP) ≥135 mmHg) will be analyzed, with the option of crossover after 12 months for patients of the sham-control group. In addition, toxicological urine analyses and pill counting are conducted, thereby assessing medication adherence. Hence, this study has the potential to answer several important questions which have repeatedly arisen [17].

21.2.2 High-Intensity Focused Ultrasound Tumor Therapeutic System

Based on the clinical treatment of different types of tumors, including the kidney with high-intensity focused ultrasound (HIFU) [18], this applied technique has been expanded in recent years. The feasibility and safety of the HIFU tumor therapeutic system (Model-JC200, Chongqing Haifu Technology Co. Ltd., Chongqing, China) for RDN was investigated in a preclinical canine model [19]. The therapeutic transducer verified an acoustic intensity at focus from 467 to 7,785 W/cm^2 (under a degassed water acoustic environment). Physical focal region has an ellipsoid shape (<2 × 2 mm). Location of target tissue was verified by using a diagnostic probe coaxially to the therapeutic beam (Fig. 21.6). For treatment, the therapeutic beam could be adjusted to 1 by 1 mm (in all three dimensions).

In a sham-controlled animal study, 3–5 color Doppler flow imaging sets were obtained for adjusting the position of the transducer in relation to the renal arteries. In total 36.3 ± 2.8 therapeutic ablations (each for 2 s) were applied within 27.4 min. In the treatment group, invasive BP was significantly reduced (–15.9/13.6 mmHg, both $p < 0.001$) after 28 days, but remained unchanged in the sham-controlled group. Accordingly, plasma noradrenaline concentration was significantly lower (–55.4 %, $p < 0.001$) on day 28 after ablation in the actively treated group, but again was unchanged in the sham-controlled group. Gross and histological examinations revealed disruption of nerve fibers in the target region, but showed also an intact endothelium and vascular smooth muscle layers. Moreover, no significant injuries along the acoustic path (e.g., skin, tissue around the target region) were observed.

Recently, the first in-man data (Chinese Clinical Trial Registry, ChiCTR-ONC-13003231) using the HIFU procedure were reported [20]. In a single-center study, 10 patients with resistant hypertension (but not consistent with the definition of ESH/ESC for dRHTN [21]) or intolerant to antihypertensive medications underwent the noninvasive HIFU-based RDN and were followed up for 6 months. By adjusting the color Doppler flow imaging, 5–6 targets longitudinally (every 5 mm), and rotationally (covering a four-quadrant ablation), and in the middle and distal segment of the renal artery were treated. Repeated acoustic energy emissions (50 × 2 s) with therapeutic power of 200–300 W were used for each target. Applied acoustic energy was 293.8 ± 43.2 kJ within 19.0 ± 0.9 min ablation time. Baseline office BP (24-h ABP) was 159 ± 9/91 ± 11 mmHg (169 ± 6/91 ± 11 mmHg) although treated with on average 4.8 ± 0.5 antihypertensive mediations. After

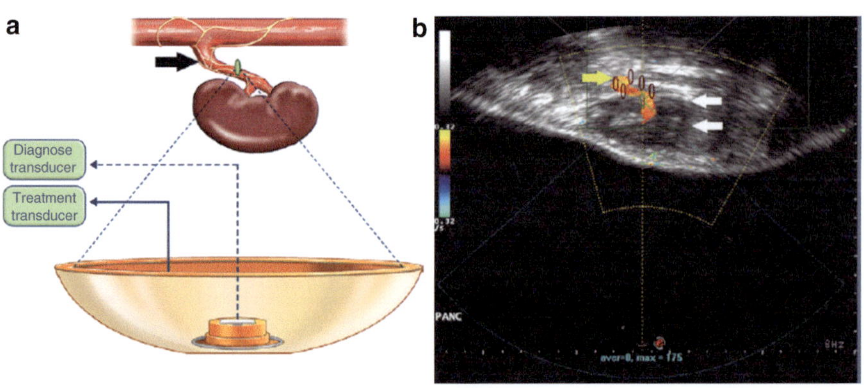

Fig. 21.6 (**a**) Illustration of RDN with HIFU tumor therapeutic system; green spot indicates focal spot of energy. (**b**) Ablated foci (*red spots*) on the renal artery (*yellow arrow*); kidney (*white arrow*) [19]

6 months, office BP was reduced by−29.2 ± 6.8/−11.2 ± 9.7 mmHg and 24-h ABP by−11.4 ± 4.8/−4.8 ± 4.8 mmHg (all $p < 0.01$), respectively. Surprisingly, no myalgia or back pain was reported after RDN. Moreover, renal artery imaging (color Doppler flow imaging or computed tomography angiography CTA in brackets showed no presence of a new hemodynamically relevant renal artery stenosis in the (relative short-term) follow-up, and renal function judged by estimated glomerular filtration rate remained unchanged.

21.2.3 Magnetic Resonance-Guided Ultrasound

Another noninvasive approach is based on magnetic resonance-guided high-focused ultrasound (MRgHiFUS), which is approved for treatment of uterine fibroids and painful bone metastases (in Europe and the USA), but also under consideration for other indications including RDN. The feasibility, safety, and efficacy were investigated in a normotensive domestic swine model ($N = 10$), since renal anatomy and morphology is similar to that of humans [22]. A clinical MR imaging-integrated focused ultrasound system (ExAblate 2000, Insightec-TxSonics, Haifa, Israel) with a transducer operating between 1.0 and 1.5 MHz was used for RDN. Target volume was based on pretreatment imaging using T2-weighted fast spin echo (FSE) sequences in three orthogonal planes. For calibration issues, 1–5 test sonications (targeting the ipsilateral longissimus lumborum muscle) were performed. After achievement of temperature elevation at target spot verified with real-time proton resonance frequency MR thermometry, focus has been moved to the originally proposed target of the periarterial tissue (Fig. 21.7). Applied acoustic energy was based

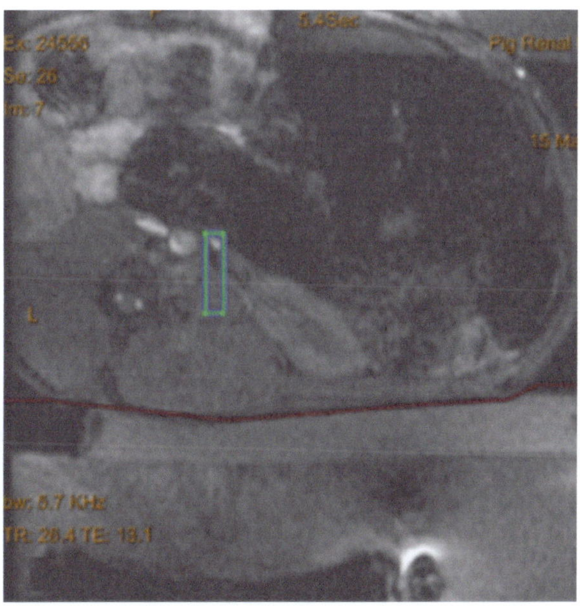

Fig. 21.7 Sonication planning image of magnetic resonance-guided high-focused ultrasound for RDN (adapted from [22])

on the established protocols for treatment of uterine fibroids. Starting at the ostium of the right renal artery (left artery served as intra-individual control) on average 9.8 ± 2.6, ablation spots (completely covering the periarterial tissue) with an acoustic energy of 2.67 ± 0.5 kJ were applied. After the intervention increased, signal intensity (due to edema in response to thermal injury) was used as a parameter of technical success, which however only was evident in 3 out of 9 treated pigs. Histopathological evaluations showed no disruption of nerve fibers, and norepinephrine concentration in the renal tissue did not clearly differ between treated (right) and untreated (left) sides (391.7 ± 110 vs. 442.2 ± 121 ng/g, $p = 0.078$). In summary, in this small animal study, MRgHiFUS failed to achieve effective RDN, which may be based on insufficient energy deposition most likely attributed to the small acoustic window and energy absorption by prominent transverse process and its adjacent fascia. In humans, however, a larger acoustic window can be assumed, and further investigations are necessary to delineate the true therapeutic efficacy in humans.

21.3 Chemical RDN with Alcohol Injection

There are several approaches for "chemical" extraluminal RDN. It has to be kept in mind that all of these techniques are of invasive nature and require, at least in part, radiation.

Ethanol is an FDA-approved drug for neurolysis and is frequently used for treatment of chronic pain (neural plexus) or spasticity (peripheral nerves) [23]. Moreover, CT-guided ethanol injection into the celiac plexus has been shown to be safe and effective for pain release due to pancreatitis and pancreas tumor, respectively [24, 25]. Beyond that, popularity of ethanol as a neurotoxic agent is driven by the facts of easy availability, inexpensiveness, and the relatively easy handling.

Based on these experiences and the underlying pathophysiology, the image-guided percutaneous ethanol injection in the surrounding tissue of renal arteries has been investigated.

21.3.1 MRI

In animal experiments (domestic pigs), the feasibility and efficacy of MR-guided ethanol injection for RDN has been tested [26]. Pre-procedural anatomy of renal arteries and skin entry was determined by axial and/or coronal fat-suppressed T2-weighted (T2w) spin echo images. Skin entry and adjustments of the 20-G needle during its path to the target (in near-real time) was done with an interactive T1w FSE sequence. Consecutively 1-ml bupivacaine-gadolinium-based contrast agent and a (600:1) mixture of 95 % ethanol and Gadovist (5 ml for the first two and 10 ml for the other four pigs) were injected. Ethanol was injected unilaterally, hence each animal served as its own control. Distribution of applied solution, as a measure of technical success (defined by homogenously periarterial spreading along the renal artery), was monitored in real time in all treated animals. Regarding efficacy, there was no significant change of norepinephrine concentration in the renal parenchyma in the first two pigs treated with 5-ml solution. In contrast, in animals treated with the increased dose application of 10 ml, there was a significant reduction of norepinephrine concentration of renal parenchyma by about 53 % (536 ± 312 vs. 254 ± 176 ng/g, $p = 0.017$) between untreated and treated side, confirmed by histologically observed neural degeneration. Regarding safety, hydronephrosis was detected in one animal treated with the increased application of 10 ml in the 4-week follow-up MRI, probably due to diffuse spread in the retroperitoneum.

21.3.2 Computed Tomography

At present, similar approaches of percutaneous ethanol application for RDN, however using CTA (due to practicable issues) instead of MRI, were evaluated in a case report [27], an animal model [28], and a first-in-human study [29].

In animal experiments (using sheep, since swine are not available in Iran), feasibility and efficacy of CT-guided ethanol injection for RDN was evaluated [28]. Using spiral CT scan, a 22-G needle was positioned from the posterolateral angle adjacent to the right renal artery, and final position was checked by injection of 10-ml 2 % lidocaine and 2-ml contrast agent. Thereafter, 99.6 % ethanol (note: the volume is not reported) was injected. Left renal artery, which is less accessible (large stomach), served as its own control. After 4 weeks, norepinephrine concentration of renal parenchyma was reduced by 40 % on average (9.73 (range 5.78–21.31) vs. 5.8 (range 1.07–15.29) ppm, $p = 0.0016$). In accordance, histological assessment revealed effective denervation, and no injury of the artery, ureter, and renal parenchyma were reported. Follow-up MRI, MR angiography, and urography showed no renal artery stenosis or other alterations.

To date, a first phase II single-arm open-label pilot trial, comprising 11 patients with "severe" dRHTN (BP >160 mmHg, despite treatment with at least three antihypertensive medications including a diuretic), assessed safety and preliminary efficacy data of CT-guided ethanol injection for RDN [29]. Prior to intervention, a CTA (slice thickness, 1 mm) was performed to assess the anatomy of renal arteries (Fig. 21.8a). Under control with CT fluoroscopy, correct placement of an 18.5-G needle next to the renal arteries was verified, and consecutively 1–2-ml of 2 % lidocaine and a mixture of 95 % ethanol with 2-ml iodine contrast agent was administered (Fig. 21.8b, c). This has the advantage that correct needle tip position can be verified as well as the appropriate distribution pattern can be visualized (Fig. 21.8d). In two cases distribution pattern was only 90° on one side, all others had at least 180°, but a distribution of 360° around the renal artery (indicative of a full four-quadrant ablation) was only evident in three cases (one of them on both sides).

Notably, antihypertensive medication was changed in all patients during the 6-month follow-up. After 6 months, office systolic BP was significantly reduced by −32.3 mmHg (baseline 195/100 mmHg, $p = 0.003$), but change of 24-h systolic ABP by −6.3 mmHg (baseline 165/94 mmHg, $p = 0.252$) did not reach statistical significance. Regarding safety, renal function showed no clear pattern (both improvement

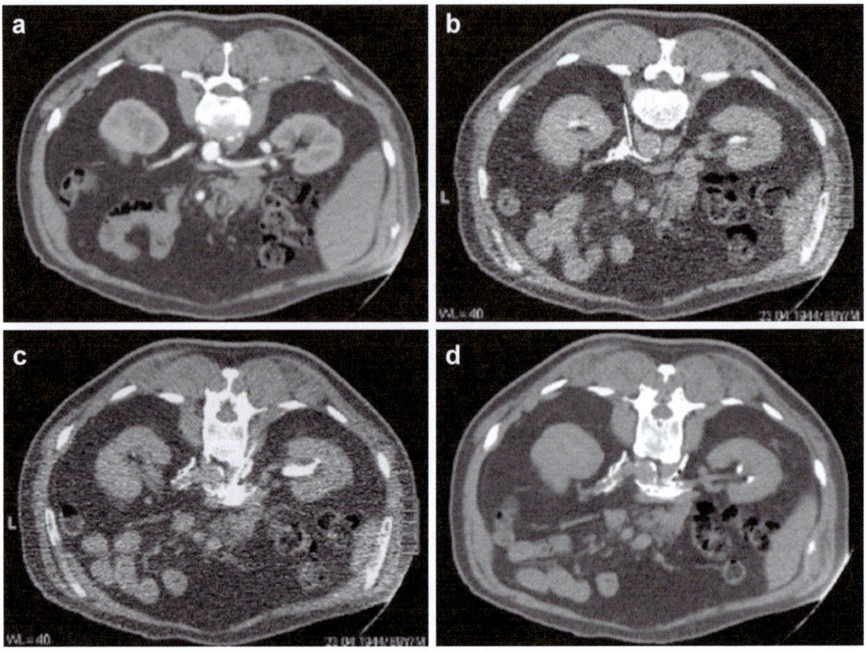

Fig. 21.8 (**a**) Planning CT angiogram for assessment of renal arterial anatomy. (**b**) Placement of an 18.5-G needle under CT fluoroscopy to the left renal artery. (**c**) Placement of an 18.5-G needle under CT fluoroscopy to the right renal artery. (**d**) Imaging of the final distribution of the radiopaque ethanol/ionidine contrast mixture (adapted from [29])

and worsening in patients with chronic kidney disease was observed, but no patient had doubling of serum creatinine or required dialysis). Pain was self-limiting within 1 day. Interestingly, four patients with prior catheter-based RDN showed also no response to CT-guided ethanol injection for RDN, and recruitment of patients with previous RDN was therefore stopped.

21.3.3 Chemical RDN with Injection of Neurotoxins and Other Agents

There are further efforts for testing other agents for RDN by local application [30]. As routinely done in animal experiment with rats, renal arteries were surgically prepared, and different agents were locally applied (via 28-G needle) to the perivascular space superior or inferior of the left renal artery. Thereafter, reflected intestines were repositioned and the abdomen was closed. After 3 days, the kidneys were removed and analyzed. Efficacy of RDN was assessed by comparing renal norepinephrine concentration in the renal tissue between un- and treated kidneys. All used agents, namely, hypertonic saline (150 µl of 10 % solution in water [1.7 M, 100 mg/mL]), salicylic acid (300 µL 10 % solution dissolved in ethanol), and guanethidine (75 µl, dissolved in glycerine at a concentration of 6.7 mg/mL), resulted in comparable norepinephrine depletion between untreated and treated kidneys (e.g., guanethidine, 84.1 ± 28.5 vs. 42.9 ± 2.1 ng/g, $p < 0.05$). Based on previous studies, only one dose of agents was used, indicating that the lowest dose of concentration necessary for "maximal" denervation is unknown.

In a subsequent study, a dose-response relationship of topical applied paclitaxel (10^{-6}–10^{-2}M) for RDN was assessed [30]. However, the feasibility of correct application of these drugs, and hence its safety and efficacy within a clinically applicable procedure (e.g., CT guided), has to be proven.

21.4 RDN of the Renal Pelvis

Another treatment approach is based on a nonvascular system that targets neither the renal artery nor the surrounding tissue of the renal artery [31].

It is proposed that the majority of afferent sensory nerves are located in the renal pelvic area with the greatest density in the pelvic wall [32], hence being easily accessible via transurethral approach. The NephroBlate™ renal denervation system (Verve Medical Inc., Santa Barbara, USA) was developed for targeting these nerves in the renal pelvis. The system consists of a monopolar radiofrequency electrode catheter and a generator (50 W) for controlling and regulating energy delivery, duration, temperature, and impedance (Fig. 21.9a). After a guidewire is placed in the renal pelvis via the working channel of a cystoscope in standard

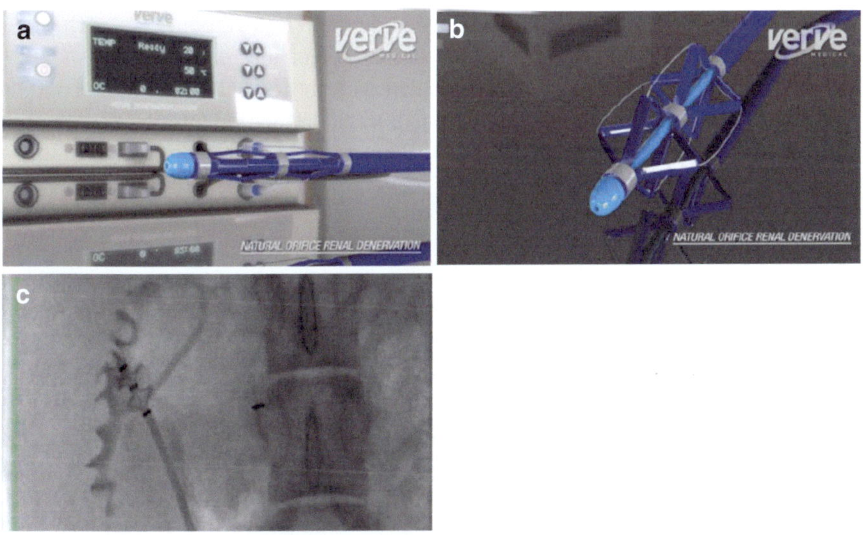

Fig. 21.9 (**a**) Verve Medical System. (**b**) Radiofrequency electrode with extended wings. (**c**) Fluoroscopic image of the radiofrequency catheter within the renal pelvis of a swine (adapted from [33])

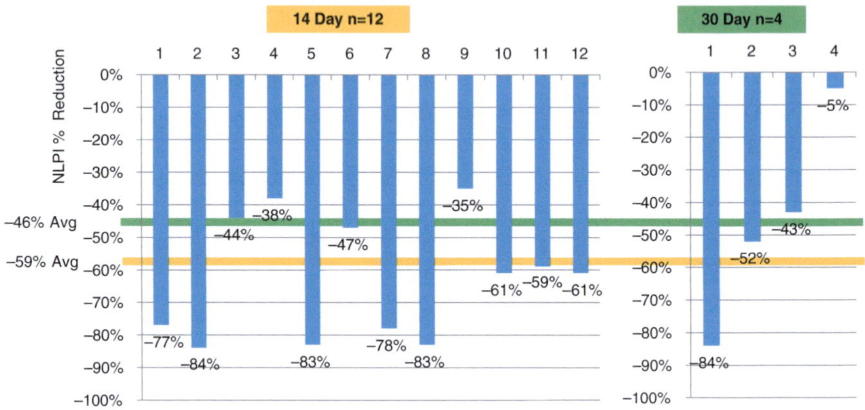

Fig. 21.10 Reduction of norepinephrine concentration from baseline after transurethral RDN; data are based on single kidneys (adapted from [33])

urological technique, the 9-F catheter can be mounted along the guidewire distal to the ureteropelvic junction and proximal to the calcites, where the wings are extended (Fig. 21.9b).

In animal experiments (domestic swine) after incision of the bladder, the catheter was advanced retrograde into the renal pelvis (Fig. 21.9c) [33]. Radiofrequency energy was applied in 16 animals and 16 other animals served as control. Of each group, three animals were euthanized immediately after RDN, five animals after 7 days, six animals after 14 days, and two animals after 30 days of RDN. For safety issues, bilateral pyelograms, ureterograms, and renal angiography were performed in the cohort with at least 7-day follow-up to detect any pathological findings. Moreover, histopathological analysis revealed damage (i.e., ablation) of the nerves in the treated area, but without parenchymal or vascular thermal injury. Consistently, norepinephrine concentration of the renal tissue was reduced in all treated animals compared to control group (Fig. 21.10).

Based on these findings, the first-in-human application was performed in three end-stage renal disease patients who underwent elective nephrectomy due to nephrolithiasis ($n=2$) and pre-renal transplantation ($n=1$) with underlying polycystic kidney disease (both kidneys were treated) [34]. Elective nephrectomy was performed one week after RDN. Histopathology showed a disruption of nerves between pelvic space and serosa (1.75 mm) in treated areas, but no alterations in the other (untreated) areas. In the next step, 4 patients with "severe" resistant hypertension (office systolic BP ≥160 mmHg (≥150 mmHg for patients with type 2 diabetes) despite being treated with ≥3 antihypertensive drugs including 1 diuretic) underwent transurethral RDN (energy delivery for 6 min, 70 °C, 5 W) within 16–25 min [34]. There was no evidence of post-procedural pain, bleeding, urologic complications (e.g., perforation or stricture), or kidney damages. At 1 month, there was a remarkable office BP reduction of 44/13 mmHg (baseline, 172/94 mmHg), and it remained stable, meaning that even after 6-month follow-up, patients were in the normotensive range.

21.5 Summary

RDN has experienced turbulent times and has not yet emerged as a clinical routine intervention in patients with dRHTN. Intensive research activities are currently performed and several alternative methods for RDN have been introduced. It has to be kept in mind that the cornerstone of any further novel approaches for RDN are primarily safety and efficacy supported by appropriate and well-conducted randomized, sham-controlled trials (including patients with true dRHTN and adequate assessment of adherence). Furthermore, new developments may also be rated on their general feasibility including predictable ablation success and operator independency, respectively. From a pathophysiological point of view and from the lessons learned in recent years, the application of noninvasive high-focused ultrasound energy may be a very promising approach for RDN. First human studies have revealed a remarkable BP reduction, without any significant safety concerns. Nevertheless, there are limitations based on the need for visualization of renal artery for targeting tracking, which may be in part difficult in, e.g., obese patients.

Other approaches are based on the imaging-guided application of "chemical" agents for RDN, but this approach has the disadvantage of being invasive. The nonvascular approach is based on targeting in particular afferent sensory nerves of the renal pelvis. These alternative approaches showed first promising results, but data are limited and do not permit any judgment of their clinical value.

So far, in humans no rigorously assessed data are available comparing different techniques regarding safety and efficacy of the various invasive and noninvasive alternative techniques of RDN. This might also be the subject of future studies.

References

1. Krum H, Schlaich M, Whitbourn R et al (2009) Catheter-based renal sympathetic denervation for resistant hypertension: a multicentre safety and proof-of-principle cohort study. Lancet 373:1275–1281
2. Symplicity HTNI, Esler MD, Krum H et al (2010) Renal sympathetic denervation in patients with treatment-resistant hypertension (the symplicity HTN-2 trial): a randomised controlled trial. Lancet 376:1903–1909
3. Bhatt DL, Kandzari DE, O'Neill WW et al (2014) A controlled trial of renal denervation for resistant hypertension. N Engl J Med 370:1393–1401
4. Kandzari DE, Bhatt DL, Brar S et al (2015) Predictors of blood pressure response in the SYMPLICITY HTN-3 trial. Eur Heart J 36:219–227
5. Sakakura K, Ladich E, Cheng Q et al (2014) Anatomic assessment of sympathetic peri-arterial renal nerves in man. J Am Coll Cardiol 64:635–643
6. ter Haar GR, Robertson D (1993) Tissue destruction with focused ultrasound in vivo. Eur Urol 23(Suppl 1):8–11
7. Neuzil P, Whitbourn RJ, Starek Z, Esler MD, Brinton T, Gertner M (2013) Optimized external focused ultrasound for renal sympathetic denervation - wave II trial. J Am Coll Cardiol 62(18_S1):B20–B20. doi:10.1016/j.jacc.2013.08.794
8. Neuzil P, Ormiston MD, Brinton TJ et al (2015) Externally delivered focused ultrasound for renal denervation. JACC Cardiovasc Interv (submitted)

9. Steigerwald K, Titova A, Malle C et al (2012) Morphological assessment of renal arteries after radiofrequency catheter-based sympathetic denervation in a porcine model. J Hypertens 30:2230–2239
10. Templin C, Jaguszewski M, Ghadri JR et al (2013) Vascular lesions induced by renal nerve ablation as assessed by optical coherence tomography: pre- and post-procedural comparison with the simplicity catheter system and the EnligHTN multi-electrode renal denervation catheter. Eur Heart J 34:2141–2148, 2148b
11. Kaltenbach B, Id D, Franke JC et al (2012) Renal artery stenosis after renal sympathetic denervation. J Am Coll Cardiol 60:2694–2695
12. Vonend O, Antoch G, Rump LC, Blondin D (2012) Secondary rise in blood pressure after renal denervation. Lancet 380:778
13. Pucci G, Battista F, Lazzari L, Dominici M, Boschetti E, Schillaci G (2014) Progression of renal artery stenosis after renal denervation. Impact on 24-hour blood pressure. Circulation journal : official journal of the Japanese Circulation Society 78:767–768
14. Ierna S, Biondi-Zoccai G, Bachis C et al (2013) Transcatheter renal sympathetic ablation for resistant hypertension: in vivo insights in humans from optical coherence tomography. Int J Cardiol 165:e35–e37
15. Karanasos A, Van Mieghem N, Bergmann MW et al (2015) Multimodality intra-arterial imaging assessment of the vascular trauma induced by balloon-based and nonballoon-based renal denervation systems. Circ Cardiovasc Interv 8:e002474
16. Schmid A, Schmieder R, Lell M et al (2016) Mid-term vascular safety of renal denervation assessed by follow-up MR imaging. Cardiovascular and interventional radiology 39:426–432
17. Mahfoud F, Bohm M, Azizi M et al (2015) Proceedings from the European clinical consensus conference for renal denervation: considerations on future clinical trial design. Eur Heart J 36:2219–2227
18. Illing RO, Kennedy JE, Wu F et al (2005) The safety and feasibility of extracorporeal high-intensity focused ultrasound (HIFU) for the treatment of liver and kidney tumours in a western population. Br J Cancer 93:890–895
19. Wang Q, Guo R, Rong S et al (2013) Noninvasive renal sympathetic denervation by extracorporeal high-intensity focused ultrasound in a pre-clinical canine model. J Am Coll Cardiol 61:2185–2192
20. Rong S, Zhu H, Liu D et al (2015) Noninvasive renal denervation for resistant hypertension using high-intensity focused ultrasound. Hypertension 66:e22–e25
21. Mancia G, Fagard R, Narkiewicz K et al (2013) 2013 ESH/ESC guidelines for the management of arterial hypertension: the task force for the management of arterial hypertension of the European Society of Hypertension (ESH) and of the European Society of Cardiology (ESC). J Hypertens 31:1281–1357
22. Freyhardt P, Heckmann L, Beck A et al (2014) MR-guided high-focused ultrasound for renal sympathetic denervation-a feasibility study in pigs. Journal of therapeutic ultrasound 2:12
23. Jang SH, Ahn SH, Park SM, Kim SH, Lee KH, Lee ZI (2004) Alcohol neurolysis of tibial nerve motor branches to the gastrocnemius muscle to treat ankle spasticity in patients with hemiplegic stroke. Arch Phys Med Rehabil 85:506–508
24. Noble M, Gress FG (2006) Techniques and results of neurolysis for chronic pancreatitis and pancreatic cancer pain. Curr Gastroenterol Rep 8:99–103
25. Kambadakone A, Thabet A, Gervais DA, Mueller PR, Arellano RS (2011) CT-guided celiac plexus neurolysis: a review of anatomy, indications, technique, and tips for successful treatment. Radiographics: a review publication of the Radiological Society of North America, Inc 31: 1599–1621
26. Streitparth F, Walter A, Stolzenburg N et al (2013) MR-guided periarterial ethanol injection for renal sympathetic denervation: a feasibility study in pigs. Cardiovasc Intervent Radiol 36:791–796
27. Streitparth F, Gebauer B, Nickel P et al (2014) Percutaneous computer tomography-guided ethanol sympathicolysis for the treatment of resistant arterial hypertension. Cardiovasc Intervent Radiol 37:513–518

28. Firouznia K, Hosseininasab SJ, Amanpour S et al (2015) Renal sympathetic denervation by CT-scan-guided periarterial ethanol injection in sheep. Cardiovasc Intervent Radiol 38:977–984
29. Ricke J, Seidensticker M, Becker S et al (2016) Renal sympathetic denervation by CT-guided ethanol injection: a phase II pilot trial of a novel technique. Cardiovasc Intervent Radiol 39:251–260
30. Consigny PM, Davalian D, Donn R, Hu J, Rieser M, Stolarik D (2014) Chemical renal denervation in the rat. Cardiovasc Intervent Radiol 37:218–223
31. Kopp UC (2015) Role of renal sensory nerves in physiological and pathophysiological conditions. Am J Physiol Regul Integr Comp Physiol 308:R79–R95
32. Marfurt CF, Echtenkamp SF (1991) Sensory innervation of the rat kidney and ureter as revealed by the anterograde transport of wheat germ agglutinin-horseradish peroxidase (WGA-HRP) from dorsal root ganglia. J Comp Neurol 311:389–404
33. Heuser RR, Mhatre AU, Buelna TJ, Berci WL, Hubbard BS (2013) A novel non-vascular system to treat resistant hypertension. EuroIntervention J EuroPCR Collab Working Group Intervent Cardiol Europ Soc Cardiol 9:135–139
34. Heuser RR, Buelna T, Gold A, Rao RR, Van Alstine W, Desai M (2014) Preclinical and early clinical experience of a non-vascular treatment for resistant hypertension. J Am Coll Cardiol 64(11_S). doi:10.1016/j.jacc.2014.07.459

Carotid Baroreceptor Stimulation 22

Luke J. Laffin and George L. Bakris

Abbreviations

BAT	Baroreceptor activation therapy
BP	Blood pressure
CBS	Carotid baroreceptor stimulation
HTN	Hypertension
SNS	Sympathetic nervous system

22.1 Introduction

Afflicting almost one third of all adults in the United States, hypertension (HTN) is a major driver of cardiovascular morbidity and mortality [1]. Unfortunately, even with over 125 antihypertensive medications available to individuals within the United States, only half of all patients with hypertension have their blood pressure (BP) adequately controlled [2]. Reasons why patients are unable to achieve goal BPs are numerous and in fact similar to the etiology of HTN itself. Common modifiable causes include, but

L.J. Laffin, MD
Section of Cardiology, Department of Medicine, University of Chicago Medicine, Chicago, IL 60637, USA

Section of Endocrinology, Diabetes and Metabolism, The ASH Comprehensive Hypertension Center, University of Chicago Medicine, 5841 S. Maryland Ave., MC 1027, Chicago, IL 60637, USA

G.L. Bakris, MD, FASN, FASH, FAHA (✉)
Section of Endocrinology, Diabetes and Metabolism, The ASH Comprehensive Hypertension Center, University of Chicago Medicine, 5841 S. Maryland Ave., MC 1027, Chicago, IL 60637, USA
e-mail: gbakris@gmail.com

C. Tsioufis et al. (eds.), *Interventional Therapies for Secondary and Essential Hypertension*, Updates in Hypertension and Cardiovascular Protection,
DOI 10.1007/978-3-319-34141-5_22

are not limited to, excess dietary salt intake, inadequate sleep, and obesity. However, even with the appropriate lifestyle modifications, the need for pharmacological therapy to lower BP is required in the vast majority of hypertensive patients.

Achieving guideline goals for BP is particularly difficult among individuals with resistant or refractory HTN. Resistant hypertension is defined as BP that remains above goal in spite of the concurrent use of three maximally tolerated antihypertensive agents of different classes, one of which is a diuretic. Refractory hypertension is defined as a subgroup of patients with resistant hypertension that have uncontrolled BP, even with maximal medical therapy (four or more drugs with complementary mechanisms given at maximal tolerated doses) under the care of a HTN specialist [3].

Guidelines published in 2014 endorsing less stringent BP goals are now in question after the results the Systolic Blood Pressure Intervention Trial (SPRINT) [2, 4]. SPRINT demonstrated significantly less cardiovascular events and improved mortality with strict BP control in a wide range of patients (including the elderly), but resulted in more medication-related adverse effects in those treated to a goal systolic BP of less than 120 mmHg. This amalgamation of factors creates quite the challenge for those managing hypertension. What is a clinician to do?

First, there must be recognition that successful BP lowering ensures all potential mechanisms for BP elevation are blocked [5]. Often overlooked, or inadequately addressed, is inhibition of the sympathetic nervous system (SNS). Adrenergic overdrive in younger patients and altered sympathetic and parasympathetic balance in older individuals may trigger elevated BPs. SNS overactivity is also likely the driving force in refractory hypertension [3], in contrast to conventional wisdom that resistant hypertension is due to persistent hypervolemia.

Pharmacologic inhibition of the SNS with centrally active alpha-2 adrenergic receptor medications, such as a-methyldopa, clonidine, and guanfacine, effectively lowers BP in most patients. However these therapies elicit intolerable, dose-dependent side effects limiting their use [6]. In response to the need for more effective BP-lowering therapies directed toward the SNS, especially in patients with resistant and refractory hypertension, device-driven therapy is an area of intense development and investigation. Renal denervation therapy, once thought to be the panacea addressing the SNS, is now in question following the negative results of SYMPLICITY HTN-3 [7]. However, the major reason for this was inadequate renal denervation as was subsequently shown, and hence, ongoing trials using a new technique and catheter will resolve this issue in the near future [8, 9].

Carotid baroreceptor stimulation (CBS) is under active intense investigation in multiple cardiovascular conditions, including hypertension, with favorable results. The following reviews the pathophysiology of CBS, procedural aspects, and the safety and efficacy.

22.2 Baroreceptors and Blood Pressure Modulation Mechanisms

Activation of the SNS is one of the major mechanisms involved in chronically elevated BPs. Sympathetic activation contributes to the development of the HTN, by promoting initial BP elevation in its early clinical stages and also by maintaining this BP elevation chronically. Adrenergic overdrive triggers not only elevated BPs, but also is a contributor to left ventricular hypertrophy and certain metabolic abnormalities detected in hypertensive patients, as well as other hypertension-related end-organ damage.

The role of sympathetic activation in HTN was determined by an experimental approach using surgical denervation of sinoaortic baroreceptors or disruption of the central relay station of the baroreflex, the nucleus tractussolitarii, which was followed by an immediate increase in BP [10].

Investigators initially attempted detecting the presence of sympathetic activation in hypertensive patients by using plasma noradrenaline levels and heart rate (HR). The results in both instances were equivocal. However, an analytical review of studies employing plasma noradrenaline as a marker of increased adrenergic drive in patients with primary hypertension demonstrated that in approximately 40 % of studies, high BP was indeed associated with elevated plasma noradrenaline values [11]. Later studies provided evidence of marked sympathetic activation occurring in hypertension by using microneurographic recording of postganglionic sympathetic neural outflow to the skeletal muscles, indicating that the adrenergic overdrive is directly proportional to the severity of HTN [12], and it is associated with other cardiovascular or metabolic diseases, such as heart failure, diabetes mellitus, and obesity [13].

There are several mechanoreceptors within the body that respond to the stretch of arterial, venous, and ventricular walls. The best understood of the reflex mechanoreceptors are those of the aorta and the carotid sinuses. At the bifurcation of the common carotid artery sit the baroreceptors of the carotid sinus. These mechanosensitive sensory nerve endings are concentrated in the lateral wall of the specialized region of the carotid artery and respond to vascular distention or "stretch." Distension occurs in the face of elevated BP or increased intravascular volume. This is the first step in the initiation of the carotid baroreflex, which is an important component in the control of both short-term and long-term fluctuations in BP. In response to this sensed distension, the baroreceptor sends a signal that travels from the carotid sinus nerve to join cranial nerve IX, eventually signaling the nucleus tractus solitarius in the medulla [14]. This is known as the afferent arm of the arterial baroreflex arc. This signal is then eventually modified in the hypothalamus. The hypothalamus is then responsible for sending signals via the efferent arm of the baroreflex arc, which results in increased parasympathetic efferent activities slowing HR and decreasing BP. It is this reflex system that not only allows individuals to respond to increased salt load or fluid intake by lowering BP, but also the same system that prevents orthostasis when standing. Ultimately, this leads to inhibition of sympathetic output, along with a decrease in the heart rate and cardiac contractility as well as the release of renin-angiotensin-aldosterone system and antidiuretic hormone, which serves to reduce intravascular volume and tone [14].

This pathophysiology serves as the basis of CBS. First reported in 1958 by Carlsten was the effect of short-term carotid sinus stimulation in patients. In five patients undergoing surgical neck dissection for cancer, electrical stimulation of the carotid sinus nerve resulted in abrupt decrease in BP [15]. As described by Scheffers in a 2010 review [16], what followed was a variety of studies exploring CBS, but given the influx of pharmacotherapy to treat hypertension in the late 1960s, and complications related to electrode placement, interest and exploration of CBS as a clinical tool was all but abandoned.

The SNS, however, has reemerged as a therapeutic target for BP control. This is, in part, due to an increasing prevalence of resistant hypertension in the late 1990s and early 2000s, relating to surges in rates of obesity rates coupled with an aging population.

CVRx ® (USA) was founded in 2001 and began conducting preclinical and clinical research focusing on baroreceptor activation therapy (BAT) [17]. After successful preclinical studies, clinical studies of the first-generation BAT device, the Rheos® carotid pacemaker system (CVRx, Inc., USA), were conducted. Three multicenter clinical investigations of BAT using the Rheos system have been performed in hypertensive subjects [18–21]. Building upon the encouraging efficacy results of the Rheos, but looking to improve the procedural safety profile, the second-generation, less invasive, and unilaterally placed Barostim neo™ system (CVRx, Inc., USA) was developed. It has been tested in a single-arm, open-label study [22] enrolling 30 patients and is now being studied in a large prospective, multinational, randomized controlled trial (ClinicalTrials.gov ID: NCT01679132).

22.3 Procedural Aspects of Device Placement

Implanting the first-generation Rheos® system (Fig. 22.1) involves an operation under general anesthesia. Electrode wires are implanted around the exterior surface of the bilateral carotid sinus walls and connected to a pacemaker generator, which is placed in a subcutaneous pocket in the pectoral region, similar to other cardiovascular implantable electronic devices [23]. Optimal positioning of the electrodes on the carotid sinus is determined during the operation itself, based on maximal reductions of heart rate and BP while delivering electrical current. The implanted pulse generator is completely programmable via radio frequency and allows controlled and customized current delivery throughout the day [24]. Electrical field stimulation of the carotid sinus nerves results in afferent signals that are interpreted as a rise in BP. This propagates the carotid baroreflex arc, resulting in efferent parasympathetic nerve activity and the downstream effects described above.

The newer Barostim neo™ (Fig. 22.1) uses the same principles and has a much smaller electrode and generator, leading to a less invasive and much shorter operating time. It is unilaterally placed, rather than bilateral, resulting in a less invasive operation, with shorter recovery time [22].

22.4 Efficacy of BAT Using the Rheos System

The three multicenter clinical investigations of BAT, using the Rheos system in hypertensive subjects, provide the preponderance of efficacy data and include the Device-Based Therapy of Hypertension (DEBuT-HT) trial, which was a European

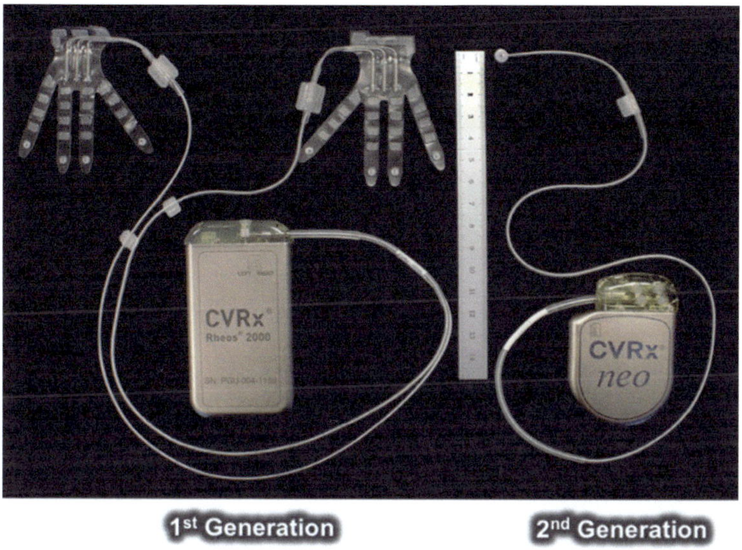

Fig. 22.1 First-generation Rheos® carotid pacemaker system (CVRx, Inc., USA) and second-generation Barostim neo™ system (CVRx, Inc., USA)

multicenter study looking at the safety and efficacy in severely hypertensive patients [20]. Trials based in the United States that address system efficacy include the initial Rheos feasibility trial [21] and the phase III Rheos Pivotal Trial [19], which includes long-term follow-up demonstrating the durable benefit of CBS [18].

The initial Rheos feasibility trial included 10 patients with resistant hypertension and resulted in significant reductions in office-measured BP, −22/−18 mmHg, with concurrent reductions in mean 24-h ambulatory BP measurements,−14/−9 mmHg [21]. Subsequently, the DEBuT-HT trial enrolled 45 patients and followed subject up to 4 years. At least a 30 mmHg sustained drop in systolic BP was noted in 72 % of patients, with 67 % of patients having a resultant systolic BP less than 140 mmHg. Interestingly, subjects continued to use a mean of 4.6 antihypertensive medications, unchanged from mean use of 4.8 medications at baseline [20].

The Rheos Pivotal Trial more recently evaluated BAT for resistant hypertension in a double-blind, randomized, prospective, multicenter, phase III clinical trial. Two hundred and sixty-five subjects with resistant hypertension were implanted and randomized (2:1) 1 month after implantation. Subjects received either CBS (Group I) for the first 6 months or delayed BAT initiation following the six-month visit (Group II). CBS generated a decrease in systolic BP of 26 mmHg for Group I and 17 mmHg for Group II at six months and a decrease of 35 mmHg for Group I and 33 mmHg for Group II at 12 months [19].

Open-label, non-randomized follow-up to assess safety and efficacy of BAT was undertaken in subjects randomized in the Rheos Pivotal Trial after they completed the initial trial [18]. Among long-term responders receiving CBS, the mean BP change was−35/−16 mmHg. Antihypertensive use was minimally reduced at the end of the randomized phase and remained lower through the follow-up. Among responders, 55 % achieved goal BPs.

In the Rheos Pivotal trial, patients also had stimulation parameters individually adjusted to provide optimal BP lowering via BAT. To this end, unilateral stimulation was applied unless bilateral stimulation resulted in more BP reduction. When investigators explored the pooled patient data based on those stimulated bilaterally ($n=80$) versus those unilaterally stimulated ($n=215$), heart rate and BP were significantly lower in the unilateral group. Further, unilateral right-sided stimulation ($n=127$) was more effective than left ($n=88$) [25].

22.5 Safety of BAT

The BP-lowering data of the first-generation device is compelling; however, the major reason the Rheos system is not currently approved relates to issues of safety immediately after the procedure. The Rheos Pivotal Trial did not meet two of the five prespecified co-primary endpoints, one of which was short-term safety. Following device implantation, only 75 % of patients were free from system- or procedure-related events [19]. This percentage is significantly less than the prespecified objective performance criterion of 82 % (which is based on historical literature on single-incision implantable cardioverter defibrillator and pacemaker implants) [26]. Of note, the majority of procedural related complications resolved in their entirety. Long-term safety and sustained efficacy of the device and therapy is much better and met prespecified endpoints [18].

In contrast to the original device, the Barostim neo is associated with far fewer short-term adverse events. Only three periprocedural complications were seen, including a generator pocket hematoma, a self-inflicted wound complication, and intermittent pain at the device site in one patient [22]. This improvement in short-term safety is promising; however, long-term follow-up from the ongoing larger trial is needed.

22.6 Efficacy of BAT

Follow-up of CBS using the Barostim neo device demonstrates similar efficacy to the Rheos system [22]. BP decreased by 26/12 mmHg over six months. Concurrent and ongoing pharmacotherapy was unchanged. Fascinatingly, 6 of 30 patients had a history of renal denervation that did not lower BP, and BAT did.

German investigators in 2015 reported that the use of unilateral BAT using the Barostim neo provided longer-term sustained BP-lowering effects. Seventeen patients with resistant hypertension demonstrated effective BP lowering after unilateral BAT placement over longer follow-up [27]. Moreover, the acute device on/off effects (i.e., increase and decrease of BP) did not depend on treatment duration

[27]. While this was an open-label single-arm evaluation, it did provide evidence of an even safer approach.

These promising BP reductions, in the setting of a better safety profile, have resulted in a large prospective, multinational, randomized, controlled trial of the smaller, unilateral system that is currently ongoing: the Barostim Hypertension Pivotal Trial (ClinicalTrials.gov ID: NCT01679132). It is anticipated that 310 subjects with resistant hypertension will be randomized to CBS or medical therapy.

22.7 Non-hypertension Trials

A trial in heart failure patients using BAT was just completed in Europe on December 23, 2015 (ClinicalTrials.gov ID: NCT01484288). The primary outcome was changes in sympathetic nervous system activity at six months from baseline. No data are available as yet; however, there are two other trials in heart failure poised to either continue or start recruiting in Europe, Barostim HOPE4HF (Hope for Heart Failure) Study (ClinicalTrials.gov Identifier: NCT01720160) and the Barostim Therapy for Heart Failure (BeAT-HF) (ClinicalTrials.gov Identifier: NCT02627196). Other trials are also listed but not recruiting. Thus, we will await yet another possible utility for BAT.

22.8 Novel Approaches to CBS

Another device is being tested that results in CBS. The MobiusHD™ device is a very flexible open cylinder placed intra-arterially in the area of the baroreceptor at the carotid bulb (Fig. 22.2). MobiusHD™ reshapes the vessel and consequently amplifies the baroreceptor signaling with every pulsatile wave; hence acute falls in BP when first placed can occur.

Two trials are ongoing using a Mobius-type device to stretch the area around the carotid bulb, Controlling and Lowering Blood Pressure with the MobiusHD™ (CALM-FIM_EUR) (ClinicalTrials.gov Identifier: NCT01911897) and Controlling and Lowering Blood Pressure with the MobiusHD™ (CALM-FIM_US) (ClinicalTrials.gov Identifier: NCT01831895). Both trials, one in Europe and the other in United States, are open-label, multicenter, first-in-man clinical trials. Eligible subjects with stage 2 resistant systemic arterial hypertension are being recruited. They must be treated with a minimum of three (3) antihypertensive drugs and consent to study participation. Potential study participants will be consented and then screened at two (2) baseline visits beginning at least 30 days prior to MobiusHD placement. Qualified patients will undergo placement of the MobiusHD under angiographic visualization and be followed for 36 months. No data are available as yet on the safety and efficacy of this approach.

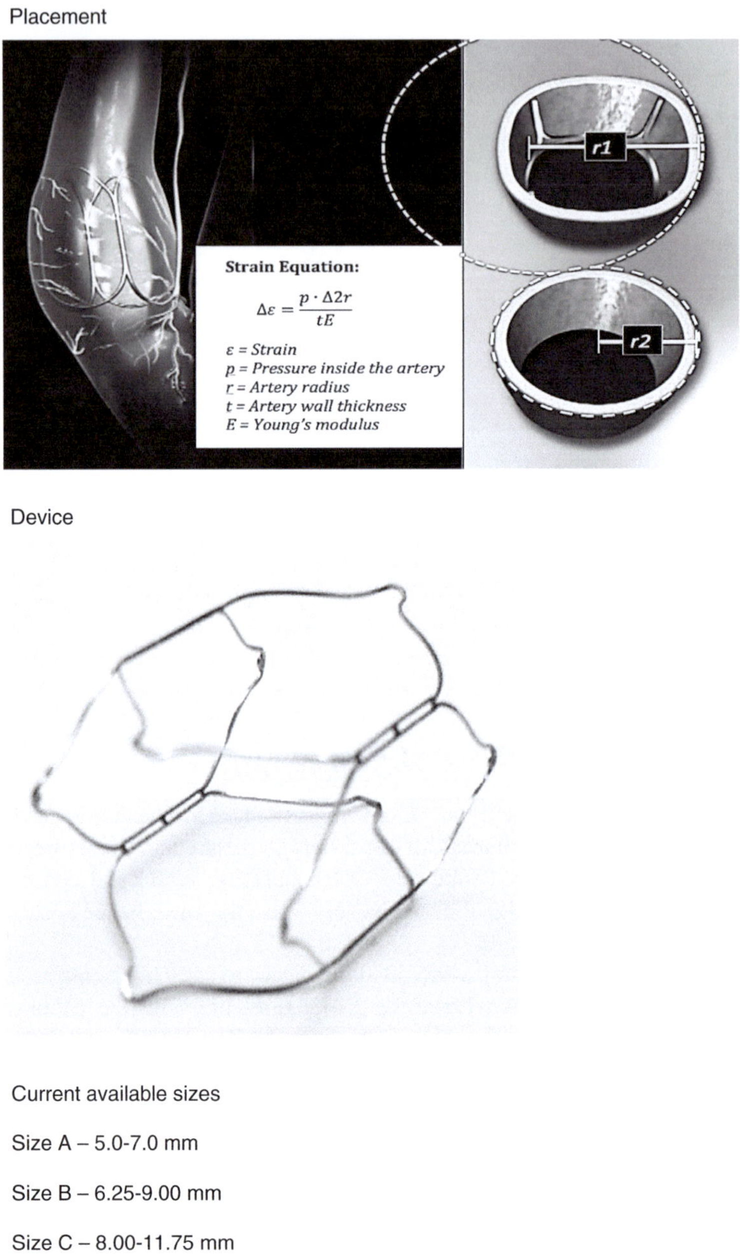

Fig. 22.2 MobiusHD placement and device

22.9 Conclusion

Our treatment of resistant HTN has advanced in many ways over the past two decades. BAT has evolved as a potential treatment for patients with resistant hypertension. CBS demonstrates great promise for the future treatment of hypertension. Current data suggest that BAT offers advantages over established pharmacologically directed strategies for treatment of primary, resistant, and refractory HTN. The effectiveness of BAT may be assessed immediately after insertion, unlike that of other devices modifying the SNS, such as renal denervation. Further, BAT devices are implantable in patients with chronic kidney disease (unlike renal denervation), who suffer a disproportionate burden of resistant hypertension. CBS using BAT or MobiusHD are currently still being evaluated and sit on the horizon as a possible intervention for patients with resistant hypertension and possibly heart failure.

References

1. Egan BM, Zhao Y, Axon RN (2010) US trends in prevalence, awareness, treatment, and control of hypertension, 1988-2008. JAMA 303(20):2043–2050
2. James PA, Oparil S, Carter BL, Cushman WC, Dennison-Himmelfarb C, Handler J et al (2014) 2014 evidence-based guideline for the management of high blood pressure in adults: report from the panel members appointed to the Eighth Joint National Committee (JNC 8). JAMA 311(5):507–520
3. Acelajado MC, Pisoni R, Dudenbostel T, Dell'Italia LJ, Cartmill F, Zhang B et al (2012) Refractory hypertension: definition, prevalence, and patient characteristics. J Clin Hypertens 14(1):7–12
4. Group SR, Wright JT Jr, Williamson JD, Whelton PK, Snyder JK, Sink KM et al (2015) A randomized trial of intensive versus standard blood-pressure control. N Engl J Med 373(22):2103–2116
5. Taler SJ (2005) Treatment of resistant hypertension. Curr Hypertens Rep 7(5):323–329
6. Briasoulis A, Bakris GL (2012) Timing and efficacy of alternative methods of sympathetic blockade. Curr Hypertens Rep 14(5):455–461
7. Bhatt DL, Kandzari DE, O'Neill WW, D'Agostino R, Flack JM, Katzen BT et al (2014) A controlled trial of renal denervation for resistant hypertension. N Engl J Med 370(15):1393–1401
8. Mahfoud F, Tunev S, Ewen S, Cremers B, Ruwart J, Schulz-Jander D et al (2015) Impact of lesion placement on efficacy and safety of catheter-based radiofrequency renal denervation. J Am Coll Cardiol 66(16):1766–1775
9. Kandzari DE, Kario K, Mahfoud F, Cohen SA, Pilcher G, Pocock S et al (2016) The SPYRAL HTN Global Clinical Trial Program: rationale and design for studies of renal denervation in the absence (SPYRAL HTN OFF-MED) and presence (SPYRAL HTN ON-MED) of antihypertensive medications. Am Heart J 171(1):82–91
10. Abboud FM (1979) Integration of reflex responses in the control of blood pressure and vascular resistance. Am J Cardiol 44(5):903–911
11. Goldstein DS (1983) Plasma catecholamines and essential hypertension. An analytical review. Hypertension 5(1):86–99
12. Grassi G, Cattaneo BM, Seravalle G, Lanfranchi A, Mancia G (1998) Baroreflex control of sympathetic nerve activity in essential and secondary hypertension. Hypertension 31(1):68–72

13. Grassi G, Seravalle G, Quarti-Trevano F, Scopelliti F, Dell'Oro R, Bolla G et al (2007) Excessive sympathetic activation in heart failure with obesity and metabolic syndrome: characteristics and mechanisms. Hypertension 49(3):535–541
14. Lohmeier TE, Hildebrandt DA, Warren S, May PJ, Cunningham JT (2005) Recent insights into the interactions between the baroreflex and the kidneys in hypertension. Am J Physiol Regul Integr Comp Physiol 288(4):R828–R836
15. Carlsten A, Folkow B, Grimby G, Hamberger CA, Thulesius O (1958) Cardiovascular effects of direct stimulation of the carotid sinus nerve in man. Acta Physiol Scand 44(2):138–145
16. Scheffers IJ, Kroon AA, de Leeuw PW (2010) Carotid baroreflex activation: past, present, and future. Curr Hypertens Rep 12(2):61–66
17. Victor RG (2015) Carotid baroreflex activation therapy for resistant hypertension. Nat Rev Cardiol 12(8):451–463
18. Bakris GL, Nadim MK, Haller H, Lovett EG, Schafer JE, Bisognano JD (2012) Baroreflex activation therapy provides durable benefit in patients with resistant hypertension: results of long-term follow-up in the Rheos Pivotal Trial. J Am Soc Hypertens 6(2):152–158
19. Bisognano JD, Bakris G, Nadim MK, Sanchez L, Kroon AA, Schafer J et al (2011) Baroreflex activation therapy lowers blood pressure in patients with resistant hypertension: results from the double-blind, randomized, placebo-controlled Rheos Pivotal Trial. J Am Coll Cardiol 58(7):765–773
20. Scheffers IJ, Kroon AA, Schmidli J, Jordan J, Tordoir JJ, Mohaupt MG et al (2010) Novel baroreflex activation therapy in resistant hypertension: results of a European multi-center feasibility study. J Am Coll Cardiol 56(15):1254–1258
21. Lovett EG, Schafer J, Kaufman CL (2009) Chronic baroreflex activation by the Rheos system: an overview of results from European and North American feasibility studies. Conf Proc IEEE Eng Med Biol Soc 2009:4626–4630
22. Hoppe UC, Brandt MC, Wachter R, Beige J, Rump LC, Kroon AA et al (2012) Minimally invasive system for baroreflex activation therapy chronically lowers blood pressure with pacemaker-like safety profile: results from the Barostim neo trial. J Am Soc Hypertens 6(4):270–276
23. Tordoir JH, Scheffers I, Schmidli J, Savolainen H, Liebeskind U, Hansky B et al (2007) An implantable carotid sinus baroreflex activating system: surgical technique and short-term outcome from a multi-center feasibility trial for the treatment of resistant hypertension. Eur J Vasc Endovasc Surg 33(4):414–421
24. Laffin LJ, Bakris GL (2015) Hypertension and new treatment approaches targeting the sympathetic nervous system. Curr Opin Pharmacol 21:20–24
25. de Leeuw PW, Alnima T, Lovett E, Sica D, Bisognano J, Haller H et al (2015) Bilateral or unilateral stimulation for baroreflex activation therapy. Hypertension 65(1):187–192
26. Iliescu R, Tudorancea I, Lohmeier TE (2014) Baroreflex activation: from mechanisms to therapy for cardiovascular disease. Curr Hypertens Rep 16(8):453
27. Halbach M, Hickethier T, Madershahian N, Reuter H, Brandt MC, Hoppe UC et al (2015) Acute on/off effects and chronic blood pressure reduction after long-term baroreflex activation therapy in resistant hypertension. J Hypertens 33(8):1697–1703

Central Iliac Arteriovenous Anastomosis for Hypertension 23

Melvin D. Lobo and Vikas Kapil

Abbreviations

BP Blood pressure
HTN Hypertension
SNS Sympathetic nervous system

23.1 Introduction

A wealth of evidence testifies to the importance of sympathetic nervous system (SNS) signalling in both the aetiology and maintenance of the hypertensive state [1]. It is therefore not surprising that the recent past has seen the introduction of a growing suite of interventional approaches that aim to modulate SNS activity in order to achieve better blood pressure (BP) control [2]. Whilst it is increasingly evident that the SNS plays a substantial role in the development of hypertension,

M.D. Lobo, MBChB, PhD, FRCP, FBHS, FESC (✉)
Barts BP Centre of Excellence, Barts Heart Centre, St Bartholomew's Hospital, London, UK

William Harvey Research Institute, Barts NIHR Cardiovascular Biomedical Research Unit, Queen Mary University, London, UK

William Harvey Heart Centre, Queen Mary University London, Charterhouse Square, London EC1M 6BQ, UK
e-mail: m.d.lobo@qmul.ac.uk

V. Kapil, MA, MRCP, PhD
Barts BP Centre of Excellence, Barts Heart Centre, St Bartholomew's Hospital, London, UK

William Harvey Research Institute, Barts NIHR Cardiovascular Biomedical Research Unit, Queen Mary University, London, UK

C. Tsioufis et al. (eds.), *Interventional Therapies for Secondary and Essential Hypertension*, Updates in Hypertension and Cardiovascular Protection,
DOI 10.1007/978-3-319-34141-5_23

somewhat overlooked has been the importance of identifying where the increased signalling derives from in the enormously complex and extensive regulatory network hierarchy, in order to better focus sympathomodulatory therapies. Furthermore, in patients with often longstanding hypertension, there has been a failure to recognise that SNS activity varies with age: for instance, renal sympathetic nervous activity is reduced in older compared to younger individuals and thus devices targeting the renal sympathetic nerves may result in lesser BP reduction [3]. The fact that a significant proportion of older patients with hypertension have arterial stiffening either as a cause or consequence of hypertension, which has significant implications for choice of antihypertensive strategy, has also been overlooked [4, 5]. Whilst pharmacological approaches to deal with hypertension of a mechanical origin are not clearly defined, a novel device technology reviewed in this chapter targets arterial/venous haemodynamics and offers a complementary approach to direct SNS modulation via therapies such as renal denervation, carotid sinus stimulation and carotid body ablation.

23.2 Background to the Coupler: Rational and Design and Procedural Detail

23.2.1 Development of the Arteriovenous Coupler

The CE-marked arteriovenous (AV) coupler is manufactured by ROX Medical and was originally developed for the treatment of advanced chronic obstructive pulmonary disease (COPD) [6, 7]. The aim of this approach was to form a fixed calibre central iliac AV anastomosis which was conceived to increase central venous oxygenation. As a result venous blood flowing through pulmonary shunts that do not usually participate in gaseous exchange, due to the parenchymal destruction in severe COPD, would have increased oxygen saturation. Thus the potentially deleterious effects of venous admixture on systemic arterial oxygen saturation and oxygen delivery would be attenuated [6]. In addition, the resultant increase in venous return would subsequently augment cardiac output and further increase oxygen delivery to the tissues [6].

23.2.2 Preclinical Data

The preclinical studies (unpublished, submitted to FDA) were reviewed by Foran and others and were conducted in sheep with coupler deployment in the aorta for up to 12 months which resulted in the creation of a fully patent anastomosis in all animals [8]. There was optimal healing of the aorta and inferior vena cava and accompanying adaptive change of venous arterialization which was to be expected. There was negligible foreign body response following device implantation, although coverage of the anastomotic struts by mature pseudointima was observed. The preclinical study concluded that deployment of the AV coupler in ovine aortas for up to 12 months resulted in a durably patent anastomosis in all animals with adequate healing and appropriate conformation of the device into the artery and the vein. No significant residual mural thrombus was noted, and a modest degree of intimal thickening observed upstream from the coupler was consistent with anticipated arterialization [8].

23.2.3 Procedure

The AV coupler is similar in appearance to a coronary stent and is also made of nickel/titanium alloy (nitinol) that exhibits shape memory (Fig. 23.1). This permits self-expansion during placement from a preloaded delivery catheter resulting in deployment into a preformed configuration (Fig. 23.2). A 40 min catheter lab procedure is required in order to implant the coupler under sterile conditions using fluoroscopic guidance and has been described in detail elsewhere [8]. In brief, a short 4 F arterial sheath is placed into the left or right common femoral artery, and a 11 F customised venous sheath is placed in the ipsilateral common femoral vein

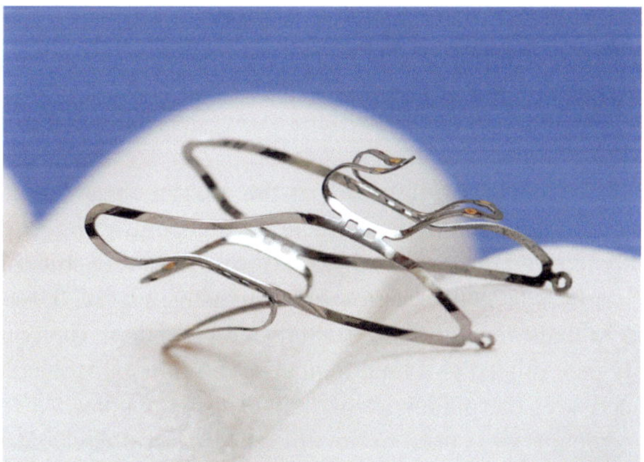

Fig. 23.1 Nitinol arteriovenous coupler device

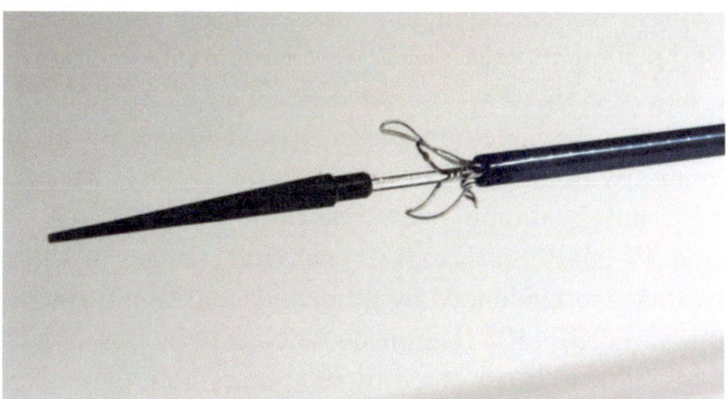

Fig. 23.2 Coupler with introducer

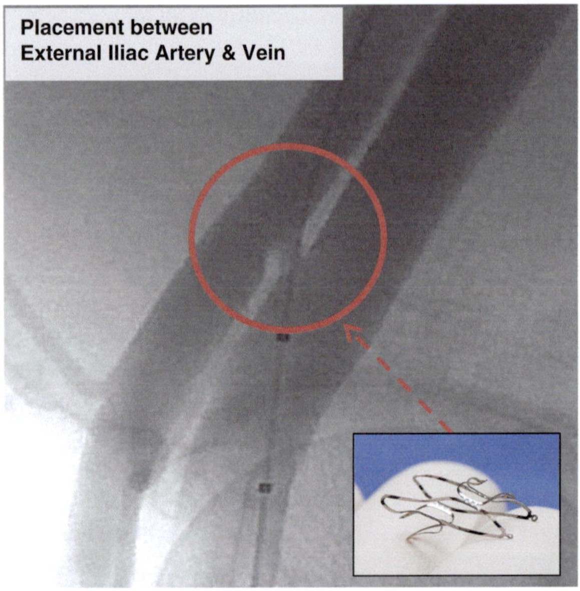

Fig. 23.3 Arteriovenous conduit post-coupler implantation visualised using contrast injection with fluoroscopy

approximately 2 cm inferior to the level of the arterial sheath insertion site. The local arterial and venous anatomy is delineated using contrast injections.

The coupler is placed between the distal external iliac vein and artery just above the level of the femoral head over a crossing wire using a spiral 0.018 in. guidewire (ROX Medical) to mark the target arterial crossing location. The coupler's anastomotic passage is then dilated to a final diameter of 4 mm using a balloon dilatation catheter advanced over the guidewire and sited in the coupler. At this point hand injected iodinated contrast is used to document successful device deployment and sizing of the anastomosis (Fig. 23.3). Post-procedural management includes standard of care practice for groin arterial and venous puncture. Femoral artery and vein haemostasis is achieved post-procedure with simple manual pressure followed by bed rest for up to 4 h. No anticoagulation or antiplatelet medication has been used to date in any of the clinical trials.

Importantly, and in contrast with a renal denervation procedure, technical success of implantation is verifiable by means of (i) direct visualisation of the arteriovenous (AV) conduit with arterial contrast injection (Fig. 23.3), (ii) palpation of a groin thrill and (iii) auscultation of a vascular bruit [9].

Opening of the AV anastomosis causes profound changes in arterial compliance and vascular resistance as evidenced by immediate and significant (15–55 mm Hg) drop in arterial systolic BP [10]. The instantaneous reduction of BP following the creation of the conduit can be reversed by temporary balloon reocclusion but then recurs with balloon deflation (Fig. 23.4). Unlike renal denervation procedures, coupler implantation is fully reversible and straightforward to achieve using a covered stent. However, coupler explantation is more complex and would require a vascular surgical approach and has not been reported to date.

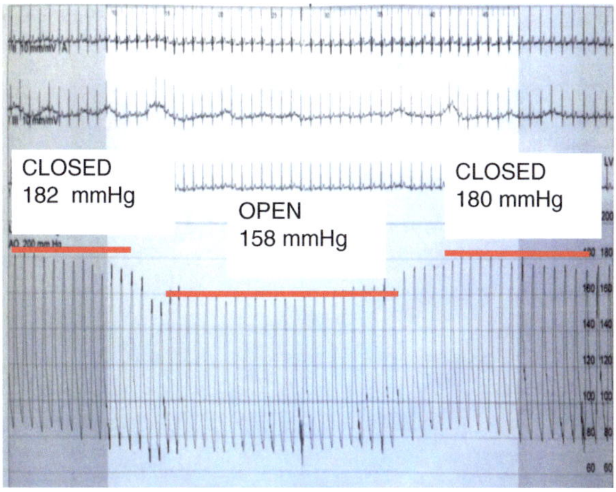

Fig. 23.4 Instantaneous change in BP with coupler opening and closure

23.3 Clinical Trial Data

23.3.1 Clinical Data: COPD

The genesis of central AV coupler therapy is rooted in an unmet need to improve outcomes in patients with advanced COPD [6]. Unfortunately initial studies in COPD cohorts demonstrated conflicting results on exercise capacity. In a proof of concept study in 12 patients with severe, hypoxic COPD, coupler implantation (sized to 5 mm diameter) resulted in a modest improvement in 6 min walking time (6MWT) after 12 weeks [7]. However, this positive effect was largely restricted to those patients whose 6MWT improved with the use of supplemental oxygen at baseline. Interestingly a nonsignificant reduction in pulmonary vascular resistance was noted and a simultaneous 20 % increase in cardiac output but high output cardiac failure was not reported in this study. In this publication, AV anastomoses were made either by end-to-side surgical anastomosis or by percutaneous AV coupler, but the final publication did not report on individual outcomes for either approach.

A subsequent proof of concept study in 15 patients with severe COPD (using the percutaneously implanted AV anastomosis sized to 5 mm diameter) failed to demonstrate improvements in the prespecified endpoints of 6MWT and quality of life measures, although new york heart association (NYHA) functional status improved slightly [11]. A substantial 40 % increase in cardiac output was noted in this study and a striking rate of study-related adverse effects: right heart failure (27 %), venous thrombosis (27 %), venous stenosis (47 %) and ipsilateral leg oedema (67 %). A total of eight patients (53 %) required closure of the AV anastomosis by means of a covered stent graft [11]. It should be noted however that this was a very high risk, maximally treated population with severe COPD resulting in established moderate pulmonary hypertension and poor mobility in whom there are no alternative strategies to improve exercise tolerance or quality of life. Currently there are no intentions to further develop coupler therapy for the COPD indication.

23.3.2 Evidence for Blood Pressure Reduction in Hypertension

23.3.2.1 Hypertensive Patients with COPD

Normotensive patients with COPD did not experience any reduction in office BP (OBP) in the aforementioned studies. However, coupler implantation resulted in significant haemodynamic changes, including BP reduction, in an open label study comprising a pooled cohort from two separate clinical trials in patients with severe COPD (ClinicialTrials.gov NCT00832611 and NCT00992680; total $n=94$). In post hoc analyses of 24 modestly hypertensive patients (mean resting OBP 145/86 mmHg), taking on average two antihypertensive drugs, insertion of the central iliac AV coupler was associated with significant and sustained OBP lowering of 13/18 mmHg at 12 months post-procedure [10, 12]. On the whole the BP lowering effects were greater in patients with more severe office hypertension: no ambulatory BP (ABP) monitoring was undertaken.

Accompanying haemodynamic changes included a 36 % reduction in systemic vascular resistance (SVR) and a 32 % increase in oxygen delivery and a 40 % increase in cardiac output ($p<0.001$ for all). Pulmonary vascular resistance was also significantly reduced by 26 %, although heart rate was unchanged. Late adverse events included four patients who developed a deep vein thrombosis which all resolved with oral anticoagulation for 3 months. As observed in prior studies, four patients also developed venous stenosis upstream from the coupler that was successfully managed with balloon venoplasty and/or stenting [10].

23.3.2.2 Patients with Resistant Hypertension

Subsequent studies have focused on evaluating the coupler in patients with hypertension given the profound vasodilator effects noted in the COPD groups. The first of these, which remains unpublished, was a prospective study of eight patients with drug resistant hypertension (dRHTN) taking on average four antihypertensive medications with a mean OBP of 175/87 mm Hg. At 6 months following coupler placement, OBP and ABP decreased by 15/16 mmHg and by 6/13 mmHg, respectively [13]. In five patients who had baseline and follow-up echocardiography, significant improvements in diastolic function and reduction of interventricular septal thickness at end diastole (IVSd) were noted [13].

23.3.2.3 The ROX CONTROL HTN Trial

The large reductions in OBP and ambulatory BP (ABP) noted in the small pilot study encouraged the manufacturer of the device to design a larger proof of concept and safety study. Results from the multicentre, randomised controlled ROX CONTROL HTN trial were reported in late 2015 [14]. In this open label study, 83 patients were randomised in a 1:1 fashion to receive usual care (medication continuation) or central iliac AV anastomosis plus usual care until the primary end point analysis (OBP and ABP) at 6 months. Patients with evidence of pulmonary hypertension and valvular heart disease and significant renal impairment (estimated glomerular filtration rate <30 mL/min) were excluded from this study. A modified *intention-to-treat* analysis was undertaken in the 77 patients with complete data, and patients randomised to usual care were offered coupler treatment after 6 months of follow-up [14].

The trial population was significantly hypertensive, although hypertension specialists were managing most patients and there was no significant difference in baseline characteristics. Severe hypertension was confirmed with OBP of 175/100 mmHg and daytime mean ABP of 160/95 mmHg despite taking on average five medications. At 6 months, OBP and 24 h mean ABP were reduced by 27/20 and 14/14 mmHg, respectively, in the coupler group ($p<0.0001$ for all changes), whilst in the control group there was no significant change in either (Fig. 23.5). In the coupler group 26 % of patients had their medications reduced from baseline, whilst in the control group 29 % of patients required an increase in antihypertensives. However, BP analysis was performed independent of medication changes which may have masked the true extent of coupler-related BP lowering [14].

In a subgroup of 16 patients who had prior renal denervation, there was highly significant OBP and ABP reduction (34/22 mm Hg and 12/15 mm Hg, respectively) at 6 months in the ten patients who had coupler therapy with no significant change for either BP measure in the six patients assigned to the control group [14]. This suggests that AV coupler therapy may be of benefit in cases where sympathomodulation has failed, raising interesting questions about underlying mechanisms of action which are addressed later in this chapter [15].

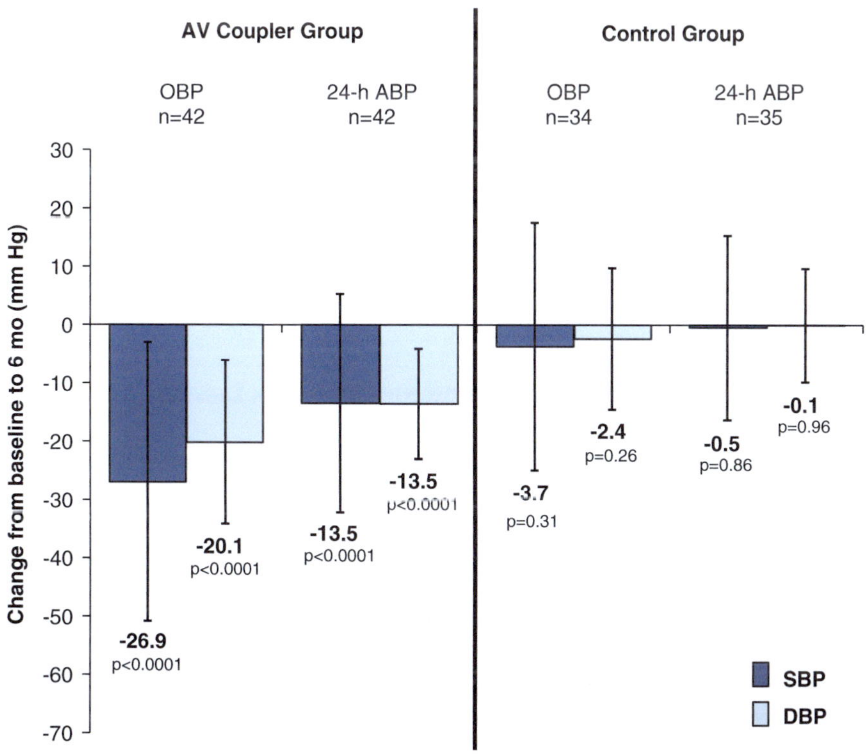

Fig. 23.5 BP reduction in ROX CONTROL HTN study. *OBP* office BP, *ABP* ambulatory BP, *SBP* systolic BP, *DBP* diastolic BP
Error bars are ± 1 Standard Deviation

Procedural adverse events were in keeping with what might be expected from a novel interventional technology and included iliac artery dissection ($n=1$), contrast reaction ($n=1$) and pain ($n=2$). Late, device-specific adverse events were exclusively related to venous stenosis resulting in ipsilateral limb oedema in 29 % of patients that was treated successfully by balloon venoplasty and stenting. It is arguable that venous stenosis would be an expected sequela of AV anastomosis, although whether or not this is an acceptable price to pay for successful BP reduction would depend on long-term outcomes from coupler therapy. However, it should be noted that in the control group, there were five hospitalisations for hypertensive crisis occurring within the primary analysis 6-month period, whilst there were none in the intervention group confirming the very high risk these patients are at.

Several study limitations were noted by the triallists, the most important and debatable of which was the lack of inclusion of a sham-control arm. Although the arguments for use of sham control are persuasive and well rehearsed, in the case of the AV coupler technology, a sham-controlled study may not be readily achievable or necessary [16]. Firstly, as soon as the anastomosis is dilated and permitting AV flow, simultaneous verification of successful implantation is possible using contrast injection [8]. The concomitant and instantaneous reduction in BP obviates meaningful contribution of the Hawthorne or placebo effect (see Fig. 23.4). Secondly, a central iliac AV anastomosis gives rise to a palpable thrill in the ipsilateral groin that is spontaneously reported by patients [8]. These caveats raise significant obstacles to the design of a meaningful sham procedure for this technology.

Other limitations of note include the lack of testing of medication adherence in the study in common with the majority of device and pharmacological intervention studies in the field of hypertension [17]. However, as stated above, changes in medication cannot account for the immediate BP reduction seen post-coupler insertion. A significant concern is that neither the immediate cardiovascular effects of the AV coupler have been assessed in detail nor have the long-term consequences been established. This is discussed further in Sect. 23.4 below.

23.4 Mechanisms of Action and Safety of the Device

23.4.1 Proposed Mechanism of Beneficial Haemodynamic Effects in Hypertension

The regulation of the circulation and thus also arterial BP is a complex matter which is beyond the scope of this chapter [18]. It has become increasingly apparent however that both mechanical aspects of circulatory control and the autonomic nervous system regulation of BP have been somewhat neglected until very recently. Whilst other therapies such as renal denervation and baroreflex activation and carotid body modulation all intervene on the SNS at different points, a central iliac AV anastomosis is thought to work by predominantly targeting mechanical aspects of the circulation although there are undoubtedly some additional effects on neurohumoral activity. Numerous mechanisms have been proposed that may be responsible for BP modulation after creation of such an AV anastomosis and have been extensively reviewed elsewhere (see Table 23.1) [19, 20].

23.4.1.1 Mechano-circulatory Aspects

Although peripheral AV fistulae (AVF) are generally undesirable in man, they are commonly created to provide vascular access in patients with end-stage renal disease (ESRD) for the purpose of haemodialysis (HD). In predialysis patients with ESRD, formation and maturation of upper limb AVFs for HD was associated with significant peripheral and central BP reduction and, in addition, a 17 % reduction in SVR and a 19 % increase in cardiac output [21, 22]. The significant observed reduction in central BP and also aortic pulse wave velocity in this study supports the notion that the creation of AVF leads to a reduction in arterial stiffness [23]. On the other hand, closure of AVF in stable HD patients post transplantation is associated with elevation in BP [24].

There is no precedent however for therapeutic use of an AV anastomosis targeting the central vasculature. The addition of a low-resistance, high-compliance central venous segment in parallel to the proximal systemic arterial circulation leads to a more substantial reduction in SVR than seen following peripheral AVF. Indeed, as discussed earlier, in hypertensive patients with COPD, creation of a 4 mm central iliac AV anastomosis resulted in BP lowering due to a 36 % reduction in SVR [10]. The 40 % rise in cardiac output that followed in these patients is due in part to

Table 23.1 Putative mechanisms whereby a central iliac AV anastomosis may lead to BP reduction

	Coupler-induced effect	Mechanism of BP lowering
Mechano-circulatory	Large reduction in SVR	Vasodilatation
	Reduced arterial stiffness	Delayed reflected wave velocity
	Reduced effective arterial volume	Transfer of blood into proximal venous circulation reduces BP without reducing total blood volume
SNS/PNS modulation	Increased venous return causing left ventricular stretch	Increased vagal tone and downregulation of sympathetic tone
	Increased right atrial pressure	Activates Bainbridge reflex to reduce renal sympathetic activity and inhibit vasopressin secretion
	Increased mixed venous oxygenation and lowered pulmonary vascular resistance	Increased arterial oxygen concentration and downregulation of chemoceptor drive with subsequent reduction in sympathetic vasomotor tone
	Increased tissue O_2 delivery, e.g. improved renal oxygenation	Reduced renal afferent signalling and reduced sympathetic vasomotor tone
Humoral	Increased venous return causing right atrial stretch	Increased atrial natriuretic peptide inhibits renal tubular sodium reabsorption
	Improved renal oxygenation	Reduced renin secretion

SVR systemic vascular resistance, *SNS* sympathetic nervous system, *PNS* parasympathetic nervous system increased venous return (equivalent to the fistula flow rate of ~1 L/min) and also due to the profound reduction in afterload leading to an increase in cardiac performance. The increase in cardiac output is not sufficient to compensate for the change in SVR and resultant engagement of neurohumoral mechanisms described below and hence BP will fall [19].

The creation of a parallel low resistance venous circuit after coupler implantation will lead to a reduction in effective arterial volume, which should attenuate the anticipated elevation in cardiac workload arising from increased cardiac volumes and output [25]. Arterial compliance (the reciprocal of arterial stiffness) will also improve as a result of reduced afterload due to restoration of the Windkessel function of the aorta. This notion is supported by the finding that a reduction in carotid-femoral pulse wave velocity following coupler implantation in a hypertensive female 4 months post AV coupler insertion was largely independent of associated BP lowering [26].

It is worth noting that reduction in effective arterial volume post-coupler insertion is not accompanied by depletion of whole body volume. This contrasts with the effects of diuretic therapy which affects the intracellular, interstitial and venous capacitance compartments and is associated with concomitant increases in SNS activity that may be responsible for attenuation of antihypertensive effect [27, 28].

23.4.1.2 Sympathomodulatory and Neurohumoral Aspects

Both SVR and pulmonary vascular resistance are significantly reduced following central AV anastomosis formation [10]. The resultant increase in flow to the cardiopulmonary circuit will stimulate release of the potent vasorelaxant atrial natriuretic peptide, which may further contribute to BP reduction by reducing renal tubular sodium reabsorption [29]. Furthermore, increased venous return will cause stimulation of right atrial baroreceptors, thus triggering the Bainbridge reflex, leading to reduced renal SNS activity and decreased vasopressin secretion causing diuresis [30, 31]. Increased venous return will also cause left ventricular stretch and consequent activation of cardiac vagal mechanoceptors and downregulation of sympathetic vasomotor tone [31].

In hypertensive patients with COPD, tissue oxygen delivery post-coupler was increased by 32% ($p<0.001$) [10]. An increase in arterial oxygen concentration should be expected due to increased venous oxygenation and improved pulmonary vascular flow following central AV anastomosis [11]. This will also result in inhibition of peripheral chemoceptor activity which has been demonstrated to have tonic hyperactivity in patients with primary hypertension [32]. Furthermore increasing renal oxygenation will downregulate afferent SNS signalling from hypoxia-sensitive renal chemoreceptors and should augment the BP lowering effects of the coupler [33, 34].

23.4.2 Safety Considerations Post-iliac AV Anastomosis

It is important to emphasise that a central iliac AV anastomosis is vastly different from a peripheral AVF both in terms of the mechano-circulatory effects and also the patient population that are exposed to these devices [35]. Furthermore a peripheral AVF is subject to repeated access for HD and not surprisingly is associated with aneurysm formation, thrombotic and bleeding complications and infection [36]. Whilst failure of vascular access for HD is commonly reported [37], to date there have been no reports of coupler migration post-implantation or of spontaneous closure of the anastomosis. A number of theoretical concerns exist however and it is possible that others may emerge in the fullness of time [38].

23.4.2.1 Increased Cardiac Output and High Output Cardiac Failure

Experiments in canines nearly one century ago demonstrated that iatrogenic large calibre AV anastomoses led to a significant, sustained reduction in BP, accompanied by deleterious high cardiac output states [39, 40]. Later observations in humans determined that in the case of spontaneous AVF development (for instance post-traumatic), the distensibility of the fistula was critical to the development of high output cardiac states which were generally reversible with fistula closure [41]. More recently, upper limb AVF formation in patients with ESRD has been associated with increased cardiac output, enlargement of cardiac chambers and deterioration in endothelial function [42]. It should be noted that upper limb AVFs for HD are not fixed in calibre and can progressively dilate with an associated increase in cardiac output. However, development of high output cardiac failure following AVF is rare and thought to only arise when fistula flow is very high (exceeding 2 L/min) and AVF flow as a proportion of cardiac output exceeds 30 % [43]. The ROX AV coupler creates a fixed calibre anastomosis that can be upsized through further balloon dilatation to a maximum diameter of 6 mm but is not capable of spontaneous expansion. With current sizing of the central iliac AV anastomosis to 4 mm in diameter, resultant flow rates of 0.8–1.2 L/min are most unlikely to result in cardiac decompensation [8].

23.4.2.2 Reduction in MAP with Preserved Pulse Pressure

Formation of a central iliac AV anastomosis results in similar reduction in both systolic BP and BP which would preserve pulse pressure and potentially reduce coronary perfusion. Long-term surveillance post-coupler implantation will be essential for safety purposes and also to demonstrate that the preservation of large pulse pressure with lower mean arterial pressure is ultimately beneficial.

23.4.2.3 Ipsilateral Venous Stenosis

Venous neointimal hyperplasia giving rise to venous stenosis is a leading cause of HD access failure in ESRD, with 2-year patency rates of only 51 %, and results in substantial morbidity and hospitalisation in ESRD patients [37, 44, 45]. Ipsilateral venous stenosis is also common following central iliac AV anastomosis and is likely to represent a venous intimal response to turbulent flow, usually occurring just upstream of where the coupler is implanted. This results in marked lower limb swelling and discomfort with associated rise in BP, although venous stenting was noted to resolve the issue in all cases [14]. It remains to be proven whether or not further iteration of the device/implantation procedure or preemptive venous stenting will be a means to obviate this complication in the future.

23.4.2.4 Ipsilateral Lower Limb Swelling

Ipsilateral limb oedema is seen in the majority of patients post-coupler therapy and is likely to arise due to venous hypertension consequent upon increased venous return and may be aggravated by concomitant use of vasodilator antihypertensives. Compression stockings are advised in all patients postprocedurally and are effective in minimising lower limb swelling.

Strategies for optimal management of persistent swelling in the absence of venous stenosis are likely to also involve the use of diuretics.

23.5 Future Directions

AV coupler therapy is in the early stages of its development as an antihypertensive strategy, and much remains to be done to build a new clinical paradigm for its use in routine practice. The emergence of this therapy has coincided with a growing recognition from the cardiovascular community that device trials of hypertension are not straightforward and that much more rigorous trial design and meticulous execution will be mandatory if any devices are to have a place in hypertension treatment guidelines of the future [46, 47]. As such a US-based pivotal trial of the ROX Coupler is in development with likely requirement for a sham-control procedure even though this may prove a challenge for reasons elucidated earlier [48].

A global registry (RH03) is now well under way with the aim of recruiting 100 patients with drug resistant hypertension (dRHTN) who will be subject to long-term surveillance for efficacy and safety (ClinicalTrials.gov: NCT01885390). The registry aims to broaden the scope of this particular device therapy and thus will permit the enrolment of other hypertension phenotypes, including those with multidrug intolerance for whom alternative treatment strategies are exceedingly limited [49]. In addition, extensive invasive haemodynamic assessment pre- and post-coupler insertion will be performed at some sites in tandem with detailed cardiac structural evaluation (with magnetic resonance imaging) to better understand the ensuing cardiac adaptations. The use of autonomic studies to evaluate sympathetic and parasympathetic function in conjunction with noninvasive, haemodynamic assessment is ongoing in RH03 patients in our centre and may shed further light on the underlying mechanisms of coupler action.

Early evidence suggests that augmented venous return post-coupler insertion may prevent vasodepressor syncope [50]. This approach is now being formally tested in a clinical trial (ClinicalTrials.gov: NCT02388087). Therapeutic use of central AV anastomosis is also under evaluation as an adjunct to AF ablation in patients with paroxysmal atrial fibrillation (ClinicalTrials.gov: NCT02243891).

Several opportunities to improve device efficacy and enhance safety are apparent. One possibility is to have a conduit of variable diameter to permit alterations in coupler flow that can be titrated against BP response and adverse effects. It would be desirable also to see procedural/device enhancements that minimise venous turbulence and subsequent neointimal hyperplasia and thereby reduce the incidence of venous stenosis. Finally, and from a converse standpoint, our understanding of the mechanism of action of the coupler would be better informed if detailed characterisation of post-coupler cardiovascular adaptations is not restricted solely to those for whom coupler therapy has been successful in reducing BP but also includes the small proportion of non-responders.

23.6 Summary

A novel device which forms a central iliac AV conduit via a proprietary anastomotic coupler now joins the armamentarium of interventional therapies to control blood pressure. At present the precise mechanisms of action are unproven although its effects are likely to be predominantly related to mechano-circulatory improvement in SVR and arterial compliance. However, given the significant effects on cardiac volumes and on central venous oxygenation, there are likely to be sympathomodulatory responses in addition. The limited clinical trial data thus far accumulated suggest the prospects for this technology are encouraging although longer-term safety and efficacy data are yet to emerge. Much larger scale randomised clinical trials, possibly sham controlled, will be mandated before this therapy can be adopted as a standard of care.

Declarations of Interest MDL has received honoraria from Medtronic Inc., St Jude Medical, ROX Medical and Cardiosonic, and the Barts Charity supports his research. MDL was PI for the ROX CONTROL HTN study.

VK is supported by the NIHR Cardiovascular BRU at Barts and the Barts Charity. He has previously received research funding from the British Heart Foundation.

References

1. Guyenet PG (2006) The sympathetic control of blood pressure. Nat Rev Neurosci 7(5):335–346
2. Ott C, Schmieder RE (2014) Invasive treatment of resistant hypertension: present and future. Current Hypertens Rep 16(11):488
3. Esler M, Jennings G, Korner P, Willett I, Dudley F, Hasking G, Anderson W, Lambert G (1988) Assessment of human sympathetic nervous system activity from measurements of norepinephrine turnover. Hypertension 11(1):3–20
4. Ewen S, Ukena C, Linz D, Kindermann I, Cremers B, Laufs U, Wagenpfeil S, Schmieder RE, Bohm M, Mahfoud F (2015) Reduced effect of percutaneous renal denervation on blood pressure in patients with isolated systolic hypertension. Hypertension 65(1):193–199
5. Williams B (2009) The aorta and resistant hypertension. J Am Coll Cardiol 53(5):452–454
6. Cooper CB, Celli B (2008) Venous admixture in COPD: pathophysiology and therapeutic approaches. COPD 5(6):376–381
7. Faul JL, Galindo J, Posadas-Valay R, Elizondo-Riojas G, Martinez A, Cooper CB (2010) An arteriovenous fistula increases exercise capacity in patients with COPD. Chest 138(1):52–58
8. Foran JP, Jain AK, Casserly IP, Kandzari DE, Rocha-Singh KJ, Witkowski A, Katzen BT, Deaton D, Balmforth P, Sobotka PA (2015) The ROX coupler: creation of a fixed iliac arteriovenous anastomosis for the treatment of uncontrolled systemic arterial hypertension, exploiting the physical properties of the arterial vasculature. Catheter Cardiovasc Interv 85(5):880–886
9. Mahfoud F, Luscher TF (2015) Renal denervation: symply trapped by complexity? Eur Heart J 36(4):199–202

10. Faul J, Schoors D, Brouwers S, Scott B, Jerrentrup A, Galvin J, Luitjens S, Dolan E (2014) Creation of an iliac arteriovenous shunt lowers blood pressure in chronic obstructive pulmonary disease patients with hypertension. J Vasc Surg 59(4):1078–1083
11. Bertog SC, Kolmer C, Kleschnew S, Franke J, Wunderlich N, Kardos P, Sievert H (2012) Percutaneous femoral arteriovenous shunt creation for advanced chronic obstructive pulmonary disease: a single-center safety and efficacy study. Circ Cardiovasc Interv 5(1):118–126
12. Brouwers S, Schoors D, Dupont A, Dolan E, Celli B, Cooper CB, Voegelmeier C, Jerrentrup A, Ficker J, Teschler H, Faul J (2012) Iliofemoral Arteriovenous Fistula Decreases Blood Pressure in Severe Copd Patients With Hypertension. J Hypertens 30:e232
13. Brouwers S, Droogmans S, Dolan E, Galvin J, Dupont A, Van Camp G, Schoors D (2013) A prospective non-randomized open label multi-center study to evaluate the effect of an iliofemoral arteriovenous fistula on blood pressure in patients with therapy-resistant hypertension. Eur Heart J 34(suppl 1):654–655
14. Lobo MD, Sobotka PA, Stanton A, Cockcroft JR, Sulke N, Dolan E, van der Giet M, Hoyer J, Furniss SS, Foran JP, Witkowski A, Januszewicz A, Schoors D, Tsioufis K, Rensing BJ, Scott B, Ng GA, Ott C, Schmieder RE, Investigators RCH (2015) Central arteriovenous anastomosis for the treatment of patients with uncontrolled hypertension (the ROX CONTROL HTN study): a randomised controlled trial. Lancet 385(9978):1634–1641
15. Brier TJ, Jain AK, Lobo MD (2015) Central arteriovenous anastomosis for hypertension: it is not all about sympathomodulation. Future Cardiol 11(5):503–506
16. Redberg RF (2014) Sham controls in medical device trials. N Engl J Med 371(10):892–893
17. Burnier M, Wuerzner G (2015) Drug adherence monitoring in clinical trials: a necessity for a correct assessment of the efficacy and safety of antihypertensive therapies. J Hypertens 33(12):2395–2398
18. Page IH (1949) Pathogenesis of arterial hypertension. J Am Med Assoc 140(5):451–458
19. Burchell AE, Lobo MD, Sulke N, Sobotka PA, Paton JF (2014) Arteriovenous anastomosis: is this the way to control hypertension? Hypertension 64(1):6–12
20. Kapil V, Sobotka PA, Saxena M, Mathur A, Knight C, Dolan E, Stanton A, Lobo MD (2015) Central iliac arteriovenous anastomosis for hypertension: targeting mechanical aspects of the circulation. Current Hypertens Rep 17(9):585
21. Korsheed S, Eldehni MT, John SG, Fluck RJ, McIntyre CW (2011) Effects of arteriovenous fistula formation on arterial stiffness and cardiovascular performance and function. Nephrol Dial Transplant 26(10):3296–3302
22. Saratzis N, Saratzis A, Sarafidis PA, Melas N, Ktenidis K, Kiskinis D (2008) Quantitative evaluation of the systemic effects of transposed basilic vein to brachial artery arteriovenous fistula: a prospective study. J Vasc Access 9(4):285–290
23. Laurent S, Cockcroft J, Van Bortel L, Boutouyrie P, Giannattasio C, Hayoz D, Pannier B, Vlachopoulos C, Wilkinson I, Struijker-Boudier H (2006) European Network for Non-invasive Investigation of Large Arteries. Expert consensus document on arterial stiffness: methodological issues and clinical applications. Eur Heart J 27(21):2588–2605
24. Unger P, Xhaet O, Wissing KM, Najem B, Dehon P, van de Borne P (2008) Arteriovenous fistula closure after renal transplantation: a prospective study with 24-hour ambulatory blood pressure monitoring. Transplantation 85(3):482–485
25. Guyton AC, Sagawa K (1961) Compensations of cardiac output and other circulatory functions in areflex dogs with large A-V fistulas. Am J Phys 200:1157–1163
26. Sobotka PA, Munnery M, Davies L, Gale NS, Cockcroft JR (2014) Creation of a fixed central arterial-venous anastomosis affects arterial stiffness and central haemodynamics: a treatment for hypertension targeting the physical properties of the arterial vasculature. Artery Res 8(4):176
27. Burnier M, Brunner HR (1992) Neurohormonal consequences of diuretics in different cardiovascular syndromes. Eur Heart J 13(Suppl G):28–33
28. Okada Y, Jarvis SS, Best SA, Bivens TB, Adams-Huet B, Levine BD, Fu Q (2013) Chronic renin inhibition lowers blood pressure and reduces upright muscle sympathetic nerve activity in hypertensive seniors. J Physiol 591(23):5913–5922
29. Rubattu S, Calvieri C, Pagliaro B, Volpe M (2013) Atrial natriuretic peptide and regulation of vascular function in hypertension and heart failure: implications for novel therapeutic strategies. J Hypertens 31(6):1061–1072

30. Hainsworth R (1991) Reflexes from the heart. Physiol Rev 71(3):617–658
31. Hainsworth R (2014) Cardiovascular control from cardiac and pulmonary vascular receptors. Exp Physiol 99(2):312–319
32. Sinski M, Lewandowski J, Przybylski J, Bidiuk J, Abramczyk P, Ciarka A, Gaciong Z (2012) Tonic activity of carotid body chemoreceptors contributes to the increased sympathetic drive in essential hypertension. Hypertens Res 35(5):487–491
33. Recordati GM, Moss NG, Genovesi S, Rogenes PR (1980) Renal receptors in the rat sensitive to chemical alterations of their environment. Circ Res 46(3):395–405
34. Winternitz SR, Oparil S (1982) Importance of the renal nerves in the pathogenesis of experimental hypertension. Hypertension 4(5 Pt 2):III108–III114
35. Agarwal AK (2015) Systemic Effects of Hemodialysis Access. Adv Chronic Kidney Dis 22(6):459–465
36. Santoro D, Benedetto F, Mondello P, Pipito N, Barilla D, Spinelli F, Ricciardi CA, Cernaro V, Buemi M (2014) Vascular access for hemodialysis: current perspectives. Int J Nephrol Renov Dis 7:281–294
37. Al-Jaishi AA, Oliver MJ, Thomas SM, Lok CE, Zhang JC, Garg AX, Kosa SD, Quinn RR, Moist LM (2014) Patency rates of the arteriovenous fistula for hemodialysis: a systematic review and meta-analysis. Am J Kidney Dis 63(3):464–478
38. Mahfoud F, Bohm M (2015) Hypertension: Arteriovenous anastomosis--next panacea for hypertension? Nat Rev Cardiol 12(4):197–198
39. Holman E (1924) Experimental studies in arteriovenous fistulas: iii. cardiac dilatation and blood vessel changes. Arch Surg 9(3):856–879
40. Holman E, Kolls AC (1924) Experimental studies in arteriovenous fistulas: ii. pulse and blood pressure variations. Arch Surg 9(3):837–855
41. Holman E (1965) Abnormal arteriovenous communications. Great variability of effects with particular reference to delayed development of cardiac failure. Circulation 32(6): 1001–1009
42. Dundon BK, Torpey K, Nelson AJ, Wong DT, Duncan RF, Meredith IT, Faull RJ, Worthley SG, Worthley MI (2014) The deleterious effects of arteriovenous fistula-creation on the cardiovascular system: a longitudinal magnetic resonance imaging study. Int J Nephrol Renov Dis 7:337–345
43. MacRae JM, Pandeya S, Humen DP, Krivitski N, Lindsay RM (2004) Arteriovenous fistula-associated high-output cardiac failure: a review of mechanisms. Am J Kidney Dis 43(5): e17–e22
44. Brahmbhatt A, Remuzzi A, Franzoni M, Misra S (2016) The molecular mechanisms of hemodialysis vascular access failure. Kidney Int 89(2):303–316
45. Feldman HI, Kobrin S, Wasserstein A (1996) Hemodialysis vascular access morbidity. J Am Soc Nephrol 7(4):523–535
46. Zannad F, Stough WG, Mahfoud F, Bakris GL, Kjeldsen SE, Kieval RS, Haller H, Yared N, De Ferrari GM, Pina IL, Stein K, Azizi M (2015) Design considerations for clinical trials of autonomic modulation therapies targeting hypertension and heart failure. Hypertension 65(1):5–15
47. Mahfoud F, Bohm M, Azizi M, Pathak A, Durand Zaleski I, Ewen S, Tsioufis K, Andersson B, Blankestijn PJ, Burnier M, Chatellier G, Gafoor S, Grassi G, Joner M, Kjeldsen SE, Luscher TF, Lobo MD, Lotan C, Parati G, Redon J, Ruilope L, Sudano I, Ukena C, van Leeuwen E, Volpe M, Windecker S, Witkowski A, Wijns W, Zeller T, Schmieder RE (2015) Proceedings from the European clinical consensus conference for renal denervation: considerations on future clinical trial design. Eur Heart J 36(33):2219–2227
48. White WB, Galis ZS, Henegar J, Kandzari DE, Victor R, Sica D, Townsend RR, Turner JR, Virmani R, Mauri L (2015) Renal denervation therapy for hypertension: pathways for moving development forward. J Am Soc Hypertens 9(5):341–350
49. Antoniou S, Saxena M, Hamedi N, de Cates C, Moghul S, Lidder S, Kapil V, Lobo MD (2016) Management of Hypertensive Patients With Multiple Drug Intolerances: A Single-Center Experience of a Novel Treatment Algorithm. J Clin Hypertens 18(2):129–138
50. Sulke N, Eysenck W, Badiani S, Furniss SS (2016) Structural cure for reflex syncope? BMJ Case Rep 20;2016. pii: bcr2015213990. doi:10.1136/bcr-2015-213990

MIX
Papier aus verantwortungsvollen Quellen
Paper from responsible sources
FSC® C105338

If you have any concerns about our products,
you can contact us on
ProductSafety@springernature.com

In case Publisher is established outside the EU,
the EU authorized representative is:
Springer Nature Customer Service Center GmbH
Europaplatz 3, 69115 Heidelberg, Germany

Printed by Libri Plureos GmbH
in Hamburg, Germany